The Cancer Patient and Supportive Care

Cancer Treatment and Research

WILLIAM L MCGUIRE, *series editor*

Livingston RB (ed): Lung Cancer 1. 1981. ISBN 90-247-2394-9.

Bennett Humphrey G, Dehner LP, Grindey GB, Acton RT (eds): Pediatric Oncology 1. 1981. ISBN 90-247-2408-2.

DeCosse JJ, Sherlock P (eds): Gastrointestinal Cancer 1. 1981. ISBN 90-247-2461-9.

Bennett JM (ed): Lymphomas 1, including Hodgkin's Disease. 1981. ISBN 90-247-2479-1.

Bloomfield CD (ed): Adult Leukemias 1. 1982. ISBN 90-247-2478-3.

Paulson DF (ed): Genitourinary Cancer 1. 1982. ISBN 90-247-2480-5.

Muggia FM (ed): Cancer Chemotherapy 1. ISBN 90-247-2713-8.

Bennett Humphrey G, Grindey GB (eds): Pancreatic Tumors in Children. 1982. ISBN 90-247-2702-2.

Costanzi JJ (ed): Malignant Melanoma 1. 1983. ISBN 90-247-2706-5.

Griffiths CT, Fuller AF (eds): Gynecologic Oncology. 1983. ISBN 0-89838-555-5.

Greco AF (ed): Biology and Management of Lung Cancer. 1983. ISBN 0-89838-554-7.

Walker MD (ed): Oncology of the Nervous System. 1983. ISBN 0-89838-567-9.

Higby DJ (ed): Supportive Care in Cancer Therapy. 1983. ISBN 0-89838-569-5.

Herberman RB (ed): Basic and Clinical Tumor Immunology. 1983. ISBN 0-89838-579-2.

Baker LH (ed): Soft Tissue Sarcomas. 1983. ISBN 0-89838-584-9.

Bennett JM (ed): Controversies in the Management of Lymphomas. 1983. ISBN 0-89838-586-5.

Bennett Humphrey G, Grindey GB (eds): Adrenal and Endocrine Tumors in Children. 1983. ISBN 0-89838-590-3.

DeCosse JJ, Sherlock P (eds): Clinical Management of Gastrointestinal Cancer. 1984. ISBN 0-89838-601-2.

Catalona WJ, Ratliff TL (eds): Urologic Oncology. 1984. ISBN 0-89838-628-4.

Santen RJ, Manni A (eds): Diagnosis and Management of Endocrine-related Tumors. 1984. ISBN 0-89838-636-5.

Costanzi JJ (ed): Clinical Management of Malignant Melanoma. 1984. ISBN 0-89838-656-X.

Wolf GT (ed): Head and Neck Oncology. 1984. ISBN 0-89838-657-8.

Alberts DS, Surwit EA (eds): Ovarian Cancer. 1985. ISBN 0-89838-676-4.

Muggia FM (ed): Experimental and Clinical Progress in Cancer Chemotherapy. 1985. ISBN 0-89838-679-9.

Higby DJ (ed): The Cancer Patient and Supportive Care. 1985. ISBN 0-89838-690-X.

Bloomfield CD (ed): Chronic and Acute Leukemias in Adults. 1985. ISBN 0-89838-702-7.

The Cancer Patient and Supportive Care

Medical, Surgical, and Human Issues

edited by

DONALD J. HIGBY
Hematology/Oncology Service
Baystate Medical Center
Springfield, Massachusetts, USA

1985 **MARTINUS NIJHOFF PUBLISHERS**
a member of the KLUWER ACADEMIC PUBLISHERS GROUP
BOSTON / DORDRECHT / LANCASTER

Distributors

for the United States and Canada: Kluwer Academic Publishers, 190 Old Derby Street, Hingham, MA 02043, USA
for the UK and Ireland: Kluwer Academic Publishers, MTP Press Limited, Falcon House, Queen Square, Lancaster LA1 1RN, UK
for all other countries: Kluwer Academic Publishers Group, Distribution Center, P.O. Box 322, 3300 AH Dordrecht, The Netherlands

Library of Congress Cataloging in Publication Data

Main entry under title:

The Cancer patient and supportive care.

    (Cancer treatment and research)
    1. Cancer--Treatment. 2. Cancer--Psychological
aspects. I. Higby, Donald J. II. Series.
[DNLM: 1. Neoplasms--therapy. W1 CA693 / QZ 266 C2163]
RC270.8.C365 1985   616.99'406   84-20656
ISBN 0-89838-690-X

ISBN 0-89838-690-X (this volume)
ISBN 90-247-2426-0 (series)

To Theresa, Sharon, Mary Clare, Susan, Elisabeth, and Donald, who keep me entertained.

Contents

Cancer Treatment and Research

Foreword

Where do you begin to look for a recent, authoritative article on the diagnosis or management of a particular malignancy? The few general oncology textbooks are generally out of date. Single papers in specialized journals are informative but seldom comprehensive; these are more often preliminary reports on a very limited number of patients. Certain general journals frequently publish good indepth reviews of cancer topics, and published symposium lectures are often the best overviews available. Unfortunately, these reviews and supplements appear sporadically, and the reader can never be sure when a topic of special interest will be covered.

Cancer Treatment and Research is a series of authoritative volumes which aim to meet this need. It is an attempt to establish a critical mass of oncology literature covering virtually all oncology topics, revised frequently to keep the coverage up to date, easily available on a single library shelf or by a single personal subscription.

We have approached the problem in the following fashion. First, by dividing the oncology literature into specific subdivisions such as lung cancer, genitourinary cancer, pediatric oncology, etc. Second, by asking eminent authorities in each of these areas to edit a volume on the specific topic on an annual or biannual basis. Each topic and tumor type is covered in a volume appearing frequently and predictably, discussing current diagnosis, staging, markers, all forms of treatment modalities, basic biology, and more.

In Cancer Treatment and Research, we have an outstanding group of editors, each having made a major commitment to bring to this new series the very best literature in his or her field. Martinus Nijhoff Publishers has made an equally major commitment to the rapid publication of high quality books, and world-wide distribution.

Where can you go to find quickly a recent authoritative article on any major oncology problem? We hope that Cancer Treatment and Research provides an answer.

WILLIAM L. MCGUIRE
Series Editor

Preface

During the course of editing 'Supportive Care in Cancer Therapy' (Martinus Nijhoff Publishers, 1983), it become apparent that several topics would have to await a second volume. Furthermore, development of new information and evolution of ideas continues. This volume continues the intent of the first to present reviews of issues relating to supportive care, and to identify areas where further definition and further research is needed.

The physician reading this volume will find the contents though-provoking. In addition to reviews authored by physicians, there are chapters authored by non-physicians, who present a different perspective and a different style of writing. Reverend Bigler writes from his long experience as a chaplain for cancer patients, and tries to identify the changes that take place in the personality of the chaplain who works with dying patients. Ms. Killion and Ms. Powell try to describe what an Oncology Nurse is, rather than what one does. Attorneys Reese and Price present a very practical summation of issues which face the cancer patient, and their chapter could easily be copied and offered to one's patients; furthermore, this chapter gives direction to the physician who is frequently called upon for advice regarding issues which lie entirely outside his/her formal training. Excellent reviews on more 'medical' subjects are here. 'Cancer in the Elderly' should provoke oncologists to re-examine their approach to the geriatric patient. If I do not specifically mention the other chapters, it is because they stand on their own merits and need no 'introduction" to the physician or nurse reader.

Again, it is hoped that this volume will not only be read for its information, but will also be used as a reference and a text. It does not stand alone, but complements the information in the first volume. In subsequent volumes, I intend to not only compile excellent reviews of subjects which are of general concern to those caring for the cancer patient, but also intend to periodically update topics in which movement is quite rapid. Finally, the contribution of non-physicians to the area of 'supportive care' cannot be underestimated, and it is helpful to the physician to see things through the eyes of those not medically trained.

I am most grateful to Ms. Corrine Cesari, who helped immeasureably in putting this book together while I was in the process of relocating. Ms. Sue Allen, my new secretary, has admirably continued Ms. Cesari's efforts. My publisher has been patient, as has Dr. McGuire. Finally, the authors of these chapters have been most cooperative, and should be proud of their accomplishments.

DONALD J. HIGBY, M.D.
Chief, Hematology/Oncology
Baystate Medical Center
Springfield, MA

List of Contributors

BERJIAN, Richard, D.O., Department of Surgery, University of Medicine and Dentistry of New Jersey, College of Osteopathic Medicine, Camden, New Jersey.

BIGLER, Lewis, M. Div., M.A., Protestant Chaplain, Roswell Park Memorial Institute, 666 Elm Street, Buffalo, New York 14263.

HIGBY, Donald J., M.D., Hematology/Oncology Service, Baystate Medical Center, 759 Chestnut Street, Springield, Massachusetts 01199.

DE VRIES-HOSPERS, H. G., M.D., Ph.D., Laboratory for Medical Microbiology, University Hospital, Groningen, The Netherlands.

KILLION, Kathleen, R.N., Research Nurse Clinician, Department of Medical Oncology, Roswell Park Memorial Institute, 666 Elm Street, Buffalo, New York 14263.

KIRSHNER, Jeffrey, M.D., Hematology Associates of Syracuse, Syracuse, New York.

POWELL, Eileen, R.N., Research Nurse Clinician, Department of Medical Oncology, Roswell Park Memorial Institute, 666 Elm Street, Buffalo, New York 14362.

PREISLER, Harvey D., M.D., Department of Medical Oncology, Roswell Park Memorial Institute, 666 Elm Street, Buffalo, New York 14263.

PRICE, W. D., J.D., Attorney at Law, Statler Building, Buffalo, New York 14212.

RAFFERTY, James, Ph.D., Department of Family Practice, School of Medicine, Wright State University, Family Health Center, Dayton, Ohio.

REESE, Peter A., J.D., Department of Computer Science, Roswell Park Memorial Institute, 666 Elm Street, Buffalo, New York 14263.

ROTSTEIN, Coleman, M.D., Division of Infectious Disease, Department of Medicine, State University of New York at Buffalo, Buffalo, New York 14215.

SPAULDING, Monica, M.D., Hematology/Oncology, Veterans Administration Medical Center, State University of New York at Buffalo, 3495 Bailey Avenue, Buffalo, New York 14215.

SPAULDING, Stephen W., M.D., Division of Endocrinology, Department of Medicine, State University of New York at Buffalo, 3495 Bailey Avenue, Buffalo, New York 14215.

VAN DER WAAIJ, Dirk, M.D., Ph.D., Laboratory for Medical Microbiology, University Hospital, Groningen, The Netherlands.

1. Bone Marrow Toxicity of Antitumor Agents

JEFFREY J. KIRSHNER and HARVEY D. PREISLER

INTRODUCTION

Bone marrow suppression is the dose-limiting toxicity for the majority of antitumor agents and may be associated with significant morbidity and mortality. In contrast to the toxic effects which antineoplastic drugs produce in some of the other organ systems, bone marrow suppression is usually predictable and dose-related. An understanding of normal hematopoiesis, cell cycle kinetics, the mechanism of action and the pharmacokinetics of the various drugs will enable the clinical oncologist to administer chemotherapy more intelligently, safely and effectively.

In this chapter, we will review current concepts of normal hematopoietic maturation, with an emphasis on *in vitro* culture techniques. The mechanisms of action of the various drugs, including new chemotherapeutic agents, will be reviewed and the effects which antineoplastic drugs produce on bone marrow will be discussed in detail. Factors associated with increased bone marrow toxicity and methods employed to decrease toxicity will also be reviewed, including an update of current investigational approaches.

1. MECHANISMS OF HEMATOPOIESIS

A schema outlining the current concepts of normal hematopoietic maturation is presented in Figure 1. The early progenitor cells are not morphologically identifiable and are operationally defined on the basis of the assays employed to quantitate these cells [1]. The pluripotent stem cell, which is capable of self-replication and giving rise to the erythroid, myeloid, megakaryocytic, and lymphoid progenitor cells, is referred to as the CFU-S (colony-forming unit-spleen), as it was initially defined as the cell which pro-

Higby, DJ (ed), The Cancer Patient and Supportive Care. ISBN 0-89838-690-X.
© *1985, Martinus Nijhoff Publishers, Boston. Printed in The Netherlands.*

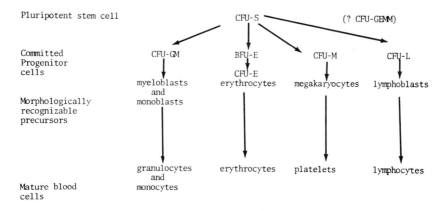

Figure 1. Normal hematopoietic maturation.

duced spleen colonies containing cells of multiple lineage when injected into a lethally irradiated mouse [2]. A similar assay does not exist for human pluripotent stem cells, but recently an *in vitro* assay has been developed which permits growth of mixed colonies in culture, containing granulocytes, macrophages, megakaryocytes, erythrocytes, and T-lymphocytes [3, 4]. The cell which gives rise to these mixed colonies may be equivalent to the pluripotent stem cell. This progenitor cell is operationally defined as the CFU-GEMM (colony-forming unit-granulocyte, erythrocyte, macrophage, megakaryocyte) [3]. It is not known if the progenitor cell responsible for these colonies is self-maintaining. The specific progenitor cells for each cell line will also clone *in vitro* and are defined as follows: the granulocyte precursor is the CFU-C (colony-forming unit-culture), historically, but is more accurately defined as the CFU-GM (-granulocyte, macrophage) since the colonies arising from this cell consist of granulocytes, macrophages, or a combination of the two cell types [1, 5]. For the erythroid series, the most immature precursor which has been identified gives rise to very large erythroid colonies referred to as 'bursts' and is called the BFU-E (burst-forming-unit-erythroid) [6]. This cell is thought to differentiate into the CFU-E (colony-forming-unit-erythroid) [7.] *In vitro* techniques have also been developed to assay progenitors of megakaryocytes (CFU-M) [8, 9], and the progenitors of both B and T lymphocytes (CFU-L) [10–12].

Whether the committed progenitor cells are capable of self-replication and thus are truly stem cells as are the CFU-S's, is unknown. Recently developed methods, including the establishment of *in vitro* long-term marrow cultures [13] and an assay to measure self-renewal capacity of progenitor cells [14], should help to answer this important question, which has obvious implications in terms of bone marrow toxicity associated with chemotherapy. In any event, the committed progenitor cells give rise to mor-

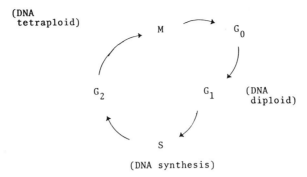

Figure 2. The cell cycle.

phologically recognizable precursor cells of each lineage, which further undergo terminal differentiation to mature blood cells (Figure 1).

2. THE CELL CYCLE

All replicating cells, including those in the bone marrow, go through an orderly sequence of events which result in cell division, referred to as the cell cycle (Figure 2) [15]. After mitosis (M), the processes which will ultimately lead to the next cell division begin again. During the G_1 phase, RNA and protein synthesis occur. In late G_1, there is a burst of RNA synthesis followed by the period of DNA synthesis (S phase). By the completion of S phase, the DNA content of the cell has doubled from diploidy to tetraploidy. The cells remain tetraploid during G_2 and are returned to the diploid state by mitosis. In addition to cells which are actively cycling, kinetically quiescent or G_0 cells exist in both normal bone marrow and in tumors. These resting cells are capable of re-entering the cell cycle resuming proliferation. Recent technological advances in flow cytometry now make it possible to quantitate the RNA and DNA content of individual cells, perhaps making possible the determination of the cell cycle status of the cells [16].

The site (or sites) of action in the cell cycle where chemotherapeutic agents exert their lethal effects is recognized for most agents. Some of these drugs, such as the antimetabolites, are capable of killing only those cells which are actively cycling and thus are referred to as cell cycle specific agents. Drugs such as cytosine arabinoside, which are effective only if cells are in the S phase of the cell cycle when exposed to the drug, are referred to as being phase and cycle specific. By contrast, alkylating agents and nitrosureas kill both resting G_0 cells and actively cycling cells and are referred to as cycle nonspecific agents.

On the basis of studies of murine hematopoiesis and on the limited number of studies of normal human hemaotpoiesis, it appears that under normal circumstances the most primitive hematopoietic cells, the CFU-S and CFU-GEMM either cycle very slowly or that the majority of these primitive cells are in G_0 [1]. This statement probably applies to the CFU-E as well. The proportion of CFU-C which are actively cycling is much higher with the suicide indices of normal bone marrow CFU-C being in the range of 20–50% [15, 17, 18]. The actual cell cycle times and the true proportion of progenitor cells which are actively cycling are unknown. The thymidine labelling index of the normal myeloblast is of the order of 50% with the labelling index of the more mature myeloid elements falling off to zero as the cells mature [15, 19]. There are essentially no data on the cell cycle characteristics of the precursors of platelets. Morphologically recognizable red cell precursors have been reported to have a relatively rapid rate of proliferation [20, 21].

The cell cycle characteristics of the various hemaotpoietic cells in part determine the effects of chemotherapeutic agents on the bone marrow. This is the case since actively dividing cells are often (but not always) more sensitive to chemotherapeutic and therefore most agents produce little effect on the marrow stem cells while producing substantial effects upon the more mature elements. It is probably this phenomenon which permits hematopoietic recovery after the production of severe marrow hypoplasia.

3. USE OF CELL CULTURES TO STUDY THE EFFECTS OF CHEMOTHERAPY

The specific target cell (or cells) in normal bone marrow which are killed by chemotherapeutic agents varies with the drug and determines the nature of hematopoietic toxicity of the agent. For example, if a drug were toxic only to the morphologically identifiable precursor (myeloblasts, promyelocytes and myelocytes) and the CFU-C were spared, administration of the drug would cause a rapid fall in the white blood cell count with a rapid recovery as the intact CFU-C differentiated into the more mature granulocytic precursor cells. On the other hand, if the pluripotent stem cells were selectively killed by an agent, delayed hematopoietic suppression would occur and would be manifest only when the more mature progenitors underwent terminal differentiation. The depth and duration of pancytopenia would depend upon the number of stem cells which were killed and their rate of recovery.

A large number of studies have been directed towards understanding the mechanism of action and effects of chemotherapeutic agents on specific precursor cells. Early work, most of which was done in murine systems, has been well reviewed by Marsh [22], and more recently by Dow [23]. Multiple assays, designed to quantitate the different progenitor cells or study their repopulating potential and various techniques of drug exposure, have been employed. For determination of drug sensitivity of murine CFU-S, the animals are treated with a drug or combination of drugs and at some later point of time, the mice are sacrificed and the number of CFU-S recovered from marrow, usually a femur, are compared to the number recovered from a control animal [22, 24]. *In vitro* assays have been employed to study the toxicity of chemotherapy on the committed progenitor cells. The cells are usually exposed to the specific drug, in a concentration which approximates that achieved clinically, then washed and cultured [22, 25]. The difference in the number of colonies recovered from the drug exposed and control groups is taken as the effect of the drug on the progenitor cell under study. Alternate methods to determine drug effects include the continuous presence of the drug in the culture system, but this method is less satisfactory, as the continuous exposure of dividing cells to certain drugs will inhibit their division, even if it in fact is ineffective in killing the cell [26]. For studies of S phase specific agents, it is prudent to also measure the suicide index, employing an incubation with ^3H-thymidine of high specific activity in order to determine the percentage of cells in S phase [26].

There are interspecies differences in progenitor cell drug sensitivity. It has been questioned as to whether one should extrapolate from the extensive murine data to the clinical situation, even when patients are treated with equivalent doses of the drug [22]. Although some discrepancies exist, much of the early work in mice has been consistent with clinical observations and predictive of toxicity for new agents.

Several patterns of *in vitro* toxicity to progenitor cells have been noted [22, 27, 28]. Non-cycle, non-phase specific agents such as the alkylators, nitrosureas, and anthracyclines, generally produce exponential dose-response curves for the various progenitor cells. By contrast, the killing of progenitor cells by S phase specific agents reaches a plateau, the level of which is dependent upon the number of progenitor cells which are in S phase during the exposure to the drug.

The ability to culture human progenitor cells from marrow and blood has obviated the problems of interspecies differences in drug sensitivity. However, the number of human studies which can be performed is obviously more limited. A specific problem at the present time is the absence of an assay for the human pluripotential stem cell. Even if the properties of the pluripotent CFU-GEMM is reflective of that of the hematopoietic stem cell, the cloning efficiency of the CFU-GEMM is too low at the present time to permit meaningful drug sensitivity studies. The effects of chemotherapy on the more mature human progenitors has also been studied in a more direct manner, by assaying the number of marrow or circulating precursor cells (usually CFU-C) at given points after the administration of the therapy [29–31].

In subsequent sections of this chapter, the effects of specific drugs on hematopoietic progenitor cells, as determined by cell techniques will be summarized and related to the clinically observed effects of the drugs on peripheral counts and bone marrow.

4. BONE MARROW TOXICITY OF SPECIFIC AGENTS

4.1 *Introduction*

The effects of most chemotherapeutic agents on granulocyte and platelet counts have been defined by Phase I and II studies and have been confirmed by clinical use of these drugs. The effects of antineoplastic agents on red cell production are less clear, perhaps because little attention has been paid to this aspect because of the ease of erythrocyte replacement. Malignant disease, per se, even without direct bone marrow involvement can decrease effective red cell production resulting in the anemia of chronic disease. The relatively long life span of the mature red blood cell also contributes to the difficulty in assessing the suppressive effects of chemotherapy on erythropoiesis. There is information available regarding the effects of some drugs on BFU-E and CFU-E *in vitro* [32, 33], but whether this information can be extrapolated to the clinical situation is unclear.

In practical terms, this does not present much of a problem in the management of patients as the fall in red cells after chemotherapy is gradual, if at all, and in contrast to the granulocytopenia and thrombocytopenia, patient's anemia can readily be managed with transfusions. The life span of a mature granulocyte is several days with a circulation time of less than 12 hours and within 13–14 days, myeloblasts mature to granulocytes [34]. Platelets survive for several days and 4–5 days are required for megakaryocytic maturation and platelet production [35]. Thus, the clinically observed depressions of granulocytes and platelets are usually observed after a period of a few days to a few weeks. The clinically relevant toxicity of specific agents on granulocytes and platelets is summarized in Table 1 [36–38]. Granulocy-

Table 1. Clinically observed effects of antineoplastic agents on bone marrow (granulocytes and platelets)

Drug Alkylating agents:	Depression of: granulocytes (G)*	Platelets (P)
Nitrogen mustard	Initially 3 d after IV dose Nadir: 14–21 d Recovery: 4–6 wk.	Less decrease than G Nadir: 20–30 d Recovery: 3–15 wk.

Table 1. (continued)

Drug Alkylating agents:	Depression of: granulocytes (G)*	Platelets (P)
Busulfan	Begins after 7–10 d. of daily po dose; Continued fall for 2 wks. after stopping Rx. Recovery: variable, may be prolonged; usually 4–8 wk.	Variable effect, usually less decrease than G.
Chlorambucil	Decrease in G after 2–3 wk of daily po dose Lymphopenia more pronounced Combined fall for 10 d after stopping Rx (may be longer) Recovery: variable, usually by 8 wk.	Variable effect, usually less decrease than G.
Cyclophosphamide	Nadir: 10–14 d after IV dose Recovery by 21–28 d Fall in G after 7–10 d of daily po dose Recovery: variable, usually bu 2 wk.	Minimal decrease, usually.
Melphalan	Nadir: 7–14 d after IV or large po dose Fall in G after 1–2 wk. of dialy po dose Recovery: variable, usually 4–6 wk.	Similar to G
Thiotepa	Nadir: 5–30 d after IV dose	Similar to G
Nitrosureas		
BCNU CCNU MeCCNU	Nadir: 3–5 wks Recovery: 4–6 wks Cmulative toxicity	Similar to G
Streptozotocin	Uncommon	Uncommon
Antimetabolites		
Methotrexate	Nadir: 7–14 d after IV Recovery: 14–21 d Fall in G with po dose, may continue for 1 wk after stopping	Similar to G
6-Mercaptopurine	Gradual decrease in G with daily po dose, may persist for several d after stopping Nadir: usually 7 d Recovery: usually within 14–21 d	Less decrease than G
6-Thioguanine	Similar to 6–MP	Similar to G
5-Fluorouracil	Nadir: 7–14 d after IV dose Recovery: usually within 21–28 d	Less decrease than G, but recovery may be slower
Ftorafur	Less than with 5-FU	Minimal
Cytosine arabinoside (Ara C)	Decrease after 5–7 d of continuous IV Continues to fall up to 7 d Recovery: 21–28 d	Similar to G
5-Azacytidine	Similar to Ara C	Similar to G

Table 1. (continued)

Drug Alkylating agents:	Depression of: granulocytes (G)*	Platelets (P)
Antibiotics		
Adriamycin	Nadir: 10–18 d Recovery: usually by 21–28 d	Less decrease than G
Daunomycin	Similar to Adriamycin	Similar to Adriamycin
Bleomycin	Usually none	None
Mitomycin	Nadir: 3–5 wks. Recovery: usually 4–6 wks, may be prolonged	Similar to G; Cumulative toxicity on P
Actinomycin D	Decrease 1–7 d after stopping daily IV dose Nadir: 1–2 wk Recovery: usually 3–4 wk	May be greater than G and occur sooner
Antimitotic agents		
Vincristine	Unusual	None. May increase P
Vinblastine	Nadir: 5–10 d Recovery: 7–14 d	Minimal
Vindesine	Nadir: 3–5 d Recovery: 6–8 d	Minimal
Miscellaneous		
Cisplatin	Nadir: 18-23 d Recovery: 21–28 d Not often dose limiting toxicity	Similar to G
L-Asparaginase	Unusual	Unusual; may inhibit synthesis of clotting factors
Decarbazine (DTIC)	Nadir: usually 10–14 d Recovery: usually by 21 d, may be delayed	Similar to G
Hydroxyurea	Rapid decrease (Nadir 7 d) and recovery (complete within 14–21 d, usually)	Less common and severe than G.
Procarbazine	May be delayed (Nadir 21–26 d) and continue 1–3 wk after stopping po dose	Less common and severe than G.
Hexamethylmelamine	Moderate, usually not dose limiting Nadir: 12–18 d Recovery: may be prolonged	Similar to G

* d = day(s)
  wk = week(s)
  Rx = therapy

Table 2. Drugs in which bone marrow suppression is the dose limiting toxicity

All of the alkylating agents (nitrogen mustard, busulfan, cyclophosphamide, chlorambucil, melphalan, thiotepa).

All of the antimetabolites (methotrexate, 6-mercaptopurine, 6-thioguanine, 5-fluorouracil, cytosine arabisnoside, 5-azacytidine).

Vinblastine
VP-16 and VM-26
Anthracyclines (adriamycin, daunomycin)
Actinomycin-D
Mitomycin
Nitrosureas (BCNU, CCNU. Me-CCNU)
Hydroxyurea
Procarbazine
Cisplatin (when administered with forced diuresis)

topenia, particularly less than 500/ul, and thrombocytopenia, particularly less than 20,000/ul, may be associated with significant infection and bleeding, respectively. The depression of granulocytes and platelets constitute the dose-limiting toxicity for the majority of chemotherapeutic drugs currently in practice (Table 2).

4.2 *Alkylating Agents*

Alkylating agents act primarily by transferring alkyl groups to cellular constituents, principally guanine in DNA, which produces irreversible cell damage [36, 39]. In general, the alkylating agents are relatively cell cycle and phase non-specific and thus do not require active cellular replication to be effective in producing cytotoxicity. Myelosuppression is the usual dose limiting toxicity for all of the alkylating agents (Tables 1 and 2).

In Table 1, the effects of the various alkylators on bone marrow are summarized [36–38]. When administered as a single I.V. or large p.o. dose as in the treatment regimens for lymphoma, Hodgkin's disease, and breast cancer, bone marrow suppression is maximal at 10–14 days with recovery several days later. Usually normal blood counts are present by day 21. The oral forms of alkylators, such as cyclophosphamide, melphalan, chlorambucil, and busulfan, are often administered daily. This results in continuous myelosuppression, but doses can be adjusted to maintain granulocyte and platelet counts at depressed but safe levels. Although the various alkylators have similar structures, mechanisms of action and some degree of cross resistance, there are specific malignancies which are more responsive to a specific drug. There are differences in the myelosuppressive effects of the various alkylators, as well. Cyclophosphamide is relatively platelet sparing and when used as a single agent, the need to decrease the dose because of granulocytepenia usually is dose-limiting. Chlorambucil is the least myelosuppressive of these agents, but produces the most marked lymphopenia, which makes it the drug of choice in the treatment of chronic lymphocytic leukemia. The duration of myelosuppression is longer after the administration of busulfan than the other alkylators and occasionally prolonged aplasia may ensue.

The observed differences in myelosuppression among the alkylating agents can be explained in part from the observations made in murine hematopoietic cultures. Cyclophosphamide and busulfan have both been demonstrated to suppress murine CFU-S, but there are qualitative and quantitative differences between the two agents [40–45]. In contrast to the complete recovery of CFU-S numbers after the administration of cyclophosphamide, CFU-S recovery after treatment with busulfan, even when administered as a large single dose, may be prolonged [45]. Busulfan depresses CFU-S and CFU-C, independent of proliferative activity [40]. It has also been demonstrated that busulfan impairs the capacity of the CFU-S to differentiate into CFU-C [41]. Of interest, is the finding that a subpopulation of CFU-S are relatively resistant to the effects of busulfan [42], which might be important in preventing the development of marrow aplasia in the majority of animals.

It is of concern that the chronic administration of alkylating agents can permanently depress the numbers of pluripotent stem cells. Despite the permanent depression of CFU-S numbers seen in mice treated with busulfan, the residual number of stem cells still exceeds the needs of the nonstressed adult animal and most of the animals treated with multiple injections of busulfan ultimately recover from the prolonged myelosuppression [46, 47]. This will be discussed in more detail later in this chapter.

The study of drug effects on murine hematopoiesis has also expanded our knowledge of the mechanisms of action of the alkylating agents. For example, Ash, et al. [48] have demonstrated that although nitrogen mustard is thought to be predominantly cycle and phase nonspecific, cells (murine CFU-S) in G_1 are most sensitive with G_2 and S phase hematopoietic cells the most resistant. Observations such as these could have theoretical clinical implications in terms of drug scheduling.

4.3 Nitrosoureas

The nitrosoureas are both alkylating and carbamylating agents which interact with both amino acids and proteins, producing DNA damage [36, 39]. They are generally cell cycle and phase nonspecific. With the exception of Streptozotocin, the dose limiting toxicity of the nitrosoureas is myelosuppression. In contrast to the myelosuppression associated with most other antineoplastic agents, bone marrow suppression from nitrosoureas is delayed, prolonged, and cumulative (Table 1) [36–38].

It has been demonstrated in mice that BCNU produces prolonged suppression of CFU-S, consistent with the prolonged panyctopenia observed clinically [49]. This also explains the delay in the decline in peripheral counts, since the more mature committed progenitor cells do not appear to be affected by the nitrosureas. Both BCNU and CCNU have been demonstrated to affect both proliferating and resting marrow cells [50]. It has been hypothesized because they are lipid soluble these drugs can freely enter cells independent of cycle status and thus provide a basis for the prolonged and delayed myelosuppression [51]. Nitrosourea analogues have been synthesized in the hopes of finding a drug with less marrow toxicity [52]. Such agents have been identified on the basis of *in vitro* studies, but to date clinical success has been rather limited [53, 54]. Attempts to limit myelosuppression by inhibiting uptake of the drug by marrow precursor cells, through the use of infusions of large amounts of glucose, have also been unsuccessful [53].

4.4 *Antimetabolites*

Although the different antimetabolites vary somewhat in their mechanisms of action, they are cell cycle and phase specific [36, 39]. There are unique and often idiosyncratic toxicities associated with the various antimetabolites (discussed elsewhere in this book), but for the most part, bone marrow toxicity is usually dose limiting (Tables 1 and 2) [36–38].

Methotrexate (MTX) is an S phase specific agent which acts primarily by the inhibition of dihydrofolate reductase which ultimately inhibits the one-carbon transfers necessary for the synthesis of thymidylic acid, an integral component of DNA [36]. Experiments in mice have demonstrated that the concentration and duration of exposure of marrow to free drug is a critical determinant of bone marrow toxicity [55]. *In vitro* experiments with human marrow have demonstrated that CFU-C are relatively resistant to MTX, even in high concentration, if the duration of exposure is short [56]. Nonetheless, myelosuppression together with mucositis is the usual dose-limiting toxicity of MTX. Pharmacologic maneuvers, which exploit differences between normal marrow progenitors and tumor cells, have been successfully employed to modify myelosuppression [57] (discussed later in this chapter).

6-mercaptopurine (6-MP) inhibits do novo purine synthesis and is also S phase specific. Myelosuppression is usually of gradual onset with relative sparing of platelets (Table 1) [58]. 6-thioguanine (6-TG) has a similar mechanism of action to 6-MP, but in addition is incorporated into DNA and RNA. Marked myelosuppression is the dose-limiting toxicity observed with 6-TG [59].

5-fluorouracil (5-FU) is also an S phase specific agent which acts primarily by inhibiting thymidilate synthetase [39]. It is also incorporated into RNA. Murine experiments have detailed morphological changes in bone marrow even after a single injection of 5-FU [60], consistent with the observed effects in patients (Table 1). It may be that bone marrow cells become resistant to the toxic effects of 5-FU if the drug is administered in reduced doses as a continuous infusion [61, 62], a possibility which one would not predict given our understanding of the mechanism of action of the drug. The N_1-2(2'-furanidyl) derivative of 5-FU, ftorafur, has a similar mechanism of action as 5-FU, but for reasons which are currently not understood, myelosuppression does not appear to be as severe [63]. Unfortunately, marked neurotoxicity may occur with this derivative [63].

Cytosine arabinoside (ara-C) is S phase specific and appears to produce cytotoxic effects through multiple mechanisms of action [36, 39]. Conversion to ara-CTP is a crucial step which is necessary for the inhibition of DNA polymerase which in turn leads to decreased DNA synthesis [64, 65]. Hematologic toxicity may be severe, depending on the route and schedule of administration [66]. Sustained drug levels of ara-C and presumed continuous exposure of the marrow progenitor cells to the drug are achieved with continuous intravenous infusion of ara-C [38]. By contrast, the intermittent subcutaneous administration of equivalent doses of ara-C, a method of administration which is employed as maintenance therapy for acute non-lymphocytic leukemia (ANLL), does not produce the sustained plasma drug levels seen with continuous IV infusion, and thus, produces significantly less myelosuppression [38]. Massive doses of ara-C can be administered intravenously if given as short infusions, spaced 12 hours apart [67]. Normal hematopoietic precursors are killed by this method of drug administration, but the myelosuppression is reversible and is comparable to that seen with continuous exposure of the drug in conventional doses.

It has been demonstrated in mice that normal CFU-S are not as sensitive to ara-C as L1210 leukemic cells [68]. It has also been demonstrated that the depression of CFU-S is reversible with an initial overshoot [49]. Given that ara-C will induce remission in ANLL, it is clear that leukemic cells must be more sensitive to the toxic effects of ara-C than normal progenitor cells. The reasons for the difference are not completely understood, but may be related to the retention of ara-CTP, with prolonged retention being associated with continual killing of the leukemic cells as they proceed from G_1 into S phase [65]. Duration of remission in ANLL has been correlated with the ability of the leukemic cells to retain ara-CTP [65].

5-azacytidine (5-aza) is employed to treat refractory ANLL and has multiple mechanisms of action, including incorporation into DNA and RNA with inhibition of protein synthesis [39]. It is an S phase specific agent, although there is some suggestion that it may be cycle nonspecific as well. As with ara-C, profound panyctopenia results after continuous intravenous administration of 5-aza, but with remission induction, normal myelopoiesis resumes. Prolonged myelosuppression has been reported with 5-aza.

4.5 Antitumor Antibiotics

The administration of the anthracycline antibiotics, currently in clinical use, adriamycin (doxorubicin) and daunomycin (daunorubicin), ultimately are limited in total cumulative dosage by cardiotoxicity. In the short term, however, myelosuppression is the dose-limiting toxicity. These agents are believed to act primarily by intercalating base pairs of DNA with inhibition of DNA-dependent RNA synthesis and are thus cell cycle nonspecific agents, although they may be more active in S phase [36, 39]. Both adriamycin and daunomycin have been shown to be toxic to normal human marrow CFU-C [69, 70], which is consistent with the marked leukopenia observed clinically. Murine experiments have demonstrated that both of these anthracyclines are less toxic to normal CFU-S than leukemic CFU-S [71], an observation which is consistent with the effects observed in treating the majority of patients with ANLL.

In addition to the search for less cardiotoxic anthracyclines, there have also been attempts to find analogues which are less toxic to normal hematopoietic progenitor cells [72, 73]. Detorubicin does appear to be less toxic to CFU-S and CFU-C in mice [72]. Both detorubicin and adriamycin as DNA complexes are less toxic to the CFU-S than are adriamycin or daunomycin. So far, these observations have not been successfully advanced to the clinical setting. The development of anthracycline analogues such as marcellomycin [73], which are less toxic to human marrow CFU-C may also have important clinical implications.

Mitomycin C has multiple mechanisms of action including alkylating agent activity and cross-linking of DNA [36, 39]. It is cell cycle nonspecific, but is most active in late G_1 and early S phases. Myelosuppression may be cumulative, particularly thrombocytopenia (Table 1) [36, 74].

Actinomycin D is a cycle nonspecific agent that acts by intercalating between DNA base pairs and inhibiting DNA-dependent RNA synthesis [36]. It is usually administered intravenously for five days and results in marrow suppression within a week after its administration is discontinued (Table 1).

In contrast to the other antitumor antibiotics, bleomycin is nonmyelosuppressive [75]. Chronic administration of bleomycin to mice has been demonstrated to result in an initial decrease in CFU-S numbers, but there is a consistent return to normal levels and the drug did not suppress more mature progenitor cells [76, 77].

4.6 *Mitotic Inhibitors*

The vinca alkaloids in clinical use, vincristine and vinblastine, have multiple mechanisms of action, but act primarily through an arrest of the mitotic spindle apparatus and are thus M phase and cycle specific agents. At high concentrations, they are also active during S and G_1 phase [36, 39]. Since dose-limiting neurotoxicity governs clinical use, it is rare to observe myelosuppression with vincristine, although in higher concentrations, the drug is toxic to human CFU-C *in vitro* [78]. In contrast, leukopenia is the usual dose-limiting toxicity associated with vinblastine, but at high dose levels neurotoxicity can occur as well [36]. Vinblastine has demonstrable toxicity to murine hematopoietic progenitor cells, but there is generally rapid recovery [79]. Vindesine, an investigational vinca alkaloid, appears to also be associated with considerable bone marrow toxicity. This agent may have antitumor activity against malignancies which are resistant to vincristine and vinblastine [80].

The epipodophyllotoxins VP-16 and VM-26 (VM-26 still being investigational) are agents which produce metaphase arrest and inhibit cell entry into mitosis [36, 81, 82]. They are G_2 and S phase specific. Bone marrow suppression is the usual dose-limiting toxicity and is schedule dependent. These agents produce an exponential decline in murine CFU-S numbers, but the normal CFU-S are more resistant than L1210 cells [83]. Clinically, there appears to be relative sparing of platelets, but there may be increased erythroid toxicity [81, 82].

4.7 *Miscellaneous Agents*

Procarbazine has multiple complex mechanisms of action, including inhibition of DNA, RNA and protein synthesis [36, 84]. It is a phase nonspecific agent with dose-limiting hematologic toxicity. Myelosuppression may be delayed for several weeks after initiating therapy with procarbazine (Table 1).

Hydroxyurea is an S phase specific agent which inhibits DNA synthesis through the inhibition of ribonucleotide reductase [36]. Bone marrow suppression is the usual dose-limiting toxicity, but is rapidly reversible. Platelets and red blood cells are affected less than white cells [85].

Dacarbazine (DTIC) inhibits purine, RNA, and protein synthesis in addition to producing some inhibition of DNA synthesis. It is a phase nonspecific agent with dose-limiting hematologic toxicity (Table 1) [36].

Cisplatin inhibits DNA synthesis and acts like an alkylating agent [86]. It is cell cycle and phase nonspecific. Now that renal insufficiency can largely be prevented with adequate hydration of the patients, hematologic toxicity may be the dose-limiting factor [87, 88]. This drug has been found to be myelosuppressive to mice in a dose-related manner and quite toxic to CFU-

S [89, 90]. There is also some evidence from human studies that cisplatin may be particularly toxic to erythroid progenitor cells [33].

Hexamethylmelamine is an S phase specific agent which inhibits incorporation of thymidine and uridine into DNA and RNA [36]. There is significant myelosuppression associated with this drug but commonly the dose needs to be lowered because of severe gastrointestinal toxicity.

4.8 *Investigational Agents*

It is beyond the scope of this chapter to detail the effects on bone marrow of all of the drugs currently under investigation as possible antitumor agents. Toxicity of new agents is delineated in preclinical and Phase I studies. It also appears that *in vitro* cultures of hematopoietic progenitor cells may also be employed to predict the toxicity for new agents.

Two agents which presently are being actively investigated as possible antineoplastic agents are m-AMSA and interferon. M-AMSA has demonstrable activity against acute leukemia and breast cancer [91, 92]. Bone marrow toxicity is considerable. The drug suppresses CFU-S and CFU-C in mice [93] and also is toxic to human CFU-C *in vitro* [94].

Interferon therapy is currently under investigation. The relative lack of clinical toxicity has been advanced as a major advantage of this form of therapy, but the dose levels which have been administered to patients have been low because of supply problems [95]. In higher doses, interferon may very well be myelosuppressive since *in vitro* cultures have demonstrated toxicity to both murine and human hematopoietic progenitor cells, including CFU-C and CFU-E [96, 97].

It is theoretically possible to test any new chemotherapeutic agent *in vitro* for toxicity to hematopoietic progenitors. Human marrow cells would probably be the most appropriate target, but even with this system, it shoould be recognized that one cannot necessarily extrapolate from the laboratory findings to what will happen when the drug is administered to a patient. There are many other factors involved in the clinical situation including the metabolism and pharmacologic disposition of the drug. For example, cyclophosphamide is inactive *in vitro* and has no demonstrable toxicity to hematopoietic progenitors unless it is metabolized in the liver. Despite these limitations, *in vitro* sutides of drug sensitivity may provide some guidelines not only in screening for new agents with antitumor effect, but also in developing agents which are less myelosuppressive.

5. CHRONIC EFFECTS OF ANTITUMOUR AGENTS ON BONE MARROW

The long-term administration of chemotherapeutic agents may result in irreversible suppression of normal hematopoiesis and/or the development of leukemia. As discussed above, prolonged myelosuppression is most often produced by the nitrosoureas and busulfan. Administration of the nitrosoureas or mitomycin may result in cumulative marrow toxicity, especially with impairment of platelet production.

Whether the number of pluripotent stem cells is limited or not is obviously of prime concern, especially when chemotherapy is administered to patients who have a chance for cure or a long life. It has been shown that the suppression of CFU-S produced by ara-C is rapidly reversible in contrast to the prolonged suppression of CFU-S seen after the administration of BCNU to mice [49]. Studies by Trainor, et al. [98, 99] in mice have demonstrated prolonged depression of CFU-S and CFU-C after the administration of busulfan, BCNU, mitomycin, chlorambucil, and L-phenylalanine mustard (melphalan). In contrast, the number of these progenitor cells consistently returned to normal after the administration of cyclophosphamide, 5-FU, 6-MP, methotrexate, and vinblastine. Studies by Dumenil, et al. [100, 101] have demonstrated that phase specific agents, such as hydroxyurea and ara-C, do not cause prolonged depression of murine CFU-S in contrast to the combination regimens which are employed to treat lymphoma. Botnick, et al. [102, 103] performed serial transfers of stem cells in mice and observed that the self-renewal potential was reduced after the administration of busulfan and to a lesser extent, melphalan. Cyclophosphamide and 5-FU did not affect the self-renewal potential. Studies by Standen and Blackett [104] with rat bone marrow employing an assay to measure erythroid and granulocytic repopulating ability, yielded similar results in that busulfan and dimethylmyleran caused a persistent decrease whereas cyclophosphamide produced a reversible decrease in repopulating ability. Taken together, these animal studies indicate that some alkylating agents have the potential to cause permanent depletion of pluripotent stem cells. The marrow stroma may also be permanently affected as suggested by the work of Fried, et al. [44], who showed that a short course of cyclophosphamide could cause long-term depression of marrow stromal function in addition to causing a decrease in the proliferative potential on murine CFU-S.

These experimental observations parallel clinical observations, since the agents which cause prolonged depletion of stem cells in animals can produce prolonged and occasionally permanent myelosuppression in man. One should not assume, however, that prolonged pancytopenia is always the result of chemotherapy since marrow involvement by tumor cells and immune-mediated mechanisms may also cause a decrease in peripheral counts and these should be excluded before one concludes that the pancytopenia is secondary to previous chemotherapy [105–107].

With prolonged survival of cancer patients, it is becoming increasingly apparent that the chronic administration of antineoplastic agents increases the incidence of leukemia [108, 109]. Secondary leukemia is seen most often in patients who have been treated for Hodgkin's disease [110, 111], ovarian [112], and breast cancer [113]. It is also observed in patients treated for multiple myeloma [114] and polycythemia vera [115], but there also appears to be an increased incidence of leukemia in untreated patients with these malignancies. Secondary leukemia has also been reported to occur after treatment for other malignancies [116, 117] as well, and has also been reported in patients with non-malignant diseases who have been treated with antineoplastic agents [118.]

Secondary leukemia has been most frequently observed after the chronic administration of alkylating agents, but has also been reported after treatment with other chemotherapeutic drugs [118]. Leukemia has also followed radiation therapy. The combination of irradiation and chemotherapy appears synergistic in producing leukemia, since as many as 10% of patients who have received combined modality therapy for Hodgkin's disease may develop leukemia [110].

ANLL is the most common type of secondary leukemia, with acute myelomonocytic leukemia (FAB-M4) being the most common subtype [108, 109]. The interval from beginning chemotherapy to the development of leukemia is variable, but is usually in the range of 3-7 years. Several features distinguish secondary from primary ANLL [108, 109]. In the case of secondary ANLL, there is frequently a preleukemic phase, with a long period of pancytopenia secondary to ineffective hematopoiesis and characteristic morphologic and cytogenetic abnormalities present in the bone marrow. Secondary ANLL appears to be very refractory to intensive chemotherapy, with remission rates below 40% [119]. With new treatment regimens employing high doses of ara-C, remission induction is improving in this subset of patients with ANLL [67]. Hopefully, these results will be confirmed in larger studies.

6. FACTORS ASSOCIATED WITH INCREASED BONE MARROW TOXICITY

Although the bone marrow toxicity of antineoplastic agents is usually predictable and dose-related, occasionally more severe, unexpected myelosuppression may occur. Multiple factors may be associated with increased bone marrow toxicity. Knowledge of some of these factors beforehand would enable one to appropriately decrease the doses of chemotherapy if severe myelosuppression is to be avoided.

The most common cause of increased myelosuppression may very well be overdosage of chemotherapy, either through incorrect calculations of doses or misunderstandings of specific regimens. It is extremely important to have

Table 3. Example of a dose modification table, for adjusting doses of myelosuppressive chemo-therapy (From CALGB Protocol 7981, Comis, et al.)

If on day of therapy			Administer the following percentage of dose
WBC/ul	and	Platelet/ul	myelosuppressive drugs*:
≥ 4,000		≥ 100,00	100%
3,500–3,999		≥ 100,000	75%
3,000–3,499		75,000–99,999	50%
2,500–2,999		75,000–99,999	25%
			0
< 2,500	or	< 75,000	delay therapy until counts increase

* If the WBC or platelet nadir (during previous course) is less than 1,000 cells/ul or 75,000 cells/ul, respectively, the calculated dose (from table) should be further decreased by 25% for this cycle.

experienced physicians, nurses, and pharmacists, if possible, all involved with the preparation and administration of chemotherapy. Since most doses of drugs are based on body surface area, it is important to weigh patients prior to each course of therapy and appropriately adjust drug dosage. Modifications of therapy, either changing the dose or the interval between doses, need to be made based on the nadir and time to recovery from the previous course. Blood counts on the day of therapy are mandatory before administering any myelosuppressive chemotherapy. Different drugs and treatment protocols call for specific types of adjustments. A general guideline is provided in Table 3 [120].

Knowledge of drug metabolism is also essential in preventing inadvertent overdosage of chemotherapy. Drugs which are metabolized in the liver such as adriamycin, should be administered at a reduced level in the presence of hepatic dysfunction [38]. The bilirubin level serves as a rough guide in determining dosage adjustments. Likewise, drugs which depend on renal excretion, such as Mtx, 6-MP, and 6-TG, need to be given at a lower dose in the presence of renal insufficiency [38].

Elderly patients are generally less able to tolerate chemotherapy than younger patients. In terms of bone marrow toxicity, marrow cellularity decreases with the age of the patient [121] and there is a suggestion that the number of hematopoietic stem cells also decreases with age [122]. In practice, for most drugs, initial doses are not usually modified for elderly patients, but in subsequent courses, doses often need to be lowered because of increased myelosuppression. Nonetheless, it is important to administer as much therapy as tolerated, even in elderly patients, as responses may be suboptimal in patients receiving less than full doses of chemotherapy [123, 124].

Myelosuppressive effects of chemotherapy may be enhanced by other factors as well. Concomitant or prior irradiation, especially to large bone marrow bearing areas of the body, increased the myelotoxic effects of most myelosuppressive agents [125]. As demonstrated by patients treated with combination irradiation/chemotherapy for Hodgkin's disease, the effects of irradiation on reduced tolerance of marrow to chemotherapy may be quite prolonged. Experiments in mice have demonstrated that irradiation depletes CFU-S and may also cause marrow stromal damage [45, 126].

The myelosuppressive effects of specific antineoplastic agents may be increased by interaction with other drugs. The best known example is the decreased metabolism of 6-MP in patients who are taking allopurinol. The dose of 6-MP should be decreased by 2/3 in these patients [36]. Other drug interactions with chemotherapeutic agents tend to be more of the idiosyncratic type and the mechanisms are not as well understood. For example, theophylline has been reported to increase the myelosuppression associated with nitrosureas [127]. Pretreatment of patients with alpha-tocopherol has been reported to increase adriamycin bone marrow toxicity [128]. Cimetidine, a frequently prescribed drug in the United States, has been demonstrated to decrease the growth of human CFU-C [128]. Byron [130] has demonstrated that there are H_2 histamine receptors present on pluripotent hemopoietic stem cells and that cimetidine competes for these receptors in a dose-dependent manner. There are also numerous reports which implicate this drug in causing varying degrees of aplastic anemia [131, 132]. Increased myelosuppression may be seen in patients receiving cimetidine, particularly with the administration of nitrosoureas. Hyperthermia has also been reported to increase the myelotoxicity *in vitro* of nitrosoureas [133].

Other phenomena may be associated with increased myelosuppression. Certain drugs, such as Mtx, accumulate in effusions and the subsequent slow re-entry of the drug into the blood may result in prolonged drug levels and increase bone marrow toxicity. Additionally, increased toxicity associated with unexplained high levels of adriamycin has been observed in several patients undergoing remissions induction therapy for ANLL [134]. These patients had normal liver function (as measured by conventional parameters) and pharmacokinetic studies are in progress to assess the frequency of this phenomenon and the reasons for its occurrence. In addition, there are certain patients whose marrow, for unknown reasons, appears to be extraordinarily sensitive to chemotherapy. Studies employing *in vitro* cultures and determinations of drug levels should improve our understanding of these problems.

7. MEASURES TO REDUCE BONE MARROW TOXICITY

Since myelosuppression is the dose-limiting toxicity for most antineoplastic agents, there have been extensive efforts to find ways to decrease bone marrow toxicity and increase the therapeutic/toxic ratio of the drugs which are employed to treat malignancies. Efforts have been directed at selectively 'rescuing' normal hematopoietic progenitor cells from the toxic effects of chemotherapy as opposed to tumor cells and at enhancing kinetic recovery of the progenitor cells after they have been suppressed.

To date, most of the success in ameliorating myelosuppression has been achieved in rescuing marrow progenitors from the effects of high dose methotrexate (Mtx), with folinic acid (leucovorin) or thymidine [57, 135]. With the former, patients are treated with high doses of Mtx and after a period of time, usually 24 hours, leucovorin is administered. For well hydrated patients with relatively normal renal function, myelosuppression is minimal with this regimen. Monitoring Mtx levels and increasing the dose of leucovorin adds a margin of safety to the regimen. Leucovorin presumably is taken up by hematopoietic progenitors and the block of dihydrofolate reductase, which has been imposed by Mtx, is bypassed [136]. Apparently the 24 hours of inhibition of DNA synthesis are tolerated by marrow cells and not by some tumor cells. Human marrow CFU-C *in vitro* have been found to be resistant to Mtx even in high doses, if the period of incubation was kept under 24 hours [56]. It has also been demonstrated *in vitro* that leucovorin can indeed reverse the killing of murine granulocytic progenitors produced by Mtx [136, 137]. While the administration of massive doses of Mtx is theoretically advantageous, it remains to be proven that high dose Mtx regimens are indeed superior to regimens which employ conventional doses of Mtx.

Mtx myelosuppression can also be prevented by supplying thymidine and purines [138]. The synthesis of these nucleosides is blocked by the depletion of reduced folates produced by Mtx. *In vitro* studies have demonstrated that thymidine in combination with a purine will protect murine CFU-C from Mtx [139]. In clinical studies, thymidine alone appears to be adequate in preventing or ameliorating Mtx-induced myelosuppression [136]. It may be that Mtx does not severely impair *de novo* purine synthesis in normal human cells or that these normal cells can utilize purine salvage pathways. The role of thymidine rescue of Mtx toxicity in the treatment of malignancies needs to be further evaluated and compared to the leucovorin rescue techniques. It is of interest that endogenous thymidine levels may vary in cancer patients, in ranges which are effective in altering CFU-C toxicity of Mtx *in vitro* [140]. These differences could theoretically explain different degrees of myelosuppression among patients treated with Mtx.

Other experimental approaches for ameliorating Mtx toxicity include the administration of carboxypeptidase [141], an enzyme which cleaves and inactivates extracellular Mtx and the administration of L-asparaginase [142], which presumably prevents the unbalanced growth induced by Mtx. There has been little effort devoted to developing methods for ameliorating the myelosuppression produced by other antineoplastic agents.

An alternative approach for ameliorating or at least shortening the duration of bone marrow suppression is the administration of agents that will enhance the recovery of progenitor cells. Since granulocytopenia is usually the most severe and life-threatening of the cytopenias, most efforts have been concentrated on raising the white blood count after myelosuppressive doses of chemotherapy. Lithium carbonate, known to be a cause of leukocytosis, has been shown to increase total neutrophil mass [143]. One of its mechanisms of action is to cause increased levels of colony stimulating activity [144–146]. Lithium has also been demonstrated to expand the pluripotential stem cell pool (CFU-S) in mice, and in murine studies, the administration of lithium reduced the length of time for recovery of normal hematopoiesis following transplantation [147].

There have been several clinical studies in which patients being treated with chemotherapy were randomized to receive or not to receive lithium [148–150]. Several groups of investigators have reported that the administration of lithium reduced the granulocyte nadir and the time to recovery for patients receiving chemotherapy [149, 150]. Other studies have failed to confirm these reports [148]. It is clear that additional factors need to be explored, such as lithium levels achieved clinically, the types of tumors being treated, and the specific drugs used to treat the tumors. Lithium has been found not to affect hemoglobin or platelet counts.

One could also theoretically take advantage of the kinetic changes produced by one drug to modify the myelosuppression resulting from the administration of another drug. For example, prior treatment of mice with cyclophosphamide has been reported to enhance the recovery of CFU-S after total body irradiation [151, 152]. In a limited clinical study, pretreatment of melanoma patients with intravenous cyclophosphamide seven days prior to high dose melphalan was associated with a more rapid recovery of granulocyte counts [153].

8. MEASURES TO DEAL WITH MYELOSUPPRESSION

Since myelosuppression is usually reversible and sometimes unavoidable if drugs are administered at clinically effective dose levels, efforts have been directed towards dealing with the effects of granulocytopenia and thrombocytopenia. With the administration of broad spectrum antibiotics, morbidity and mortality from chemotherapy induced granulocytopenia has significantly decreased. In patients who are neutropenic for prolonged periods of time, such as those receiving therapy for ANLL, prophylactic therapy with cotrimoxazole appears to have decreased the incidence of infectious episodes [154]. Granulocyte transfusions are now readily available in most medical centers, and may be of some value in treating the neutropenic patient who fails to respond to broad spectrum antibiotics. The role for laminar air flow rooms and nonabsorbable oral antibiotics is unclear. Platelet transfusions are also readily available in most hospitals and should be given to patients whose platelets fall below 20,000/ul secondary to chemotherapy.

There has been recent interest in cryopreserving bone marrow from patients prior to treatment with unusually large doses of chemotherapy and then using this marrow as an autotransplant [155–157]. To date, success has been rather limited and has been precluded in part by a high incidence of severe hepatic and renal toxicity associated with the administration of 'megadose' chemotherapy. Occasional patients have benefited from this procedure, but the success of this approach may be limited by the general resistance of many of the solid tumors to chemotherapy.

9. CONCLUSION

This review of bone marrow toxicity associated with antitumor agents is not exhaustive. It does not, for example, address the far more complex problem of synergistic and additive effects which might be expected to occur with combination chemotherapy. Because of the complexities of the latter, our understanding of their influence on marrow function can to date only be reached by empiric means. However, a thorough understanding of the effects of each agent on the myeloid organ allows a more rational approach to devising safe combinations.

Oncologic chemotherapists tend to think in terms of standard doses, schedules, and regimens, which are modified downward based on pre-treatment variables (age, lean body weight, previous treatment history) and on actual observation of the toxicity of a course of treatment. But is this not a logical blind alley? Undoubtedly, as we develop better methods to determine the subcellular pharmacology of both host tissue and tumor, it is likely that combinations will be devised to match the particular patient and his/her tumors; studies currently directed towards dissecting the effects of a given agent on the elements of myelopoiesis are a primitive albeit real beginning to this end.

Likewise, as has already been learned through autologous transplantation experiments, escalation of drug doses permitted by passing or ameliorating marrow toxicity uncover new dose-limiting toxicities to the mucosa, liver, and other organs. As there is still a rationale to strive for the ability to deliver increased doses of drugs, we must begin to study the variables affecting toxicities in these tissues and methods for reducing them.

ACKNOWLEDGEMENT

This study is supported in part by USPHS Grant CA-5834 from the NCI.

REFERENCES

1. Metcalf D: Hemopoietic colonies. *in vitro* cloning of normal and leukemic cells. Berlin, Springer-Verlag, 1977.
2. Till JE, McCullough EA: A direct measurement of the radiation sensitivity of normal mouse bone marrow. Radiat Res 14:213–222, 1961.
3. Fauser AA, Messner HA: Identification of megakaryocytes, macrophages, and eosinophils in colonies of human bone marrow containing neutrophilic granulocytes and erythroblasts. Blood 53:1023–1027, 1979.
4. Messner HA, Izaguirre CA, Jamal N: Identification of T-lymphocytes in human mixed hemopoietic colonies. Blood 58:402–405, 1981.
5. Bradley TR, Metcalf D: The growth of mouse bone marrow cells *in vitro*. Aust J Exp Biol Med 44:287–299, 1966.
6. Axelrad AA, McLeod DL, Shreeve MM, Heath DS: Properties of cells that produce erythrocytic colonies *in vitro*. In: Hemopoiesis in Culture, Robinson WA (ed), Washington, DC, US Gov't Printing Office, 1974, p 226.
7. Stephenson JR, Axelrad AA, McLeod DL, Shreeve MM: Induction of colonies of hemoglobin-synthesizing cells by erythropoietin *in vitro*. Proc Natl Acad Sci USA 68:1542, 1971.
8. Mazur E, Hoffman R, Chasis J, Marchesi S, Bruno E: Immunofluorescent identification of human megakaryocyte colonies using antiplatelet glycoprotein antiserum. Blood 57:277–286, 1981.
9. Nakeff A, Daniels-McQueen S: *in vitro* colony assay for a new class of megakaryocyte precursor: Colony-forming unit megakaryocyte (CFU-M). Proc Soc Exp Biol Med 151:587–590, 1976.
10. Claesson MM, Rodger MD, Johnson GR, Whittinham S, Metcalf D: Colony formation by human T lymphocytes in agar medium. Clin Exp Immunol 28:526, 1977.
11. Fibach E, Gerassi E, Sachs L: Induction of colony formation *in vitro* by human lymphocytes. Nature 259:127–129, 1976.
12. Izaguirre CA, Minden MD, Howatson AF, McCulloch EA: Colony formation by normal and malignant human B-lymphocytes. Br J Cancer 42:430, 1980.
13. Dexter TM: Hematopoiesis in long-term bone marrow culture. Acta Haemat 62:299–305, 1979.
14. Buick RN, Till JE, McCulloch EA: Colony assay for proliferative blast cells circulating in

myeloblastic leukemia. Lancet 1:862–863, 1977.

15. Tannock IF: Cell kinetics and chemotherapy: A critical review. Cancer Treat Rep 62:1117–1133, 1978.

16. Gray JW, Dean PN, Mendelsohn ML: Quantitative cell-cycle analysis. In: Flow Cytometry and Sorting, Melamed MR, Mullaney PF, Mendelsohn ML (eds), New York, Wiley, 1979, p 383–408.

17. Iscove NN, Till JE, McCulloch EA: Proliferative state of human granulopoietic cells. Blood 36:828, 1970.

18. Liu YK, Stallard SS, Koo V, Dannaher CL: The proliferative states of circulating granulopoietic stem cellsin man. Scand J Haematol 22:258–262, 1979.

19. Cronkite EP, Fliedner TM, Bond VP, et al: Dynamics of hemopoietic proliferation in man and mice studied by tritiated thymidine incorporation into DNA. Ann NY Acad Sci 77:803–820, 1959.

20. Killmann SA: Cell classification and kinetic aspects of normoblastic and megaloblastic erythropoiesis. Cell Tissue Kinetics 3:217–228, 1970.

21. Kesse-Elias M, Harriss EP, Gyftaki E: In vitro study of DNA synthesis time and cell cycle time in erythrocyte precursors of normal and thalassaemic subjects using ^{3}H- and ^{14}C-thymidine double labelling technique. Acta Haematol 38:170–177, 1967.

22. Marsh JC: The effects of cancer chemotherapeutic agents on normal hematopoietic precursor cells: A review. Cancer Res 36:1853–1882, 1976.

23. DowLW: Sensitivity of normal and neoplastic cells to chemotherapeutic agents in vitro. Adv Intern Med 25:427–452, 1980.

24. Blackett NM, Marsh JC, Gordon MY, Okell SF, Aguado M: Simultaneous assay by 6 methods of the effect on hemopoietic precursor cells of adriamycin, methyl CCNU, 60 Co gamma rays, vinblastine, and cytosine arabinoside. Exp Hematol 6:2–8, 1978.

25. Greenberg PL, Vankersen I, Mosny S: Cytotoxic effects of 1-beta-D-arabinofuranosylcytosine and 6-thioguanine in vitro on granulocytic progenitor cells. Cancer Res 36:4412–4417, 1976.

26. Preisler HD, Epstein J: A comparison of two methods for determining the sensitivity of human myeloid colony-forming units to cytosine arabinoside. Br J Haematol 47:519–527, 1981.

27. Brown CB, Carbone PP: Effects of chemotherapeutic agents on normal bone marrow growth in vitro. Cancer Res 31:185–190, 1971.

28. Bruce WR, Meeker BE, Valeriote FA: Comparison of the sensitivity of normal hematopoietic and transplanted lymphoma colony-forming cells to chemotherapeutic agents administered in vitro. J Natl Cancer Inst 37:233, 1966.

29. Labedzki L, Illiger J, Drebber G, et al: Monitoring of aggressive chemotherapy by circulating myeloid stem cells. Exp Hematol 7 (Suppl 6):140, 1979.

30. Lohrmann HP, Schreml W, Fliedner TM, Heimpel M: Reaction of human granulopoiesis tohigh dose cyclophosphamide therapy. Blut 38:9–16, 1979.

31. Lohrmann HP, Schreml W, Lang M, et al: Changes of granulopoiesis during and after adjuvant chemotherapy of breast cancer. Br J Haematol 40:369–381, 1978.

32. Nowrousian MR, Schmidt CG: Differential sensitivity of murine bone marrow hematopoietic stem cells to cisplatin. Exp Hematol 9:23, 1981.

33. Rothman SA, Weich JK: Cisplatin toxicity for erythroid precursors. N Engl J Med 304:360, 1981.

34. Golde DW, Cline MJ: Production, distribution, and fate of granulocytes. In: Hematology, Williams WJ (ed), New York, McGraw-Hill, 1977, p 699–706.

35. Aster RH: Production, distribution, life-span, and fate of platelets. In: Hematology, Williams WJ (ed), New York, McGraw-Hill, 1977, p 1210-1220.

36. Carter SK, Livingston RB: Drugs available to treat cancer. In: Principles of Cancer Treat-

ment. Carter SK, Glatstein E, Livingston RB (eds), New York, McGraw Hill, 1981, p 111-145.

37. Greenwald ES: Cancer Chemotherapy. Second edition. Flushing, NY: Medical Examination Publishing Company, 1973.

38. Henderson ES: The granulocytopenic effects of cancer chemotherapeutic agents. In: Drugs and hematologic Reactions, Dimitrov NV and Nodine JH (eds), New York, Grune & Stratton, 1974, p 207-221.

39. Pinedo HM. Cancer Chemotherapy Annual 2. New York: Elsevier, 1980.

40. Delmonte L: Effect of myleran on murine hemopoiesis. I. Granulocytic cell line specificity of action on progenitor cells. Cell Tiss Kinet 11:347-358, 1978.

41. Delmonte L: Effect of myleran on murine hemopoiesis. II. Direct and host-mediated action on proliferative capacity and differentiation bias of spleen colony-forming units (CFU-S). Cell Tiss Kinet 11:359-367, 1978.

42. Delmonte Lb: Effect of myleran on murine hemopoiesis. III. Changes in the density distribution of spleen colony forming (CFU-S) and agar gel colony-forming cells (CFU-C). Cell Tiss Kinet 11:369-375, 1978.

43. Dunn CDR, Elson LA: The comparative effect of busulfan ('myleran') on hematopoietic colony-forming units in the rat. Cell Tiss Kinet 3:131, 1970.

44. Fried W, Barone J: Residual marrow damage following therapy with cyclophosphamide. Exp Hematol 8:610-614, 1980.

45. Fried W, Kedo A, Barone J: Effects of cyclophosphamide and of busulfan on spleen colony-forming units and on hematopoietic stroma. Cancer Res 37:1205-1209, 1977.

46. Botnick LE, Hannon EC, Hellman S: Multisystem stem cell failure after apparent recovery from alkylating agents. Cancer Res 38:1942-1947, 1978.

47. Morley A: Residual marrow damage from cytotoxic drugs. Aust NZ J Med 10:569-571, 1980.

48. Ash R, Chaffey JT, Hellman S: The effect of nitrogen mustard on the survival of murine hematopoietic stem cells. Cancer Res 32:1695-1702, 1972.

49. Preisler HD, Henderson ES: Effects of cytosine arabinoside and 1,3-bis (2-chloroethyl)-1-nitrosurea on hematopoietic precursors in the mouse. J Natl Cancer Inst 47:971-977, 1971.

50. Haas RJ, Rohruber W, Netzel B, et al: Effects of CCNU on hematopoiesis in rats. Cancer Treat Rep 63:377-383, 1979.

51. Byfield JE, Galalro-Jones P, Murnane J, et al: Transport-dependent cytotoxicity of water versus lipid soluble alkylating agents: Origins of cumulative marrow toxicity. Proc Amer Ass Cancer Res 20:136, 1979.

52. Panasci LC, Fox PA, Schein PS: Structure activity studies of methylnitrosurea antitumor agents with reduced murine bone marrow toxicity. Cancer Res 37:3321-3328, 1977.

53. Panasci LC, Comis R, Ginsberg S, et al: Phase I trial of chlorozotocin: Attempted amelioration of myelotoxicity by glucose administration. Cancer Treat Rep 65:647-650, 1981.

54. Schein PS, Bull JM, Doukas D, et al: Sensitivity of human and murine hematopoietic precursor cells to 2-[3-(2-chloroethyl)-3-nitrosureido] D-glucopyranose and 1,3-bis(2-chloroethyl)-1-nitrosurea. Cancer Res 38:1070-1074, 1978.

55. Pinedo HM, Chabner BA: The role of drug concentration, duration of exposure, and endogenous metabolites in determining MTX cytotoxicity. Cancer Treat Rep 61:709-715, 1977.

56. Koizumi S, Yamagani M, Ueno Y, Miura M, Taniguchi N: Resistance of human bone marrow CFU-C To high dose methotrexate cytotoxicity. Exp Hematol 8:635-640, 1980.

57. Frei E, Blum RH, Pitman SW, et al: High dose methotrexate with leucovorin rescue. Rationale and spectrum of anti-tumor activity. Am J Med 68:370-376, 1980.

58. Burchenal JH, Murphy ML, Ellison RR, et al: Clinical evaluation of a new antimetabolite, 6-mercaptopurine, in the treatment of leukemia and allied diseases. Blood 8:965–999, 1953.
59. Le Page GA, Whitecar JPJ: Pharmacology of 6-thioguanine in man. Cancer Res 31:1627, 1971.
60. Radley JM, Scurfield G: Effects of 5-fluorouracil on mouse bone marrow. Brit J Haematol 43:341–352, 1979.
61. Fraile RJ, Baker LH, Buroker TR, Horwitz J, Vaitkevicius VK: Pharmacokinetics of 5-fluorouracil administered orally, by rapid infusion and by slow infusion. Cancer Res 40:2223–2228, 1980.
62. Lokich J, Bothe A, Fine N, Perri J: Phase I study of protracted venous infusion of 5-fluorouracil. Cancer 48:2565–2568, 1981.
63. Hall SW, Valdivieso M, Benjamin RS: Intermittent high single dose ftorafur. A phase I clinical trial with a pharmacology-toxicity correlation. Cancer Treat Rep 61:1495–1498, 1977.
64. Kessel D, Hall TC, Rosenthal D: Uptake and phosphorylation of cytosine arabinoside by normal and leukemic human blood cells in vitro. Cancer Res 24:459–463, 1969.
65. Rustum YM, Preisler HD: Correlation between leukemic cell retention of 1-β-darabinosyl-cytosine-5′-triphosphate and response to rherapy. Cancer Res 39:42–49, 1979.
66. Frei E III, Bickers JN, Hewlett JS, et al: Dose schedule and anti-tumor studies of arabinosyl cytosine (NSC 63878). Cancer Res 29:1325–1332, 1969.
67. Early AP, Preisler HD, Slocum H, Rustum YM: High dose cytosine arabinoside for acute leukemia and refractory lymphoma: Clinical efficacy and pharmacology. Cancer Res (in press).
68. Wodinski I, Swiniarski J, Kensler CJ: Spleen colony studies of leukemia L1210. I. Differential sensitivities of normal and leukemic bone marrow colony-forming units to single and divided dose therapy with cytosine arabinoside. Cancer Chemother Rep 51:423, 1967.
69. Buick RN, Messner HA, Till JE, et al: Cytotoxicity of adriamycin and daunomycin for normal and leukemia progenitor cells in man. J Natl Cancer Inst 62:249–252, 1979.
70. Spiro TE, Mattelaer M, Eflra A, Stryckmans P: Sensitivity of myeloid progenitor cells in healthy subjects and patients with chronic myeloid leukemia to chemotherapeutic agents. J Natl Cancer Inst 66:1053–1059, 1981.
71. Razek A, Valeriote F, Vietti T: Survival of hematopoietic and leukemia colony-forming cells in vivo following the administration of daunorubicin or adriamycin. Cancer Res 32:1496–1500, 1972.
72. Huybrechts M, Trouet A: Comparative toxicity of detorubicin and doxorubicin, free and DNA-bound for hemopoietic stem cells. Cancer Chemother pharmacol 5:79–82, 1980.
73. Issell BF, Ginsberg SJ, Tihon C, Rudolph AR, Commis RL: Combining the in vitro human tumor and bone marrow clonogenic assays in cancer therapy development. Proc Am Soc Clin Oncol, 1982.
74. Crooke ST, Bradner WT: Mitomycin C: A review. Cancer Treat Rev 3:121–140, 1976.
75. Blum Rh, Carter SK, Agre K: A clinical review of bleomycin – a new antineoplastic agent. Cancer 31:903–914, 1973.
76. Bogliolo GV, Massa GG, Solvero AF, Lanfranco EO, Pannacciulli IM: Sensitivity of spleen colony-forming units to chronic bleomycin. Brit J Cancer 40:489–492, 1979.
77. Briganti G, Levi G, Spalletta E, Galloni L, Mauro F: Effect of bleomycin on mouse haematopoietic colony-forming cells in culture (CFUC). Cell Tiss Kinet 3:145–151, 1980.
78. Goldberg J, Zamkoff KW, Tice D, et al: The in vitro effects of vincristine on blood CFU-C in the blastic phase of chronic granulocytic leukemia. Blood 54:220A (Suppl 1), 1979.
79. Winton EF, Vogler WR, Parker MB, Kincade JM: Temporal correlation of the marrow's

production of granulopoietic stimulatory activity and granulocyte regeneration after vinblastine. Exp Hematol 9:619–627, 1981.

80. Blum RH, Dawson DM: Phase I trial of vindesine in man. Proc Amer Assoc Cancer Res 17:108, 1976.

81. Creaven PJ, Newman SJ, Selaury OS, Cohen MH, Primack A: Phase I clinical trials of weekly administration of 4'-demethylepipodo phyllotoxin-9-(4,6-O-ethylidene-β-glucopyranoside) (NSC-14-540; VP-16-213). Cancer Chemother Rep 58:901–907, 1974.

82. Rozencweig M, Von Hoff DD, Henney JE, Muggia FM: VM-26 and VP-16–213: A comparative analysis. Cancer 40:334–342, 1977.

83. Vietti TJ, Valeriote FA, Kalish R, Coulter D: Kinetics of cytotoxicity of VM-26 and VP-16–213 on L1210 leukemia and hematopoietic stem cells. Cancer Treat Rep 62:1313–1320, 1978.

84. Spivak SD: Procarbazine. Ann Intern Med 81:795–802, 1974.

85. Thurman WG, Bloedow C, Howe CD, et al: A phase I study of hydroxyurea. Cancer Chemother Rep 29:103, 1963.

86. Rozencweig M, Von Hoff DD, Slavik M, Muggia FM: Cis-diamminedichloroplatinum (II). A new anticancer drug. Ann Intern Med 86:803–812, 1977.

87. Chary KK, Higby DJ, Henderson ES, Swinerton KD: Phase I study of high dose cis-dichlorodiammineplatinum (II) with forced diuresis. Cancer Treat Rep 61:367, 1977.

88. Lippman AJ, Helson C, Helson L, et al: Clinical trials of cis-diamminedichloroplatinum (NSC-119875). Cancer Chemother Rep 57:191–200, 1973.

89. Jenkins VK, Perry RR, Goodrich WE: Effects of cis-diamminedichloroplatinum (II) on hematopoietic stem cells in mice. Exp Hematol 9:281–287, 1981.

90. Wierda D, Pazdernik TL: Toxicity of platinum complexes on hemopoietic precursor cells. J Pharmacol Exp Ther 211:531–538, 1979.

91. Legha SS, Keating MJ, Zauder AR, McCredie KB, Bodey GP, Freireich EJ: 4'(9-Acridinylamino) methansulfon-m-anisidide (AMSA): A new drug effective in the treatment of adult acute leukemia. Ann Intern Med 93:17–20, 1980.

92. Von Hoff DD, Mowser D, Gormley P, et al: Phase I study of methanesulfonamide N-(4-(9-acridinylamino)-3-methoxyphenyl)-(m-AMSA) using a single dose schedule. Cancer Treat Rep 62:1421–1426, 1978.

93. Zauder AR, Maddux B, Spitzer G, et al: Evaluation of toxicity of AMSA on murine bone marrow. Proc Am Assoc Cancer Res 21:275, 1980.

94. Spiro TE, Socquet M, Delforge A, Stryckmans P: Chemotherapeutic sensitivity of normal and leukemic hematopoietic progenitor cells to N-4-(9 acridinylamino)-3-methoxyphenyl-methaneosulforamide, a new anticancer agent. Natl Cancer Inst 66:615–618, 1981.

95. Gutterman JU, Blumenschein GR, Alexanian R, et al: Leukocyte interferon induced tumor regression in human metastatic breast cancer, multiple myeloma, and malignant lymphoma. Ann Intern Med 93:399–406, 1980.

96. Balkwill FR, Oliver RT: Growth inhibitory effects of interferon on normal and malignant human haemopoietic cells. Int J Cancer 20:500–505, 1977.

97. Greenberg PL, Mosny SA: Cytotoxic effects of interferon in vitro on granulocytic progenitor cells. Cancer Res 37:1794–1799, 1977.

98. Trainor KJ, Morley AA: Screening of cytotoxic drugs for residual bone marrow damage. J Natl Cancer Inst 57:1237–1239, 1976.

99. Trainor KJ, Seshadri RS, Morley AA: Residual Marrow injury following cytotoxic drugs. Leukemia Res 3:205–210, 1979.

100. Dumenil D, Sainteny F, Frindel E: Some effects of chemotherapeutic drugs on bone marrow stem cells. I. The long-term effects of phqse-specific drugs on mouse bone marrow stem cells. Cancer Chemother Pharmacol 2:197–201, 1979.

101. Dumenil D, Sainteny F, Frindel E: Some effects of chemotherapeutic drugs on bone mar-

row stem cells. II. Effect on non-Hodgkin's lymphoma chemotherapy on various hemopoietic compartments of the mouse. Cancer Chemother Pharmacol 2:203–207, 1979.

102. Botnick LE, Hannon EC, Hellman S: A long lasting proliferative defect in the hematopoietic stem cell compartment following cytotoxic agents. Int J Radiat Oncol Biol Phy 5:1621–1625, 1979.

103. Botnick LE, Hannon EC, Vigneulle R, Hellman S: Differential effects of cytotoxic agents on hematopoietic progenitors. Cancer Res 41:2338–2342, 1981.

104. Standen GR, Blackett NM: Effect of daily administration of cytotoxic drugs on the erythroid and granulocytic repopulating ability of rat bone marrow. Acta Haematol 63:252–256, 1980.

105. DiFino SM, Lachant NA, Kirshner JJ, Gottlieb AJ: Adult idiopathic thrombocytopenic purpura. Clinical findings and response to therapy. Am J med 69:430–442, 1980.

106. Kim HD, Boggs DR: A syndrome resembling idiopathic thrombocytopenic purpura in 10 patients with diverse forms of cancer. Am J Med 67:331–337, 1979.

107. Kirshner JJ, Zamkoff KZ, Gottlieb AJ: Idiopathic thrombocytopenic purpura and Hodgkin's disease: Report of two cases and a review of the literature. Am J Med Sci 280:21–28, 1980.

108. Auclerc G, Jacquillat C, Auclerc MF, Weil M, Bernard J: Posttherapeuric acute leukemia. Cancer 44:2017–2025,1979.

109. Casciato DA, Scott JL: Acute leukemia following prolonged cytotoxic agent therapy. Medicine 58:32–47, 1979.

110. Coleman CN, Williams CJ, Flint A, Glatstein EJ, Rosenberg SA, Kaplan HS: Hematologic neoplasia in patients treated for Hodgkin's disease. N Engl J Med 297:1249–1252, 1977.

111. Rosner F, Grunwald H: Hodgkin's disease and acute leukemia: Report of eight cases and review of the literature. Am J Med 58:339–353, 1975.

112. Reimer RR, Hoover R, Fraumeni JF, Young RC: Acute leukemia after alkylating agent therapy for ovarian cancer. N Engl J Med 297:177–181, 1977.

113. Rosner F, Carey RW, Zarrabi MH: Breast cancer and acute leukemia: Report of 24 cases and review of the literature. Am J Hematol 4:151–172, 1978.

114. Rosner F, Grunwald H: Multiple myeloma and Waldenstrom's macroglobulinemia terminating in acute leukemia. Review with emphasis on karyotypic and ultra-structural abnormalities. NY Stage J Med 80:558–570, 1980.

115. Landaw SA: Acute leukemia in polycythemia vera. Sem in Hematol 13:33–48, 1976.

116. Zarrabi MH, Rosner F, Bennett JM: Non-Hodgkin's lymphoma and acute myeloblastic leukemia: Report of 12 cases and review of the literature. Cancer 44:1070–1080, 1979.

117. Zarrabi MH, Grunwald HW, Rosner F: Chronic lympkhocytic leukemia terminating in acute leukemia. Arch Intern Med 137:1059–1064, 1977.

118. Grunwald HW, Rosner F: Acute leukemia and immunosuppressive drug use: A review of patients undergoing immunosuppressive therapy for non-neoplastic diseases. Arch Intern Med 139:461, 1979.

119. Preisler HD, Lyman GH: Acute myelogenous leukemia subsequent to therapy for a different neoplasm: Clinical features and response to therapy. Am J Hematol 3:209–215, 1977.

120. Comis RL, Schein PS, Hoth D, Holland J: Cancer and Leukemia Group B Protocal #7981. A phase III study: Comparison of FAM versus MA in locally advanced or metastatic gastric cancer, 1979.

121. Williams WJ: Hematology in the aged. In: Hematology, Williams WJ (ed), New York, McGraw-Hill, 1977, p 49–54.

122. Mauch P, Botnick L, Hellman S: Decline in bone marrow proliferative capacity as a function of age. Blood 58 (Suppl 1):113A, 1981.

123. Bonadonna G, Valagussa P: Dose-response effect of adjuvant chemotherapy in breast can-

cer. N Engl J Med 304:10–15, 1981.

124. Frei E III, Canellos GP: Dose: A critical factor in cancer chemotherapy. Am J Med 69:585–594, 1980.

125. Sacks EL, Goris ML, Glatstein E, Gilbert EH, Kaplan HS: Bone marrow regeneration following large field radiation: Influence of volume, age, dose, and time. Cancer 42:1057–1065, 1978.

126. Chamberlain W, Barone J, Kedo A, Fried W: Lack of recovery of murine hematopoietic stromal cells after irradiation induced damage. Blood 44:385–392, 1974.

127. Zeltzer PM, Feig SA: Theophylline induced lomustine toxicity. Lancet 2:960–961, 1979.

128. Alberts DS, Peng YM, Moon TE: Alpha-tocopherol pretreatment increases adriamycin bone marrow toxicity. Biomed EXP 29:189–191, 1978.

129. Fitchen JH, Koeffler HP: Cimetidine and granulopoiesis: Bone marrow culture studies in normal man and patients with cimetidine – associated neutropenia. Brit J Haematol 46:361–366, 1980.

130. Byron JW: Cimetidine and bone marrow toxicity. Lancet 2:555–556, 1977.

131. Klotz SA, Kay BF: Cimetidine and agranulocytosis. Ann Intern Med 88:579–580, 1978.

132. Posnett DN, Stein RS, Graber SE, Krantz SB: Cimetidine-induced neutropenia. A possible dose-related phenomenon. Arch Intern Med 139:584–586, 1979.

133. O'Donnel JF, McKoy WS, MaKuch RW, Bull JM: Increased *in vitro* toxicity to mouse bone marrow with 1,3-bis (2-chloroethyl)-1-nitrosurea and hyperthermia. Cancer Res 39:2547–2549, 1979.

134. Preisler HD, Gessner T: Intergroup AML Study, 1981.

135. Bertino JR: Rescue techniques in cancer chemotherapy: Use of leucovorin and other rescue agents after methotrexate treatment. Sem in Oncol 4:203–216, 1977.

136. Pinedo HM, Zaharko DS, Bull JM, Chabner BA: The reversal of methotrexate cytotoxicity of mouse bone marrow cells by leucovorin and nucleosides. Cancer Res 36:4418–4424, 1976.

137. Schreml W, Lohrmann HP: Effect of high dose methotrexate with citrovorum factor on human granulopoiesis. Cancer Res 39:4195–4199, 1979.

138. Howell SB, Ensminger WD, Krisham A, Frei E: Thymidine rescue of high dose methotrexate in humans. Cancer Res 38:325–330, 1978.

139. Straw JA, Talbot DC, Taylor GA, Harry KR: Some observation on the reversibility of methotrexate toxicity in normal proliferating tissues. J Natl Cancer Inst 58:91–97, 1977.

140. Howell SB, Mansfield SJ, Taetle R: Significance of variation in serum thymidine concentration for the marrow toxicity of methotrexate. Cancer Chemother Pharmacol 5:221–226, 1981.

141. Chabner BA, Johns V, Bertino JB: Enzymatic cleavage of methotrexate provides a method for prevention of drug toxicity. Nature 239:395–399, 1972.

142. Capizzi RL: Improvement in the therapeutic index of methotrexate by asparaginase. Cancer Chemother Rep 6:37, 1975.

143. Rothstein G, Clarkson DR, Larsen W, Grosser BI, Athema JW: Effect of lithium on neutrophil mass and production. N Engl J Med 298:178–182, 1978.

144. Harker WG, Rothstein G, Clarkson D, et al: Enhancement of colonystimulating activity production by lithium. Blood 49:263–267, 1977.

145. Joyce RA, Chervenick PA: The effect of lithium on release of granulocytes colony stimulating activity *in vitro*. Adv Exp Med Biol 127:79–86, 1980.

146. Richman CM, Kinnealey A, Hoffman PC: Granulopoietic effects of lithium on human bone marrow *in vitro*. Exp Hematol 9:449–455, 1981.

147. Doukas MA, Coppola MA, Niskanen EO, Quesenberry PJ: *In vitro* and *in vivo* effect of lithium on a primitive hemopoietic stem cell. Blood 58:108A (Suppl 1), 1981.

148. Belch AR, Ronald AR, Feld R, Pater JC: Efficacy of lithium during remission induction of

acute myelogenous leukemia (AML). Blood 58:135A(Suppl 1), 1981.

149. Greco FA, Brereton MD: Effect of lithium carbonate on theneutropenia caused by chemotherapy: A preliminary clinical trial. Oncology 34:153, 1977.

150. Stein RS, Beaman C, Ali MY, Hansen R, Jankins DD, June'an HG: Lithium carbonate attenuation of chemotherapy-induced neutropenia. N Engl J Med 297:430–435, 1977.

151. Abrams RA, McCormack K, Bowles C, Deisseroth AB: Cyclophosphamide treatment expands the circulating hematopoietic stem cell pool in dogs. J Clin Invest 67:1392–1399, 1981.

152. Blackett NM, Aguado M: The enhancement of hematopoietic stem cell recovery in irradiated mice by prior treatment with cyclophosphamide. Cell Tiss Kinet 12:291–298, 1979.

153. Hedley DW, McElwain TJ, Millar JL, Gordon MY: Acceleration of bone marrow recovery by pre-treatment with cyclophosphamide in patients receiving high dose melphalan. Lancet 2:966–968, 1978.

154. Gurwith MJ, Brunton JL, Lank BA, Harding GKM, Ronald AR: A prospective controlled investigation of prophylactic trimethoprim/sulfamethoxazole in hospitalized granulocytopenic patients. Am J Med 66:248–256, 1979.

155. Douer D, Champlin RE, Ho WG, et al: High dose combined modality therapy and autologous bone marrow transplantation in resistant cancer. Am J Med 71:973–976, 1981.

156. Spitzer G, Dicke KA, Litam J, et al: High dose combination chemotherapy with autologous bone marrow transplantation in adult solid tumors. Cancer 45:3075–3085, 1980.

157. Tobias JS, Weiner RS, Griffiths CT, et al: Cryopreserved autologous marrow infusion following high dose cancer chemotherapy. Eur J Cancer 13:269–277, 1977.

2. Chemotherapy and Gonadal Function

MONICA B. SPAULDING and STEPHEN W. SPAULDING

1. THE TESTIS

1.1 Normal Testicular Development and Physiology

The testes have both hormonal and reproductive functions. One major hormonal function, the synthesis and secretion of testosterone, is performed by Leydig cells, the interstitial cells which lie between the seminiferous tubules. In utero, interstitial cell function is important for genital development, but testosterone secretion decreases before birth and after a brief increase in secretion during infancy, returns to relatively low levels until the onset of puberty. At that time, the hypothalamus becomes progressively less sensitive to inhibition by testosterone. The hypothalamus begins to stimulate the pituitary to release bursts of luteinizing hormone (LH) during sleep, which in turn increases nocturnal testosterone secretion from the Leydig cells. Later in puberty, bursts in LH secretion from the pituitary occur throughout the day, inducing the Leydig cells to maintain a tonically higher level of testosterone secretion. The increase in androgen secretion results in the development of secondary sex characteristics such as growth of facial and body hair, enlargement of the external genitalia, laryngeal growth (with deepening of the voice), and muscular development.

Spermatogenesis, the reproductive function of the testes, takes place in the seminiferous tubules. Seminiferous tubules are present at birth, but they lack a lumen and are lined only by primary germ cells and Sertoli cells. As puberty begins, secretion of follicle stimulating hormone (FSH) from the pituitary increases gradually but progressively. The rising levels of FSH combined with the increased levels of testosterone from the Leydig cells cause the primary germ cells to develop into sperm.

Within the seminiferous tubules, sperm pass through six stages requiring an interval of some 75 days to develop from spermatogonia through spermatocytes to mature spermatozoa. The Sertoli cells support and nourish the

Higby, DJ (ed), The Cancer Patient and Supportive Care. ISBN 0-89838-690-X.
© 1985, Martinus Nijhoff Publishers, Boston. Printed in The Netherlands.

germinal epithelium in this developmental process. The Sertoli cell is a target organ for FSH in the male. In response to FSH, the Sertoli cell makes an androgen binding protein (ABP) which serves as a transport protein and reservoir for testosterone. The process of spermatogenesis requires both FSH and testosterone; testosterone is required for initial phases of spermatogenesis, while FSH is responsible for the terminal development and maturation of the spermatid. The Sertoli cells also secrete a substance designated 'inhibin' which exerts negative feedback on FSH secretion from the pituitary.

1.2 *Pathophysiology*

If the testes are damaged and both spermatogenic and Leydig cell function are lost, both FSH and LH titers rise. If there is selective damage to the germinal tissue alone, only FSH levels rise, because of a lack of 'inhibin' feedback. On the other hand, selective damage to the Leydig cells will reduce testosterone levels: LH levels will rise while FSH levels remain normal. If, in evaluation of a patient, one finds that either of the serum gonadotropin levels is elevated, one can establish that primary gonadal failure has occurred either at the level of the Sertoli or Leydig cell. If both gonadotropin levels are low, primary pituitary failure may have occurred which, in turn, causes the germinal epithelium to involute: fibrosis and hyalination of the seminiferous tubules occur and testosterone secretion by the Leydig cell ceases.

Testicular function is determined by several means: physical examination to assess secondary sex characteristics, measurements of testosterone (free and total), evaluation of seminal fluid and finally, testicular biopsy. Obviously, the stage of sexual development is important. The prepubertal male lacks secondary sex characteristics, has low levels of testosterone, and a testicular biopsy will show immature germinal cells lining seminiferous tubules which lack a lumen. During puberty (which normally occurs between ages 9 to 16 in boys), the levels of testosterone rise from levels of less than 20 ng/dl to over 400 ng/dl (Fig. 2). The concomitant increase in testicular size reflects maturation of the seminiferous tubules. A freshly-collected semen specimen in a pubertal or postpubertal male will normally have a sperm count greater than 30 million spermatozoa/ml. Normal motility is greater than 50%, two hours after ejaculation. Testicular biopsies will reveal active spermatogenesis in all stages of development. The periphery of the tubules will be lined by Sertoli cells filled with glycogen while between the tubules, clusters of Leydig cells are frequent. Determination of serum prolactin levels is also important: elevated levels can inhibit gonadal function.

Finally, it is important to note that various elements of the pituitary-testicular axis can be affected by depression [1], malnutrition [2], or fasting [3]. Obviously, these conditions commonly exist in patients with tu-mors, and can complicate the interpretation of the effects of therapy in patients with a malignancy.

1.3 *Radiation Therapy*

The effect of radiation on the human testis has been recognized for some time: germ cell proliferation is impaired while Sertoli cell morphology and Leydig cell function are maintained. Damage to germinal tissue is dose-dependent but a given dose administered fractionally over a period of time will cause more damage than the same amount of irradiation given on a single occasion. It is recognized that cells at different stages in development show different sensitivities: the early spermatogonium is more sensitive than the later spermatocyte, which in turn is more sensitive than the radio-resistant mature spermatozoan. Heller [4] reported on the changes observed in the sperm count of normal men after they received a single dose of irra-diation to the testes. With low doses (15 to 100 rads), the sperm count declined 50 days after the radiation. With larger doses, the sperm count declined earlier, indicating that damage had occurred to spermatogenic cells in the later stages of development and to the spermatocytes, whereas the smaller doses had affected only spermatogonia. With single X-ray doses of up to 600 rads, some recovery of spermatogenesis can be expected but may take up to five years. At 600 rads and above, azoospermia was noted with-out apparent recovery.

The testes are more sensitive to irradiation given in fractionated doses. In dogs, for instance, a total dose of 475 rads given at a rate of 3 R/day causes complete and permanent azoospermia, whereas a single dose of 2000 R causes depression of the sperm count but not permanent azoospermia [5]. Similar observations have been made with regard to brief vs protracted courses of chemotherapy. X-ray therapy can affect the gonads even when they are not in the direct field of irradiation. This observation is clinically important: irradiation can also reach the testes by scatter when large field irradiation therapy is being given. Thus when the inverted inguinal field treatment is given to patients with Hodgkin's disease, an average daily dose of 12 rads is given to the testes [6]. In a group of 10 men with Hodgkin's disease receiving irradiation to this field, there was a total testicular dose of 140–300 rads given over 14–26 fractions. Despite the use of a testicular shield, all of these men became azoospermic for prolonged periods of time following their treatment. Since many patients with hematologic malignan-cies receive both chemotherapy and irradiation, shielding of the testes and careful attention to radiation ports is important to reduce the combined antigonadal effects of chermotherapy and radiation.

1.4 *Single Agent Chemotherapy*

Alkylating agents, particularly chlorambucil and cyclophosphamide, are the chemotherapeutic agents most consistently noted to have adverse effects on the male gonad, predominantly on spermatogenesis (Table 1).

1.4.1 *Chlorambucil.*

Richter [7] reported the effects of chlorambucil on eight adult males, aged 19 to 30, with various lymphomas. All eight had evidence of normal testicular function before treatment. The patients were treated with daily oral chlorambucil in doses of 0.1 mg/kg to 0.4 mg/kg. The effect of chlorambucil was monitored by evaluation of spermatic fluid, hormone assays and testicular biopsies. As the cumulative dose of chlorambucil approached 400 mg. there was progressive oligospermia, but there were no other changes in the spermatic fluid; both volume and sperm motility remained normal. There were never more than 20% abnormal forms in the qualitative semen analysis. At doses above 400 mg., azoospermia developed. Testicular biopsies were performed in four patients. In those with azoospermia, the biopsies showed peritubular fibrosis and absence of germinal cells. Sertoli cells persisted in the seminiferous tubules, as did the Leydig cells in the interstitium. In the patients with oligospermia, the biopsies showed arrest of spermatogenesis at the spermatid stage and less severe peritubular fibrosis. Recovery from the azoospermia was not observed in these patients as all had received further chemotherapy.

Cheviakoff [8 subsequently reported that some men who had received more than 400 mg. of chlorambucil can recover spermatogenesis. Of his five patients, four were azoospermic and one was oligospermic at cessation of therapy. Two regained normal sperm counts more than 30 months after therapy had been completed. A third reportedly had fathered a child 40 months after cessation of therapy, although his sperm count remained low. Sperm counts in the remaining two who had received more than 2 gm of chlorambucil were still low more than 40 months after therapy. The length of time before there were signs of recovery was linked to the total dose of the alkylating agent.

Both chlorambucil and cyclophosphamide have been used frequently as immunosuppressive agents in the treatment of nephrosis. This nonmalignant disorder (the 'minimal lesion' nephrotic syndrome), is generally responsive to corticosteroids, but alkylating agent therapy is used in those individuals who develop intolerable toxic side effects (from the cortisone) or whose renal status does not improve with the corticosteroid therapy.

1.4.2 *Cyclophosphamide.*

Fairly, Barrie and Johnson [9] reported adverse effects on spermatogenesis in adult males receiving cyclophosphamide (Cytoxan®) for the nephrotic syndrome. Of 31 patients being treated with doses

Table 1. Chemotherapy and Gonadal Function

Drug	Total dose or duration of therapy	Males	Females	Author
Cyclophosphamide 1½–3 mg/kg/day	<365 mg/kg total	4 prepubertal: ↓ sperm count (previous orchopexy); 6 pubertal: 3 ↓ sperm counts; 1 postpubertal: ↓ sperm count	2 prepubertal-one has ovarian cyst; 1 pubertal; 2 postpubertal, normal temperature curves	Lentz 1977
+ all studies done when postpubertal	<365 mg/kg	2 prepubertal: azoospermia; 2 pubertal: 1 is azoospermic; 3 postpubertal: all azoospermic	2 prepubertal-normal temperature curve; 1 pubertal – has child; 5 postpubertal - one had polycytic ovaries - others had normal temperature curves	
Cyclophosphamide 50–100 mg/d off therapy for 1–5.3 years	2–12 months	Ages: 4.7–15.4; 4 prepubertal: Normal hormone profile; 7 pubertal: 3 had ↓ FSH & LH with ↓ sperm coount 4 with normal hormone profiles but ↓ sperm count in 2	Ages: 4.3–14.1; No change in FSH, LF, 17 B estradiol, 17 a hydroxyprogesterone & progesterone	Parra 1978
Cyclophosphamide 3 mg/kg/d off therapy for 2–28 months	>6 months	Ages: 17–48; 8 males – testicular biopsies showed no germinal epithelium in 6; no mature spermatozoa in 2	Ages: 16–44; All developed amenorrhea during therapy-menses resumed in 6	Kumar 1972
Cyclophosphamide 2.5–5 mg.kg/day off therapy for 1.5–5.5 years	1.5–6 months	23 patients; 16 prepubertal-testicular biopsies in 3 showed focal atrophy of germinal epithelium; 7 pubertal - ↓ spermatogenesis in all - ↑ FSH in 5/6	8 prepubertal – only 3 are pubertal with normal menses; 4 postpubertal had no mentrual irregularities during treatment	Penisi 1975
Cyclophosphamide 2 mg/kg/day or 500–1000 mg/m²	1–29 months	Ages: 23/12–124/12; FSH & LH levels normal for ages	Ages: 4 5/12–17 8/12; No FSH or LH abnormalities menses normal	De Groot 1974

of 50–100 mg/day, all developed either low sperm counts or azoospermia. Azoospermia was noted as early as four months after therapy was initiated, but a depression in the sperm count was noted after only three weeks of therapy. Kumar [10] performed testicular biopsies on eight males who had received cyclophosphamide for steroid resistant nephrotic syndrome 2–28 months after completion of cyclophosphamide therapy. All eight patients had evidence of testicular atrophy with absence of mature spermatozoa and in the most severe cases, total disappearance of germ cell precursors with only Sertoli cells remaining in the seminiferous tubules.

Following therapy with cyclophosphamide, as with chlorambucil, spermatogenesis may return [11] but recovery takes some time. In a study of 26 adult men treated with cyclophosphamide (2–5 mg/kg/day) for periods ranging from 5–34 months, all were found to be azoospermic after six months of therapy [12]. In those who had taken cyclophosphamide for less than 18 months, recovery of spermatogenesis had occurred in 9 of 14 patients after followup of 49 months. In patients treated for more than 18 months, recovery of spermatogenesis occurred in only 3 of 12 patients. Testicular biopsies obtained in the latter group of patients had shown tubular fibrosis and no spermatogonia were seen during the period of azoospermia. However, since some did in fact recover, it is clear that not all spermatogonia had been ablated.

1.4.3 *Azathioprine.* Azathiprine, an antimetabolite whose major use is as an immunosuppressive agent in patients undergoing renal transplants, has been reported to cause azoospermia and testicular atrophy. However, long-term renal insufficiency itself, like many other chronic diseases, appears to affect fertility [13]. Phadke [14] performed testicular biopsies on patients undergoing dialysis. He found sperm maturation arrested at the spermatocyte and reduced tubular cellularity. Leydig cells appeared normal. After receiving renal transplants, 11 patients, all on azathioprine and prednisone, had testicular biopsies showing adequate cellularity and normal spermatogenesis. Thus it would appear that the majority of such fertility and potency changes are probably secondary to chronic renal insufficiency rather than to the use of this antimetabolite.

1.4.4 *Other Chemotherapeutic Agents.* Data on other chemotherapeutic agents used as single agents is limited. The only other alkylating agent clearly recognized as causing germinal tissue damage is busulfan [15]. BCNU has been reported to cause gynecomastia [16], but the mechanism is unknown. Gonadal function in patients with this finding was normal. Nitrogen mustard (mechlorethamine) has been administered together with chlorambucil to young males with nephrosis [17]. This combination did not appear to have any more effect on the male gonad than chlorambucil alone. No anti-metabolites have been shown to affect gonadal function at doses used clinically. Neither of the mitotic inhibitors, vincristine or vinblastine, has been reported to have any effect on male germinal tissue, although vincristine has been recognized to cause impotence via neurologic toxicity [18]. There have been no reports of gonadal toxicity from the antibiotics: adriamycin, bleomycin, danurobucin, mithramycin or mitomycin.

Procarbazine, a methyl hydrazine derivative, has been shown to induce germinal aplasia in primates [19]. Biopsies from the testes of monkeys receiving procarbazine for prolonged periods of time showed normal Sertoli cells with abnormal seminiferous tubules. While there is no clinical data concerning its possible anti-gonadal effect when used as a single agent in the treatment of various malignancies, there are reasons to suspect such an effect from studies of combination chemotherapy (see 1.4.5).

1.4.5 *Effects on the Prepubertal Male.* The effect of alkylating agents on the prepubertal testes could theoretically be different from the adult, since the germinal epithelium is in a resting state and tubules are nonfunctioning. Nineteen young men, all postpubertal when evaluated, had been treated with cyclophosphamide for nephrotic syndrome: some were prepubertal during therapy [20]. Six of eight treated with more than 365 mg of cyclophosphamide/kg were found to be azoospermic. The occurrence of azoospermia was not related to whether the patients were prepubertal, pubertal or postpubertal during their course of therapy, but to the total dose of cyclophosphamide they had received. At doses less than 365 mg of cyclophosphamide, (11 of the 19 subjects) azoospermia was not observed. FSH was elevated in five out of six patients with proven azoospermia. Four also had low serum testosterone but only one had an increased LH value, so the levels of testosterone might have reflected normal variation rather than an effect of cyclophosphamide on Leydig cell function. Hormonal studies done on another group of prepubertal males treated for periods ranging from 2 to 12 months revealed elevated FSH levels in three who received the drug during a period of early sexual development [21]. The initial studies had been done nine months to 2.7 years after completing therapy, and were repeated along with semen analyses in two of these boys, four and six months after discontinuation of cyclophosphamide. At the time of the second determination, FSH levels remained elevated; one boy was azoospermic and one had severe oligospermia.

In contrast, none of eight prepubertal males aged 2 to 12½, treated with cyclophosphamide for various nonmalignant conditions, showed any changes from the expected serum gonadotropin levels [22]. Three of the males were in early puberty when evaluated, the other five were prepubertal.

The duration of therapy was brief (1½ 6o 8 months) and the drug was given by an intermittent intravenous schedule to most, so that the benign outcome noted in this study cannot be directly compared to other studies on the prepubertal male given cyclophosphamide.

Chlorambucil can also be harmful to the nonfunctioning germinal tissue of the prepubertal male [17]. Ten males given chlorambucil for one to 12 months prior to puberty, were found to have reduced or absent spermatogenesis when examined at age 16 or older. The effect on other secondary sex characteristics was variable. Axillary and pubic hair development were normal. but the penis was small in four patients and the testes were small in two. In all patients, the serum testosterone levels were normal even when there was evidence of poor secondary sex development. The FSH levels were elevated in four patients and LH was increased in only one.

Thus, in summary, single agent therapy with alkylating agents often impairs spermatogenesis. The likelihood of recovery is related to the total dose, duration of therapy and duration of time since therapy was discontinued. While long-term alkylating agent therapy can produce frank testicular atrophy, testosterone and LH levels in such patients have generally been normal. Reports of Leydig cell dysfunction due to single agent chemotherapy have been uncommon.

1.5 Combination Chemotherapy

Combination chemotherapy has resulted in dramatic improvement in survival statistics in hematologic malignancies. With prolonged survival, however, has come the unhappy recognition of long-term toxicity, particularly the effects of chemotherapeutic agents on several aspects of sexual function. This was reported by Sherins and DeVita [23] in 16 males previously treated for lymphomas who has been off chemotherapy and in remission for periods ranging from two months to seven years. They had all received alkylating agents, either cyclophosphamide or nitrogen mustard, in addition to other drugs including vincristine, methylhydrazine, methotrexate and prednisone. Semen analysis showed that ten of the men were azoospermic. Testicular biopsies showed total germinal aplasia in most, but two had biopsy evidence of some germinal activity. Four others were oligospermic or had normal semen analysis, but these had been in remission and off chemotherapy the longest. The evidence of damage to germinal epithelium and time it took to recover, could be roughly correlated with the amount of alkylating agent received by each patient. Libido and potency were not affected in these patients.

In 15 of these men, gonadotropin secretion and Leydig cell function were also evaluated [24]. Follicle stimulating hormone was more than four times normal in ten of those 15 men. Luteinizing hormone levels were normal in all. Those five men in whom both FSH and LH were normal, had evidence of a return of normal spermatogenesis by seminal fluid analysis and/or testicular biopsy. Thus the pituitary gland appears to respond to germinal tissue depletion by increased FSH secretion due to the loss of the negative feedback effect of 'inhibin'. Although testosterone levels were below normal in two patients, LH levels were not elevated and there was no other evidence for Leydig cell dysfunction.

Thirty-two patients treated with multiagent chemotherapy for disseminated lymphoma were studied by Roser [25]. After treatment, 31 of the 32 had an elevated FSH and there was azoospermia in all of the 15 patients examined. Sixteen patients were taken off chemotherapy following remission of their tumor. Ten of these patients had received cyclophosphamide (with vincristine and prednisone). Within three years of followup, seven had regained a normal FSH. The three with persistently elevated FSH had persisting azoospermia. In contrast, of six patients treated with the alkylating agent nitrogen mustard, plus procarbazine (with vincristine and prednisone) only one had regained a normal sperm count after 50 months of followup. The other patients all had persistent azoospermia and increased serum levels of FSH. This study suggests that procarbazine may increase damage to the germinal epithelium in addition to that due to another alkylating agent. Five patients in this study were also noted to have elevated levels of LH in association with decreased levels of testosterone in three, suggesting a degree of Leydig cell damage as well.

Leydig cell function may be affected by MOPP combination chemotherapy in the adolescent male. Sherins et al. [23] gave MOPP (nitrogen mustard, vincristine, procarbazine and prednisone) to 19 young men: thirteen were pubertal and showed secondary sex characteristics at the time of treatment, while six were prepubertal. Clinically detectable gynecomastia occurring 12 to 34 months after treatment were noted in nine of the 13 pubertal boys. The FSH was markedly elevated in 8 of the 9, and LH levels were increased in 7 of the 9. In the boys with gynecomastia, testosterone levels were in the low range. This is the first study to suggest that combination chemotherapy might also cause Leydig cell injury, at least in the adolescent testes, although Whitehead has questioned this [26]. Interestingly, the 6 younger boys, prepubescent when treated, were found to have FSH, LH, testosterone and estrogen levels which were normal for their age. Gynecomastia is often noted transiently in the normal adolescent, but in the Sherins study may have been a clue to dysfunction of the Leydig cell, probable due to a decrease in the serum testosterone/estrogen ratio. Elevated estrogen levels have been noted in some prepubertal males treated with cyclophosphamide alone, but this elevation did not result in clinical gynecomastia [21] and its significance was not clear.

Although early studies suggested that chemotherapy resulted in no change in libido or sexual performance, Chapman [27] evaluated 74 young men receiving similar combination therapy (nitrogen mustard, procarbazine, vinblastine and prednisone) for Hodgkin's disease. The occurrence of azoospermia was universal and only four of 74 patients regained spermatogenesis (followup one to 62 months) in this study. FSH levels were elevated in all. Although testosterone levels were normal, LH levels were increased, suggesting partially impaired Leydig cell function. One-quarter had hyperprolactemia. Despite normal testosterone levels, a major decline in libido and sexual activity was recorded in some of the patients, which may, of course, have been related to other stress factors, rather than to alterations in endocrine function. In any event, sexual counselling and possibly sperm cryopreservation should be considered as part of the treatment plan.

There is evidence, however, that gonadal function may be abnormal in males with Hodgkin's disease or other metastatic cancer, prior to treatment. Chapman [28] studied 47 men (age range 16 to 61) with Hodgkin's disease before any treatment was initiated. Semen analysis in 37 patients showed that in 43%, the sperm count was below 50 million/ejaculate (i.e. an 'inadequate' sperm count). In six of 39 men FSH levels were elevated (15%); in 16 of 40, LH levels were elevated (40%); and in five of 27, testosterone levels were below normal (19%). In this population of patients, after therapy was begun, sperm counts and fertility decreased, and after the third cycle of MOPP therapy (nitrogen mustard, vinblastine, procarbazine, and prednisone) all were sterile. As sperm counts decreased, FSH levels rose. Testicular biopsies before treatment were obtained in nine patients. One was normal, one showed active spermatogenesis, and six showed focal or larger areas of hyalinization and absence of tubular epithelium.

Chapman also reviewed eleven other males with Hodgkin's disease (ages 19 though 38) before beginning therapy, and confirmed that sperm counts were decreased and motility was impaired in some of these patients. Testosterone levels were lower in these untreated Hodgkin's disease patients than in a control group of twenty normal men; LH was inappropriately low in these patients, suggesting that both testicular and pituitary function were abnormal unrelated to treatment. The patients described by Chapman ranged in extent of disease from Stage IA to IVB, and pretreatment gonadal abnormalities were found even in some patients with limited disease.

Heber and Chlebewski [29] studied testosterone levels (total and free) and serum LH in 44 patients with metastatic cancer. Twelve patients had decreased testosterone with increased LH levels and 12 others had normal testosterone levels but increased LH, suggesting primary hypogonadism as a consequence of their advanced disease. An additional group of nine patients with both decreased testosterone and LH levels had more weight loss.

Whether the weight loss and malnutrition secondary to malignant disease leads to the hypogonadism, or whether the hypogonadism is due in some part to the malignant process and results in protein wasting and catabolism because of the testosterone deficiency, cannot be determined by these studies.

The effects of chemotherapy on gonadal function have been previously described in patients with lymphoma treated with combinations including an alkylating agent and sometimes procarbazine. Recently, a combination of drugs, lacking both alkylating agents and procarbazine, has been found to be equally active in advanced Hodgkin's disease [30]. None of the drugs in the combination 'ABVD' (adriamycin, bleomycin, vinblastine and DTIC), has been shown to interfere with gonadal function when used as a single agent. In a group of patients with advanced Hodgkin's disease (Stage IIB, IIIA&B) receiving both this drug combination (ABVD) and low dose irradiation (2000 R) to involved fields, only 12.5% of the patients treated had azoospermia at the end of therapy, as opposed to 100% in a similar group treated with MOPP and radiation therapy.

The duration of the azoospermia induced by combination chemotherapy in Hodgkin's disease is unknown. Serial sperm counts have shown a recovery of spermatogenesis in only a few patients even more than four years following therapy [30, 25]. However, Stricher [32] reported two patients who had fathered children six and 11 years after MOPP therapy. In each case, paternity was confirmed by blood and HLA typing. Such reports suggest that eventual recovery of spermatogenesis may occur in these patients.

The dramatic changes in survival seen in the patients with malignant lymphomas has resulted in the accumulation of considerable data on the gonadal damage induced by combination chermotherapy used for these diseases. Information concerning possible effects of other chemotherapeutic combinations is still sparse because the increase in survival in other malignant diseases has not been so marked. Two exceptions are childhood lymphoblastic leukmia (ALL) and testicular malignancies. At least 50% of the children with acute lymphoblastic leukemia can be cured by various combinations of chemotherapeutic agents, most of which do not contain alkylating agents.

Most children with ALL are treated with a combination of prednisone, vincristine, 6-mercaptopurine and methotrexate. Blatt [33] followed 14 boys prospectively, both while they were receiving that combination and following discontinuation of therapy. At the time therapy was started, one was sexually mature, nine were prepubertal, and four were intrapubertal. All of the boys recieved cranial irradiation to a dose of 2400 R. No evidence of testicular or pituitary dysfunction could be obtained. Testosterone and FSH levels were normal throughout the course of treatment and physical examination showed evidence of normal sexual maturation.

Forty-four boys with ALL treated at the Children's Hospital in Manchester, England were also evaluated [34]. All underwent testicular biopsies, 23 following therapy, 21 while still receiving therapy. Five were found to have leukemic infiltrates. A tubular fertility index (TFI) based on the percentage of seminiferous tubules found to contain identifiable spermatogonia was calculated for the other patients. A decrease in the TFI was found to correlate with: 1) the toal dose of cyclophophamide received, 2) a dose of cytosine arabinoside greater than 1 gm/m^2, and 3) inversely with the time off therapy before biopsy was obtained.

This was the first study linking cytosine arabinoside to germinal tissue damage in the absence of concurrent therapy with alkylating agents; an additional study of testicular histology in adult males receiving cytosine arabinoside and 6-thioguanine as antileukemic therapy has also shown a reduction in spermatogenesis, the extent of reduction depending upon the duration of therapy [35].

In nonseminomatous testicular cancer the prognosis has improved because of newer techniques in surgery such as retroperitoneal node dissection, the use of tumor markers to identify early recurrence, and effective chemotherapy with Cis-DDP, bleomycin and vinblastine. In general, the retroperitoneal node dissection disrupts sympathetic nerve pathways, causing a loss of emission and a dry ejaculate. Lange [36] retested 60 patients who underwent radical lymphadenectomy. Fifty percent had a return to normal of their sperm volumes within 2–36 months after surgery. Twelve other patients received sympathomimetic drugs, resulting in normal ejaculation in 58%. Twenty-four were eventually treated by chemotherapy with cis-platinum, vinblastine and bleomycin. None of those evaluated less than one year after chemotherapy had a return of normal sperm count. However, of ten patients off chemotherapy for more than two years, all were found to have normal spermatogenesis. It appears that in testicular cancer, chemotherapy has only a temporary effect on spermatogenesis, with cis-platinum, an alkylating agent, being the most likely agent involved.

1.6 Evaluation and Therapy for The Effects of Chemotherapy on Male Gonadal Function

The possibility of teratogenic changes developing in germ cells which survive the effects of chemotherapy remains of concern although there is little solid data (however there is some experimental data to support such suspicions, vida infra, Section 2.5). If one decides to assist a patient who has apparently become infertile following chemotherapy, the initial clinical evaluation should include questions concerning libido, the presence of erections before arising in the morning, noctural emissions and changes in secondary sex characteristics (body hair, shaving frequency, gynecomastia, etc.). Obviously, chemotherapy may not be to blame. In addition to changes due to the malignancy itself, exposure to agents such as furadantin, marijuana, alcohol, lead and insecticides like dibromochloropropane, ethylene dibromide and carbaryl should be noted. A past history of orchitis, testicular injury or retrograde ejaculation should be noted, as should apparent evidence of prior fertility. Increased scrotal temperature (large varicoceles, jockey shorts, steam baths or jobs requiring prolonged sitting) may also be implicated.

Physical examination may reveal hypospadias or varicoceles, and a description of body hair, gynecomastia and testicular volume and consistency should all be recorded before therapy, to permit an accurate assessment of possible effects of chemotherapy. Evaluation of several samples of ejaculate will indicate whether the average volume (1–7 cc), sperm count (over 30,000,000/cc), morphology (over 60% normal) and motility (over 50% at two hours) are normal.

Blood tests should include determination of both total and free levels of testosterone and the pituitary hormones LH, FSH, as well as prolactin to determine whether there is evidence of endocrine deficiency, and if so, at what level it exists.

Several forms of therapy have been employed to treat infertile men when sperm are present but the count is low. However, neither testosterone rebound therapy nor clomiphene treatment are effective in more than 10% of the cases and improvement is transient when it is seen. There is little data concerning the efficacy of such therapy in men suffering from infertility following chemotherapy for malignancy: 'watchful waiting' has been the usual approach. A fall in FSH can be a hopeful sign. If gynecomastia or other clinical manifestations of androgen deficiency are troublesome, treatment with testosterone enanthate can be effective [37].

Recently-developed analogs of gonadotropin-releasing hormone may hold promise for a form of prophylaxis: pretreatment with [D-leu^6]-des-Gly-NH$_2^{10}$pro-ethylamide GnRH protects mice from cyclophosphamide-induced testicular damage [38].

2. THE OVARY

2.1 Normal Ovarian Development and Physiology

Unlike the male, in whom there is constant renewal of spermatogonia following puberty, the number of oocytes in a woman's ovary is fixed at birth, where they lie enveloped in a layer of pregranulosa and pretheca cells which form the primordial follicles. During childhood, some oocytes undergo a partial cycle of follicle maturation and then atresia. None of the follicles discharge ova and no corpora lutea develop. Of the two million ova present at birth, there are only 400,000 left by the time true ovulation begins at puberty.

In the adult woman, the factors causing certain follicles to mature during any particular cycle have not been identified, but as a rule only one follicle matures completely and actually ovulates in each cycle.

Unlike the tonic levels of sex hormones and gonadotropins in the adult male, sex hormone and gonadotropin levels undergo monthly cycles in the sexually mature woman. The gonadotropin FSH acts on the granulosa cells, causing fluid to accumulate around the ovum, forming the Graafian follicle. Many of the cells surrounding the ovum synthesize steroids. Both the granulosa cells and the theca interna cells synthesize estradiol. Rising FSH and LH levels appear to be responsible for promoting estrogen secretion. As the estrogen level in the serum increases, it causes a further release of LH. This 'LH surge' results in ovulation.

Following the rupture of the follicle, the granulosa cells, surrounding thecal cells and blood vessels mingle to form the corpus luteum. During its usual 14-day life, it produces estadiol and progesterone.

Several years before menopause, there is a decrease in estradiol and progesterone and a compensatory increase in LH and FSH secretion from the pituitary. Following menopause, the ovary is virtually devoid of follicles and consequently does not secrete significant amounts of estrogen. Serum LH and FSH levels rise further because of the absence of sex steroid feedback. Thus, unlike the testis, when the ovary loses its germ cells, the pituitary commonly increases the secretion of both gonadotropins. It should be recognized that even if gonadotropin levels remain normal after therapy, primordial follicle loss could remain undetected until premature menopause develops.

2.2 Radiation Therapy

Irradiation given to the ovary can result in cessation of normal function. The sensitivity of the ovary to X-ray therapy depends primarily upon the age of the woman receiving it; women nearer to the menopause are more sensitive to irradiation because there are fewer oocytes left. Although there are no primary germ cells that can replenish the oocytes destroyed, the germ cells of the ovary are more radioresistant than those of the testis: while a dose of 600 rads to the ovaries of women aged 40 or more can cause permanent sterility [39], a dose four times greater has only a 50% probability of inducing sterility in a young woman.

The ovarian function of 18 prepubertal females who had received abdominal radiation (2500 to 300 rads over 25 to 44 days) for childhood tumors, was reported by Shalet et al. [40]. At the time of evaluation, 12 were over the age of 13 (the mean age of menarche in Great Britain) and none had menstruated. In addition to finding low serum estrogen levels, high FSH and LH were found, confirming that ovarian failure had resulted from the prepubertal treatment.

Patients with Hodgkin's disease in whom abdominal involvement is suspected or confirmed, generally receive radiation therapy, either to an upper abdominal port covering the para-aortic nodes, or to an inverted port which covers para-aortic, iliac and pelvic lymph nodes. In patients receiving upper abdominal radiation, the ovaries receive only scatter irradiation, although it generally amounts to about 150 rads/ovary. In four women receiving such therapy, Thomas [41] found no evidence of significant ovarian damage. Serum gonadotropins were normal and the menstrual histories were unremarkable. Because the ovaries lie directly in the field of radiation for the inverted 'Y' port, a surgical oophoropexy is performed before treatment. The ovaries are either moved laterally to the pelvic brim or medially to lie in front of and behind the uterus. In twelve women who underwent medial oophoropexy prior to the treatment, Thomas found that despite the surgical procedure, the dose to the ovaries still ranged from 650 to 3500 rads. All of his patients, ranging in age from 18 to 36 at the time of treatment, became amenorrheic. Three patients regained their menses and one became pregnant, confirming that the ovarian damage caused by irradiation is not necessarily permanent. Six other patients, who underwent oophoropexies but received no infra-diaphragmatic irradiation, had no menstrual irregularities and four subsequently became pregnant. The substantial contribution of radiation therapy to the development of ovarian damage must be remembered in the evaluation of patients receiving combined therapy.

2.3 *Single Agent Chemotherapy*

Chemotherapeutic agents can interfere with ovarian function, although the female generative system appears to be somewhat less sensitive than that of the male (Table 1). Alkylating agents, which are radioninetic, can cause damage to the ovaries similar to that caused by irradiation. The severity of the effect is related to the total dose, to the duration of therapy and to the proximity of treatment to the menopause.

2.3.1 *Cyclophosphamide.* The occurrence of amenorrhea in patients receiving cyclophosphamide was first noted when the agent was used as an immunosuppressive in the treatment of lupus erythematosis [42] and rheumatoid arthritis [43]. Fosdick treated 54 patients with rheumatoid arthritis with daily oral cyclophosphomide. Thirty-three women took cyclophosphamide for six months or more. Six women had early cessation of menses accompanied by hot flashes. A few years later, Miller et al. [44] described a

young girl with a mixed connective tissue disease who received cyclophos-phamide (1–2 mg/kg/day) for 30 months who showed a variety of side effects from the drug, including alopecia, lymphopenia, impaired antibody production and hemorrhagic cystitis. Post mortem examination showed that her ovaries totally lacked ova and follicles. Only stromal cells remained.

Warne et al. [45] were able to study 22 women receiving cyclophospham-ide for either progressive glomerulonephritis or rheumatoid arthritis. All the women had had normal pubertal development and were having regular menses at the time treatment was instituted. Nineteen of the 22 developed amenorrhea which began one to 33 months (mean 16.9 months) after the institution of therapy. In two, the amenorrhea turned out to be due to preg-nancy, but in the others, the amenorrhea was attributed to the alkylating agent. The amenorrhea developed more quickly in women over age 35. Fourteen of the 17 women with amenorrhea were found to have a hormonal pattern consistent with ovarian failure: urinary gonadotropins were elevated and urinary estrogens were low. Six patients underwent ovarian biopsies; none had evidence of follicular maturation and ova were seen in only two biopsy specimens, which were abnormal in appearance and surrounded by flattened thecal cells. Despite this evidence of ovarian damage, one of these women subsequently became pregnant, indicating that the changes are not invariably irreversible. However, the time before the ovaries recover may be prolonged. Only one of the twelve patients demonstrated to have ovarian failure had return of normal menses, 31 months after completion of cyclo-phosphamide therapy.

Cyclophosphamide used in the treatment of nephrosis also has a variable effect on the ovary. Pennisi [46] found no gonadal toxicity in seven prepu-bertal girls treated with daily doses of 2–3 mg/kg of cyclophosphamide for 2–3 months. All had normal FSH and LH levels throughout therapy. Three, now postpubertal and off therapy, developed normal menses. Four other patients treated with the same dose schedule while postpubertal likewise had no menstrual irregularities. Three have subsequently become pregnant. There have been similar results in other studies [20, 22, 21]. The same doses of alkylating agents which impair spermatogenesis in males cause no men-strual irregularities in females (Table 1).

2.3.2 *Other Chemotherapeutic Agents.* Busulfan has long been recognized to cause irregular menses and even amenorrhea [15, 47]. Autopsy studies in patients treated with long-term busulfan show extensive ovarian fibro-sis [48]. Chlorambucil, thio-tepa and L-phenylalanine mustard are three other alkylating agents reported to interfere with normal ovarian function. Thio-tepa was the first chemotherapeutic drug used as an adjunct to surgery in the National Surgical Adjuvant Breast Project (NSABP). The drug was given for only a brief period following surgery. Eighteen of 49 premenopausal petients treated with thio-tepa became amenorrheic shortly after taking the drug, whereas only one of 37 premenopausal placebo-treated patients became amenorrheic [49].

The NSABP conducted a larger trial with L-phenylalanine mustard (L-PAM) as the surgical adjuvant. The drug was given for nine months (6 mg/d q6wks × 4) in these patients. Rose and Davis [50] reported that five premenopausal women became amenorrheic within six months of starting L-PAM. The amenorrhea was accompanied by a decrease in the plasma estrogens and a rise in gonadotropins. Further evidence for a direct antiovarian effect of L-PAM was provided by plasma measurements. This steroid is made in equal amounts by the ovaries and adrenals in the premenopausal patient but is secreted mostly by the adrenal in the post-menopausal patients. During the L-PAM chemotherapy, plasma androstanedione levels decreased more in the premenopausal women than in postmenopausal women, suggesting that the ovarian secretion of this steroid had been impaired by chemotherapy.

2.4 Combination Chemotherapy

Combination chemotherapy in the pre-menopausal patient with breast cancer has also been found to affect ovarian function. The combination of cyclophosphamide (100 mg/m^2 qd × 14), 5-FU (600 mg/m^2) and methotrexate (60 mg/m^2) given monthly × 12 was used by Bonnadonna [51] in a study of post-mastectomy chemotherapy in 207 patients. The development of amenorrhea was age-related, occurring in almost all patients over the age of 40. When amenorrhea occurred in younger patients, normal cycles recurred after therapy was stopped in more than half the affected patients. A similar adjuvant protocol [52], consisting of 5-FU, adriamycin, cyclophosphamide and BCG, was shown to cause amenorrhea in 2/3 of the 55 patients treated. In these patients, primary ovarian failure was confirmed by the presence of low plasma estrogen, abnormally high levels of FSH and LH, and excessive response to LH-releasing hormone. In both of these combinations, cyclophosphamide is suspected of being most likely responsible for the toxic effect on the ovary.

Patients treated for Hodgkin's disease with any combination which includes an alkylating agent may also develop ovarian failure. Ezdinli and Stutzman [53] reported that two of 31 female patients treated with chlormabucil alone became amenorrheic. Sobrinho [54] studied 10 women with Hodgkin's disease treated with nitrogen mustard and chlorambucil. All became amenorrheic; six of these had postmenopausal levels of FSH and LH. Chapman [55 reported on 41 women observed for 16 months following the completion of chemotherapy for Hodgkin's disease. Forty had received standard nitrogen mustard, vinblastine, procarbazine and prednisone (MOPP) therapy and one had received chlorambucil-VPP therapy. All had normal ovarian function before treatment (by history and hormone level determinations; three had ovarian biopsy), indicating that Hodgkin's disease per se caused no adverse effect on gonadal function. Following therapy, 17% had normally functioning ovaries, 34% failing ovaries and 49% complete ovarian failure.

In the group whose ovaries failed completely, FSH and LH levels were elevated and estradiol levels were low (in the postmenopausal range). All but three of these women had symptoms of estrogen deficiency with hot flashes and irritability, decreased or absent libido. In many cases, these symptoms were incorrectly assumed to be unavoidable side effects of chemotherapy. The symptoms had, in some cases, led to the breakup of families and social relationships. The group with the failing ovaries had irregular menses and episodic flushing, irritability and fatigue. As chemotherapy continued and ovarian dysfunction progressed, libido diminished. Biochemical studies on these women showed increasing gonadotropins and inadequate levels of luteal-phase progesterone. Circulating estradiol levels tended to decrease as treatment continued. Basal body temperatures in these patients were compatible with sporadic ovulation. Ovarian biopsies were obtained after therapy on six women who were undergoing surgery for other reasons. Three of the biopsied ovaries were from women who had shown clinical and hormonal evidence of failed ovaries. Two of these biopsies showed atrophy with but two primordial follicles. Even in the three other women, (two with functioning ovaries and one with failing ovaries), the biopsies showed only two to four primoridal follicles. In contrast, the three biopsies obtained before therapy had shown 18 to 55 primordial follicles, normal corpora lutea and developing secondary follicles.

In summary, the older the patient is at the time of combination chemotherapy, the more likely is permanent ovarian failure. When X-ray therapy is added to the regimen, the chances of ovarian failure are substantially increased. A preliminary report of an attempts at 'protecting' ovarian function by the administration of oral contraceptives before starting combination chemotherapy for Hodgkin's disease has been published [56]. Obviously, evident hormonal deficiency following chemotherapy should receive therapy, if there are no clinical contraindications.

Combination chemotherapy for childhood leukemia has also been evaluated for its effect on gonadal function. Siris, Leventhal and Vaitukaitus [57] examined its effect on pubertal development and reproductive function in 34 girls, whose diagnosis of acute leukemia was made between the ages of 2 and 16 years. All had received a combination of chorticosteroid, vincristine, methotrexate and 6-mercaptopurine (POMP) with 2400 R of cranial irradiation and intra-thecal chemotherapy. Nine of these patients had also received cyclophosphamide. Ovarian function and the hypothal-amic-pituitary-ovarian axis were studied by history, by evaluation of sexual development, and by measurement of FSH, LH and estradiol.

Seventeen patients were prepubertal at the time of diagnosis. Nine of these underwent normal menarche, including five who began their menstural cycles while receiving chemotherapy. At the end of chemotherapy, one eight year old and one 12-year old were still prepubertal. Five of the remaining 6 children were progressing normally through puberty. One child, who was receiving additional chemotherapy with a cyclophosphamide-containing regimen, had evidence of delayed pubertal development and inappropriately low FSH and LH levels. Of the ten girls who had received chemotherapy during puberty (over 10 years of age but menses had not begun), seven matured normally and three had decreased levels of FSH and LH and did not undergo menarche during the period of observation. Of the seven girls who received chemotherapy postpubertally, five had no hormonal abnormalities when studied. The other two had prolonged secondary amenorrhea during their treatment and while amenorrheic, had elevated FSH and LH levels and low estradiol. Menses returned spontaneously in both, indicating that the ovarian failure they incurred was temporary.

Although many of these girls received cyclophosphamide, its use did not appear to result in ovarian dysfunction. Rather, delayed maturation and decreased levels of FSH and LH were found. While the cause for this reduced secretion of gonadotropins was not established, regulation of gonadotropic function by the central nervous system could have been affected, since the girls were frequently quite ill. The use of cranial irradiation is a routine part of the therapy for ALL and doubtless contributed to the impaired hypothalamic-pituitary-ovarian function; the dose of 2400 rads received by these children has also been noted to decrease growth hormone levels [56].

2.5 Teratogenic and Mutagenic Effects

Chemotherapy with folic acid antagonists and 6-MP during pregnancy, particularly during the first trimester, causes abortions and fetal anomalies [57]. Alkylating agents may terminate early pregnancies but have not produced a dramatic increase in fetal malformations [58]. The temporary occurrence of azoospermia or amenorrhea in patients treated for malignant diseases has raised concerns about the outcome of pregnancy in those who regain their fertility.

There have been several studies evaluating both the incidence of normal pregnancies and the risk of abnormalities in the offspring of those who have previously received chemotherapy or chemotherapy combined with irradiation therapy, but the number of subjects studied has not been large enough to permit a definitive statement concerning the possibility of an increase in fetal wastage or malformation over that found in the general population.

Van Thiel [24] studied 50 women who had received methotrexate and actinomycin D for trophoblastic disease. All were in remission when studied. Of 88 subsequent pregnancies, 71 were normal; there were two stillbirths and 15 resulted in spontaneous abortions. As the expected rate of spontaneous abortions is about 10%, this incidence could be within normal limits.

Holmes and Holmes [60] reviewed the medical records of 624 patients who had received treatment for Hodgkin's disease at the University of Kansas from 1944 to 1975. Twenty-nine female patients in this group had become pregnant and 19 male patients had fathered children for a total of 93 pregnancies. Eighty-two prenancies went to term and there were 76 normal offspring (including two sets of twins) and eight with congenital abnormalities. Of the 10 abortions, seven were spontaneous and three were therapeutic. There was one tubal pregnancy. Because the time span included in this chart review was so long (31 years), the patients had received a variety of treatments. For evaluation of treatment, the patients were divided into two groups: those who had received radiation only, and those who had received both chemotherapy and radiation. There was no difference in the rates of spontaneous abortions in either group or between these patients and a control group of their siblings. In the general population, approximately 9.6% of pregnancies result in minor abnormalities in offspring and 3.3% result in major abnormalities. Overall, the incidence of eight abnormal offspring in a group of 82 pregnancies was similar to the general incidence rate and also to that found in the offspring of the sibling controls (26 abnormalities in 209 live births). However, five of the abnormal offspring occurred in the 14 pregnancies in women who had received combined therapy. This incidence was significantly greater than that found in the women who had received irradiation alone (3/15) and in the general population (15%), although the numbers involved are small.

More recently, Horning [61] reviewed the reproductive function in 103 women (less than 40 years of age) treated for Hodgkin's disease at the Stanford Medical Center. Nineteen patients had received total lymphoid irradiation (TLI), 50 were given TLI and chemotherapy and 34 received chemotherapy alone. All those receiving pelvic irradiation had undergone a midline oophoropexy. Twenty women became pregnant after treatment with a total of 28 pregnancies. There were no spontaneous abortions, birth defects or developmental abnormalities in these children. Overall, 34 women were sexually active and used no form of birth control so that 59% (20/34) were fertile. Age at treatment and the resumption of menses without menopausal symptoms were significant factors in predicting recovery of fertility. Those who had received both pelvic irradiation and chermotherapy were most likely to have mensutral abnormalities, menopausal symptoms and decreased reproductive potential.

Li et al. [62] reviewed a larger group of patients who had received diverse treatments for an assortment of malignancies. Of 293 pregnancies in 146 patients, there were 242 live births, seven stillbriths, 19 therapeutic and 25 spontaneous abortions. There were four major birth defects (1.9%) and 16 minor birth defects (6.6%) among the progeny, a rate not significantly different from the normal population.

Although there is no clear increase in teratogenesis following antineoplastic treatment clinically, it is clear that both irradiation and chemotherapy can cause germ cell damage. In mice, the number of abnormal sperm can be increased by as little as 30 rads of X-ray. Similarly when mice were treated with a number of chemotherapeutic agents and sperm analysis was made at one, four and 10 weeks following exposure, a number of abnormalities were found [63]. The alkylating agents thio-tepa, mitomycin and myeleran caused the most marked abnormalities. Although antimetabolites also caused abnormalities, the number was less and the effects generally disappeared within 10 weeks of stopping therapy. These results are comparable to those in man, in which the most lasting germ cell effect appears to be due to alkylating agents rather than to antimetabolites.

Concern about possible mutagenicity cannot be entirely assuaged even though the current data do not show a major increase in congenital abnormalities in the first generation: genetic damage may not be evident for several generations. 6-mercaptopurine has been shown to cause chromosomal breaks, fragmentation and gaps in the chromosomes of treated patients. When the drug is given to mice during their breeding period and the offspring of that mating are subsequently mated, there is a marked decrease in the litter size and the number of live offspring from the second generation mating [64]. Histologic examination of the ovaries of embryonic mice whose mother had received 6-mercaptopurine before pregnancy, revealed a decrease in the number of oocytes and ovarian follicles. To date, there is no clinical information on the fertility of the offspring of mothers who had previously received 6-mercaptopurine or its analog.

3.0. OVERVIEW

There have been several recent reviews of the subject of the effect of chemotherapy on gonadal function [65, 66]. In summary, the alkylating drugs appear to be responsible for the greatest amount of gonadal injury, but cytosine arabinoside, procarbazine and other agents also appear to have damaging effects.

Total dose is an important variable in predicting anti-gonadal effects, whereas data on the duration of treatment is not as clearcut. Pubertal or prepubertal gonads may be less susceptible to damage, although long-term effects, both on the patients and their offspring, remain to be assessed. In the female, increasing age is clearly related to increasing risk of immediate gonadal dysfunction. Sperm banking may be an approach to the loss of fertility following chemotherapy in the male, although diminished sperm count and function are often present even before therapy is begun. Treatment for specific hormone deficiencies should be instituted following chemotherapy, if not otherwise contraindicated.

REFERENCES

1. Brambilla F, Smeraldi E, Sachetti E, et al: Deranged anterior pituitary responsiveness to hypothalamic hormones in depressed patients. Arch Gen Psychiatry (35):1231–1238, 1978.
2. Smith SR, Chhetri MK, Johanson AJ, et al: The pituitary-gonadal axis in men with protein-calorie malnutrition. J Clin Endocrinol Metab 41:60–69, 1975.
3. Klibanski A, Breitins IZ, Badger T, Little R, McArthur JW: Reproductive function during fasting in men. JCEM 53:258–263, 1981.
4. Heller CG, Heller GV, Warner GA, Rowley MJ: Effect of graded doses of ionizing radiation on testicular cytology and sperm count in man. Rad Res 35:493–494, 1968.
5. Casarett GW: Pathologic changes after protracted exposure to low dose radiation. In: Late Effects of Radiation. Fry RM, Grahn D, Griem ML, Rust JH (eds): London, Taylor and Frances Ltd. 1970, pp 85–100.
6. Speiser B, Rubin P, Casarett G: Aspermia following lower truncal irradiation in Hodgkin's disease. Cancer 32:692–698, 1973.
7. Richter P, Calamera JC, Morgenfeld MC, et al: Effect of chlorambucil on spermatogenesis in the human with malignant lymphoma. Cancer 25:1026–1030, 1970.
8. Cheviakoff S, Calamera JC, Morgenfeld M, Mancini RE: Recovery of spermatogenesis in patients with lymphoma after treatment with chlorambucil. J Reprod Fertil 33:155–177, 1973.
9. Fairley KR, Barrie JU, Johnson W: Sterility and testicular atrophy related to cyclophosphamide therapy. Lancet 1:568–569, 1972.
10. Kumar R, Biggart JD, McEvoy J, McGeown MG: Cyclophosphamide and reproductive function. Lancet 1:1212–1214, 1972.
11. Quereshi MSA, Pennington JH, Goldsmith JH, Cox PE: Cyclophosphamide therapy and sterility. Lancet 2:1290–1292, 1972.
12. Buchanan JD, Fairley KF, Barrie JU: Return of spermatogenesis after stopping cyclophosphamide therapy. Lancet 2:156–157, 1975.
13. Lindgardh G, Andersson L, Osterman B: Fertility in men after renal transplantation. Acta Chir Scand 140:494–497, 1974.
14. Phadke AG, MacKinnon KJ, Dossetor JB: Male fertility in uremia: restoration by renal allografts. Can Med Assoc J 102:607–608, 1970.

15. Galton DAG, Till M, Wiltshaw E: Busulfan: summary of clinical results. Ann N Y Acad Sci 68:967–973, 1958.
16. Shorer AE, Oken NM, Johnson GJ: Gynecomastia with nitrosurea therapy. Cancer Treat Rep 62:574–576, 1978.
17. Guesry P, Lenoir G, Broyer M: Gonadal effects of chlorambucil given to prepubertal and pubertal boys for nephrotic syndrome. J Pediatr 92:299–303, 1978.
18. Holland JF, Scharlau C, Gailani S, Krant MJ: Vincristine treatment of advanced cancer: a cooperative study of 392 cases. Cancer Res 33:1258–1264, 1973.
19. Sieber S, Correa P, Dalgard D, Adamson R: Carcinogenic and other adverse effects of procarbazine in nonhuman primates. Cancer Res 39:2124–2134, 1978.
20. Lentz RD, Bergstein J, Steffes WM, et al: Postpubertal evaluation of gonadal function following cyclophosphamide therapy before and during puberty. J Pediatr 91:385–394, 1977.
21. Parra A, Santos D, Cervantes C, et al: Plasma gonadotropins and gonadal steroids in children treated with cyclophosphamide. J Pediatr 92:117–124, 1978.
22. DeGroot GW, Faiman CA, Winter JSD: Cyclophosphamide and the prepubertal gonad: a negative report. J Pediatr 84:123–125, 1974.
23. Sherins RJ, Olweny CLM, Ziegler JL: Gynecomastia and gonadal dysfunction in adolescent boys treated with combination chemotherapy for Hodgkin's disease. N Engl J Med 299:12–16, 1978.
24. Van Thiel DH, Ross GT, Lipsett MB: Pregnancies afterx chemotherapy of trophoblastic neoplasms. Science 169:1326–1327, 1970.
25. Roeser HP, Stocks AE, Smith AJ: Testicular damage due to cytotoxic drugs and recovery after cessation of therapy. Aust NZ J Med 9:250–254, 1978.
26. Whitehead E, Shalet SM, Blackledse G, Todd I, Crowther B, Beardwell CG: The effects of Hodgkin's disease and Combination chemotherapy on gonadal function in the adult male. Cancer 1:49(3):418–422, 1982.
27. Chapman RM, Sutcliffe SB, Rees LR, et al.: Cyclical combination chemotherapy and gonadal function. Lancet 1:285–289, 1979.
28. Chapman RM, Sutcliffe SB, Malpas JS: Male gonadal dysfunction in Hodgkin's disease. A prospective study. J Am Med Assoc 245:1323–1328, 1981.
29. Heber D, Chlebowski RT: Hypogonadism in male patients with metastatic cancer prior to treatment. Clin Res 29:293A, 1981.
30. Santoro A, Bonadonna R, Zucali R, et al: Therapeutic and toxicologic effects of MOPP vs ABVD when combined with RT in Hodgkin's disease. Proc 17th Ann Meeting Am Soc Clin Oncol 22:522, 1981.
31. Van Thiel DH, Sherins RJ, Meyers GH, Jr, DeVita VT, Jr: Evidence for a specific seminiferous tubular factor affecting follicle-stimulating hormone secretion in man. J Clin Invest 41:1009–1019, 1972.
32. Stricker S, Crosby K, Carey RW: Paternity after chemotherapy-induced sterility in Hodgkin's disease [letter]. N Engl J Med 19:1173, 1981.
33. Blatt J, Sherins RJ, Poplack DG: Evidence of normal testicular function in boys following chemotherapy for acute lymphoblasic leukemia. N Engl J Med 304:1121–1124, 1981.
34. Lendon M, Palmer MK, Morris Jones PH, et al: Testicular histology after combination chemotherapy in childhood for acute lymphoblastic leukemia. Lancet 2:439–441, 1978.
35. Maguire LC, Dick RF, Sherman BM: Effect of anti-leukemic therapy on gonadal histology in adult males. Proc Am Assoc Cancer Res and Am Soc Clin Oncol, 1979, p 365.
36. Lange PH, Marayan P, Vogelzang NJ, et al: Changing concepts about fertility after treatment for nonseminomatous germ cell resticular tumor (NSGCT). Proc Am Assoc Cancer Res and Am Soc Clin Oncol, 1981, p 431.
37. Friedman NM, Plymate SR: Leydig cell dysfunction and gynecomastia in adult males

treated with alkylating agents. Clin Endocrinol 12:553–556, 1980.

38. Glode LM, Robinson J, Gould SF: Protection from cyclophosphamide-induced testicular damage with an analogue of gonadotropin-releasing hormone. Lancet 1:1132–1134, 1981.

39. Lushbaugh CC, Casarett GW: The effects of gonadal irradiation in clinical radiation therapy: a review. Cancer 37:1111–1120, 1976.

40. Shalet SM, Beardwell CG, Morris Jones PH, et al: Ovarian failure following abdominal irradiation in childhood. Br J Cancer 33:655–658, 1976.

41. Thomas PRM, Winstanley D, Peckham MJ, et al: Reproductive and endocrine function in patients with Hodgkin's disease: effects of oophoropexy and irradiation. Br J Cancer 33:226–231, 1976.

42. Fries J, Sharpi GC, McDevitt HO, Holman HR: Cyclophosphamide therapy in connective tissue disease. Clin Res 18:134, 1970.

43. Fosdick WM, Parsons JL, Hill DF: Long-term cyclophosphamide therapy in rheumatoid arthritis. Arthritis Rheum 11:151–161, 1968.

44. Miller J, Williams G, Leissring J: Multiple late complications of therapy with cyclophosphamide including ovarian destruction. Am J Med 50:530–535, 1971.

45. Warne GL, Fairley KF, Hoobs JB, Martin FIR: Cyclophosphamide-induced ovarian failure. N Engl J Med 289:1159–1162, 1973.

46. Pennisi AJ, Brushkin CM, Liberman FE: Gonadal function in children with nephrosis treated with cyclophosphamide. Am J Dis Child 129:315–318, 1975.

47. Belohorsky B, Siracky J, Sandor L, Kaluber E: Comments on the development of amenorrhea caused by Myleran cases of chronic myelosis. Neoplasma 7:397–402, 1960.

48. Smalley RV, Wall RL: Two cases of busulfan toxicity. Ann Intern Med 64:154–164, 1966.

49. Fisher B, Slack N, Katrych D, Wolmark N: Ten year follow-up results of patients with carcinoma of the breast in a co-operative clinical trial evaluating surgical adjuvant chemotherapy. Surg Obstet Gynecol 140:528–534, 1975.

50. Rose DP, Davis TE: Ovarian function in patients receiving adjuvant chemotherapy for breast cancer. Lancet 1:1174–1176, 1977.

51. Bonadonna G, Rossi A, Valagussa P, Banfi A and Veronesi U: The CMF program for operable breast cancer with positive axillary nodes. Cancer 39:2904–1915, 1977.

52. Samaan N, deAsis DN, Buzdar AU, Blumenschein GR: Pituitary-ovarian function in breast cancer patients on adjuvant chemo-immunotherapy. Cancer 41:2084–2087, 1978.

53. Ezdinli EZ, Stutzman L: Chlorambucil therapy for lymphomas and chronic lymphocytic leukemia. J Am Med Assoc 191:444–450, 1965.

54. Sorbrinho LG, Levine RA, DeConti RC: Amenorrhea in patients with Hodgkin's disease treated with antineoplastic agents. Am J Obstet Gynecol 109:135–139, 1971.

55. Chapman RM, Sutcliffe SB, Malpas JS: Cytotoxic-induced ovarian failure in women with Hodgkin's disease. J Am Med Assoc 242:1877–1881, 1979.

56. Chapman RM, Sutcliffe SB: Protection of ovarian function by oral contraceptives in women receiving chemotherapy for Hodgkin's disease. Blood 58:849–851, 1981.

57. Siris ES, Leventhal BG, Vaitukaitis JL: Effects of childhood leukemia and chemotherapy on puberty and reproductive function in girls. N Engl J Med 294:1143–1146, 1976.

58. Nicholson HO: Cytotoxic drugs in pregnancy. J Obstet Gynecol 75:307–312, 1968.

59. Schein P, Winokus SH: Immunosuppressive and cytotoxic chemotherapy: long-term complications. Ann Intern Med 82:84–95, 1975.

60. Holmes GE, Holmes FF: Pregnancy outcome of patients treated for Hodgkin's disease. A controlled study. Cancer 41:1317–1322, 1975.

61. Horning SJ, Hoppe RT, Kaplan HS, Rosenberg SA: Female reproductive potential after treatment for Hodgkin's disease. N Eng J Med 304:1277–1382, 1981.

62. Li FP, Fine W, Jaffe N, Holmes G, Holmes F: Offspring of patients treated for cancer in

childhood. JNCI 62:1193–1197, 1979.

63. Wyrobeck J, Bruce W: Chemical induction of sperm abnormalities in mice. Proc Nat Acad Sci USA 72:4425–4429, 1975.

64. Reimers T, Sluss P: 6-mercaptopurine treatment of pregnant mice: effects on second and third generations. Science 201:66–67, 1978.

65. Shalet SM: Effects of chemotherapy on gonadal function of patients. Cancer Treatment Reports 7:141, 1980.

66. Shilsky RL, Lewis BJ, Sherins RJ, Young RC: Gonadal dysfunction in patients receiving chemotherapy for cancer. Ann Int Med 93:109–114, 1980.

3. Viral infections in cancer patients

COLEMAN ROTSTEIN

INTRODUCTION

Viruses are intracellular organisms that multiply only inside cells and are absolutely dependent on the host cell for protein synthesis and energy-producing functions. Over 400 distinct viruses are capable of causing human infection. Infection caused by these agents involves an interaction of host defense mechanisms, the organism, and the environment; all of which are similar to features of infectious processes seen with other organisms. Yet, viral diseases have certain unique features. Viruses produce infection at a higher frequency than they produce disease [1]. Infection refers to the multiplication of the virus within the host and is determined by factors that govern exposure to the virus and the susceptibility of the host. Disease represents the host response to infection when it evokes a recognizable pattern of clinical symptoms. Viruses are also unique in that they have variable incubation periods, exhibit periods of latency and can spread along peripheral nerves (eg, herpes zoster).

Herpetoviridae (herpes simplex, cytomegalovirus, Epstein-Barr and varicella-zoster virus) seem to have a predilection for cancer patients, and are therefore detected more frequently in this type of immunocompromised host than in immunocompetent individuals. These viral agents cause a spectrum of illnesses ranging from subclinical infection to lethal disease. Hepatitis B virus [2, 3] and human wart virus [4] also have higher prevalence among cancer patients than in the general population. Other viruses, such as rhinoviruses, enteroviruses and influenza, produce disease in cancer patients at a rate comparable to the population at large, although influenza appears to cause slightly higher mortality rates (2 to 3% above expected) among patients with malignant neoplasms [5].

Higby, DJ (ed), The Cancer Patient and Supportive Care. ISBN 0-89838-690-X.
© 1985, Martinus Nijhoff Publishers, Boston. Printed in The Netherlands.

IMMUNOLOGIC RESPONSE TO VIRAL INFECTION

Various immune responses are mobilized by the human host in response to viral infection. These responses include: activation of macrophages by T lymphocytes, cytotoxic effect of T lymphocytes on virus-infected cells, antibody production, and release of interferon [1, 6]. The immune response to most viral infections, particularly those in which viral transmission transpires by cell-to-cell contact (eg, herpes virus) rather than by release of virus into the extracellular environment, appears to be cell-mediated [7, 8]. T lymphocytes and macrophages respond to virally directed antigens that appear on the cell membrane of the infected host cells causing the production of biological mediators which are chemotactic for inflammatory cells. The mediators attract other lymphocytes which exert a toxic effect on infected host cells and also produce lymphotoxin that inhibits viral replication. Once the infected cells are eliminated, there is a diminution in the inflammatory response.

The prevention of the spread of viruses from the extracellular space and the blood is largely dependent on neutralization by humoral antibody [1, 8]. Infections characterized by viremia produce the most marked humoral antibody response and the resulting immunity is usually of long duration. Antibodies of the IgG, IgM, and IgA classes have been described which neutralize the ability of extracellular viruses to infect their target cells by limiting the invasion of the viruses into the intracellular milieu, where viral replication takes place [1, 9]. Complement may also be involved [7]. Antibody production by B lymphocytes plays a more prominent role in resistance to future infection and a minor role in recovery from viral infections [10].

Interferon is produced by lymphocytes and fibroblasts in response to viral infection. There are three major classes of interferon (alpha, beta, and gamma) which can be distinguished by their cellular origin (leukocytes, fibroblasts and lymphocytes), by the agents which induce their synthesis, and by their biologic, antigenic and physiochemical properties [11]. Interferon is an early response of the infected cell that limits the spread of infection to adjacent cells. It has been shown to be produced in herpes zoster vesicles in immunocompromised hosts where elevated interferon titers correlated with localization of the disease and recovery [6].

ALTERATION OF HOST DEFENSE MECHANISMS

The above described immune responses are necessary to prevent and combat viral diseases in immunocompetent hosts. In cancer patients, many

Table 1. Viral Infections Associated with Cancer

Disease Entity	Altered Defense Mechanism	Viral Agent
Hodgkin's Disease	CMI*	varicella-zoster, herpes simplex, hepatitis B, cytomegalovirus, human wart virus
Non-Hodgkin's Lymphoma	CMI	varicella-zoster, herpes simplex, hepatitis B, cytomegalovirus, Epstein-Barr virus, human wart virus
Acute Lymphocytic Leukemia	CMI	varicella-zoster, herpes simplex, hepatitis B
Chronic Lymphocytic Leukemia	HI+	varicella-zoster, herpes simplex
Multiple Myeloma	HI	enteroviruses, herpes simplex, varicella-zoster
Oat Cell Carcinoma	CMI	varicella-zoster
Iatrogenic Disease: Cytotoxic Drugs	CMI, HI	varicella-zoster, herpes simplex, hepatitis B, cytomegalovirus
Corticosteroids	CMI	varicella-zoster, herpes simplex
Radiation	CMI	varicella-zoster, herpes simplex

* CMI = cell-mediated immunity
+ HI = humoral immunity

of the immune responses may be altered by the underlying malignant disease itself or by therapy used to treat the malignant disease, resulting in susceptibility to viral infection. Table 1 summarizes many of the viral diseases which may be seen in immunocompromised cancer patients, together with the corresponding alterations in host immunity.

Hodgkin's disease serves as an excellent example of the alteration in host immune response secondary to the underlying malignancy. Hodgkin's disease causes a defect in cell-mediated immunity (CMI) in the host. Lymphocytopenia is present and is more severe with diffuse disease [12]. The abnormality in CMI in patients with Hodgkin's disease is correlated with diminished in vitro lymphocyte transformation to antigens and mitogens, and diminished transformation in mixed lymphocyte culture. When skin testing is performed to assess CMI, approximately 100% of immunocompetent individuals will respond to one or more of the antigens employed; whereas, only about 66% of the patients with Hodgkin's disease will respond. Similarly, only 65% of patients with Hodgkin's disease can be sensitized to dinitrochlorobenzene, while 96% of normal persons can be sensitized [12, 13]. Skin test reactivity in Hodgkin's disease correlates with the presence or absence of systemic symptoms. Patients with B symptoms (fever, night sweats, pruritis and/or weight loss) have less skin reactivity than asymptomatic patients [12]. As a result of defective CMI, patients with Hodgkin's disease are predisposed to intracellular viral pathogens such as herpes zoster and herpes simplex. Interestingly, patients who have malignancies other than those of the reticuloendothelial system and who have early disease that has not been immunosuppressed by cytotoxic drugs, have normal CMI when evaluated by skin testing [14].

Pharmacologic agents have profound effects on both humoral immunity and CMI. Some drugs have a specific effect because of their mechanism of action. Antimetabolites affect mainly cells in the proliferative phase, while alkylating agents affect cells in all phases, but especially those in the precursor stage [15]. Cyclophosphamide, an alkylating agent, is one of the most potent immunosuppressive agents available [16]. Cyclophosphamide is cytotoxic to both rapidly proliferating and resting lymphoid cells. It suppresses both the primary and secondary humoral immune responses, as well as the delayed hypersensitivity reaction of CMI.

6-mercaptopurine inhibits the development of the primary antibody response after antigenic stimulation and delayed hypersensitivity [16]. It exerts maximum inhibition of antibody response if administered during the early proliferative phase of the immune response, that is, during the first 48 hours after challenge with the antigen.

Methotrexate, a folic acid antagonist, can suppress the primary antibody response, the secondary antibody response and the development of delayed hypersensitivity. It is most effective if given 48 hours after antigenic stimulation. Folinic acid, a methotrexate antagonist, can alter the toxic effects of the drug, but not its immunosuppressive properties [16].

Cytosine arabinoside, an inhibitor of DNA synthesis, partially suppresses primary and secondary antibody responses and delayed hypersensitivity, since its effect is only on proliferating cells and is limited by its short half-life [16].

The vinca alkaloids and actinomycin D have little immunosuppressive activity [16].

Other agents such as radiation and corticosteroids also have effects on the host's immune responses. Radiation, when given as total body irradiation, induces lymphocytopenia within a few minutes to hours and suppresses both humoral immunity and CMI [17]. Delayed hypersensitivity responses are suppressed if radiation for bronchial carcinoma, head and neck tumors and breast carcinoma with large tumor load is given before antigen exposure [18]. Local irradiation has been found to reduce lymphocyte responses to phytohemagglutinin, concanavalin A, and pokeweed antigen to approximately 55% of their baseline values until about 2 months after the completion of radiation therapy [19].

Corticosteroids are potent immunosuppressive agents [20]. They can influence every aspect and stage of lymphocyte function. The effects of corticosteroids on lymphocyte populations may result in alterations in host defenses. These effects on lymphocytes can be characterized as follows: 1) effects on the traffic movement and circulatory capabilities of these cells; 2) direct and indirect effects on their functional capabilities; and 3) effects on the production of soluble mediators involved in the immune response [21]. Corticosteroids cause lymphocytopenia and monocytopenia that is maximal at 4-6 hours after drug administration [22]. This effect is more pronounced in circulating T lymphocytes. Corticosteroids interfere with cellular interactions of the immune response, and suppress *in vitro* blastogenic responses and lymphocyte cytotoxicity [21]. It is well known that corticosteroids abolish cutaneous delayed hypersensitivity reactions [21].

Many of the above mentioned agents used in combination to treat patients with malignancy produce profound immunosuppression, and thus enhance the susceptibility of the host to viral infection. Certain general statements may be made about these viral infections in cancer patients [10]:

a) Viruses that produce latent or persistent infections are the ones most frequently associated with disease states in these patients.
b) The herpesvirus group is the major cause of infections in these patients. Varicella-zoster, herpes simplex 1 and 2, and cytomegalovirus are the most virulent; Epstein-Barr virus is less virulent.
c) The more severely depressed the CMI in the host, the more severe a viral infection will be.

HERPES SIMPLEX VIRUS (HSV) INFECTIONS

Epidemiology

Herpes simplex virus is a double-stranded DNA virus enclosed within a lipid-containing laminated envelope. HSV replication occurs within the cell nucleus and is associated with lysis of the productive cell. Humans are the only natural reservoir for HSV [23]. There is no known animal vector. Spread of HSV occurs by direct contact with infected secretions – oral secretions most commonly in the case of HSV-1 and genital secretions in the case of HSV-2. At any given time, 0.26–5.0% of population is excreting HSV-1 or HSV-2 [24]. The epidemiology of HSV is such that 80–100% of lower socioeconomic class people have antibodies to the virus, whereas 30–50% of the upper socioeconomic class have antibodies to the virus [25, 26]. Recurrent infections are very common with HSV, due to endogenous reactivation of the virus despite the presence of circulating antibody. Seventeen to forty-two percent of the general population have recurrent lip lesions triggered by stress, sunlight, fever, trauma, or other factors [27].

In cancer patients, HSV infections are usually localized and self-limited with clinical manifestations differing little from intact hosts. Individuals such as bone marrow transplant recipients or those receiving antineoplastic agents which cause defects in cell-mediated immunity or breaks in the natural mucocutaneous barrier are prone to more serious or unusual forms of HSV infections [28, 29]. Most infections seem to be due to ractivation of the virus.

Although HSV most commonly affects the oropharynx and upper respiratory tract in cancer patients, it may also cause pneumonia [29], disseminated skin eruption [28], esophagitis [30–32], gastritis [33], visceral organ dissemination [34, 35], meningoencephalitis [36], chronic cutaneous ulcerations [37], colitis [38], and perianal ulcerations [39]. The incidence of HSV isolation from the oropharynx in patients with myeloproliferative and lymphoproliferative disorders is reported at 16% as compared to a rate of only 2% in a control population [40]. In these same populations, a higher titer of HSV antibodies was present than in the controls, possibly indicating that a defect in cell-mediated immunity may play a role in the occurrence of HSV infections rather than humoral immunity.

Although historically HSV infections were felt to be more common in patients with lymphoma [28], Aston et al. found a similar incidence in patients with acute leukemia (33%) and lymphoma (38%) [40]. In another study, viral shedding was found to be similar in the two groups as well [41]. HSV may also occur in a variety of other neoplasms [42].

Clinical Manifestations

As mentioned above, HSV most commonly affects the oropharynx and upper respiratory tract [28, 41]. These cutaneous lesions are usually clinically evident. Vesicular eruptions may be more severe in patients with malignant diseases [28]. Occasionally chronic ulcerations occur [37].

Herpetic esophagitis is a condition which is probably more prevalent than is clinically appreciated; the esophagus may well be the visceral organ most frequently involved by HSV infection [42]. Among 55 autopsies with evidence of esophageal ulcers, 14 were due to HSV [30]. Four of these cases were seen in patients with malignant neoplasms. The typical macroscopic pattern revealed punched-out ulcers in the upper and middle thirds of the esophagus with confluent lesions in the distal third. Candidal esophagitis was frequently co-existent. A clinical antemortem diagnosis of herpetic esophagitis should be entertained in cancer patients complaining of dysphagia and retrosternal pain unresponsive to antifungal agents. The clinical suspicion of HSV esophagitis can be confirmed with endoscopy and subsequent biopsy and/or brush cytology [31, 32].

Perianal HSV infections occur among homosexuals with acquired immune deficiency syndrome (AIDS) with Kaposi's sarcoma [39]. A discussion of acquired immune deficiency syndrome is beyond the scope of this article.

Cutaneous dissemination (Kaposi's varicelliform eruption) of HSV is uncommon, with only 1 case described in a review of 20 cases of HSV infections in hematologic malignancies [28]. Visceral dissemination is usually unrecognized antemortem and therefore knowledge of these cases is derived from autopsy series [34]. No cases of herpes virus pneumonia were diagnosed antemortem in a recent report [29]. Dyspnea and cough were the commonest initial symptoms. It was suggested that localized herpes virus pneumonia appeared to result from direct spread of the virus from the upper to the lower respiratory tract, whereas diffuse pneumonia appeared to be caused by dissemination (most likely hematogenous) from genital or oral lesions. The factors that determine whether severe localized disease, cutaneous dissemination, or visceral dissemination will occur in a patient, are still undefined.

Diagnosis

Mucocutaneous HSV infections are very common and can thus be easily recognized clinically, but can be confused with the oral lesions of candidiasis, drug toxicity, or Stevens-Johnson syndrome. Verification of the presence of HSV in mucocutaneous lesions can be obtained with scrapings from suspect skin lesions. These scrapings from the base of the lesions are smeared, fixed with ethanol or methanol, and stained with Giemsa (Tzanck smear), Wright, or Papanicolaou preparation. The presence of multinucleated giant cells indicates infection with HSV or varicella-zoster virus. Intranuclear inclusions can be seen as well in Papanicolaou-stained smears.

Isolation of HSV from lesions can be performed. Vesicles within the first 24–28 hours have the highest titers of virus [43] and specimens should be collected early. Once obtained and placed into viral transport media, the specimens are then inoculated promptly into tissue cultures such as rabbit kidney cells or human diploid fibroblasts [44]. Specimens may be frozen at −70 °C until processed. Cytopathic effects appear rapidly (24–48 hours) in the cell monolayer if the virus inoculum is high. Typing of the isolates can be accomplished with immunofluorescence [45]. This technique can be used for rapid identification and typing of HSV in clinical specimens. Biologic methods such as pock size on egg chorioallantoic membranes or temperature sensitivity have also been used to type isolates [46]. In the future, DNA hybridization will probably be used to detect HSV DNA in clinical specimens and to differentiate HSV-1 from HSV-2 [47]. Monoclonal antibodies to HSV look promising for typing HSV as well [48].

Serological techniques to assay antibody titer may be helpful in diagnosing primary HSV infections, but are rarely of value in recurrent infections or in differentiating between HSV types [46]. During primary infections, a four-fold or greater rise in titer is observed between acute and convalescent sera. In recurrent infections such rises may or may not be seen.

HSV infections of visceral organs can be diagnosed by histological examination of tissue and culture; tissue obtained by biopsy and stained with hematoxylin and eosin show evidence of ballooning degeneration of cells, ground glass nuclei with eosinophilic intranuclear inclusions (Cowdry Type A bodies), and multinucleated giant cells [30]. Cultures may be performed as described above. Electron microscopy may demonstrate viral particles from cutaneous and visceral herpetic lesions.

Treatment

The treatment of HSV infections in cancer patients has improved dramatically in the last few years, primarily because of the availability of acyclovir (acycloguanosine). The treatment of various HSV infections will be reviewed with some comments about the action and toxicity of each of the antiviral agents.

The bulk of HSV infections seen in cancer patients are of mucocutaneous origin. In immunocompromised hosts, acyclovir has been used for both prophylaxis [49–51] and therapy [52–54]. Acyclovir prophylaxis has been demonstrated to prevent oral HSV infections in patients with acute leukemia who had prechemotherapy complement-fixation titers of 1:16 or greater [51]. Eleven of the fifteen patients receiving placebo developed HSV infections, whereas none of the fourteen receiving acyclovir developed HSV infection or viral shedding. Nevertheless, six of the fourteen patients on acyclovir prophylaxis subsequently had reactivated HSV infection one to six months after they completed the study.

Acyclovir is a nucleoside analogue with a high degree of activity against HSV and varicella-zoster virus. Cells infected with HSV produce viral thymidine kinase which phosphorylates acyclovir to acyclovir monophosphate [55]. Acyclovir is phosphorylated much more rapidly by viral thymidine kinase than by cellular enzymes, resulting in a 40–100 times increase in acyclovir monophosphate in infected cells. Subsequent phosphorylation by cellular enzymes causes production of acyclovir triphosphate. Viral DNA polymerases are inhibited at considerably lower concentrations of acyclovir triphosphate than cellular DNA polymerases. Acyclovir triphosphate may also inhibit DNA synthesis by serving as a substrate for these enzymes, leading to premature chain termination of viral DNA [56].

Acyclovir is approximately 160 times more active than vidarabine against HSV-1 [57]. HSV-2 is also quite susceptible to acyclovir. Yet, HSV develops resistance to acyclovir by several mechanisms [58]. Viral mutations resulting in a marked decrease in production of thymidine kinase are most commonly found [58]. Viruses producing no thymidine kinase have been isolated from patients receiving acyclovir [59].

Acyclovir is remarkably low in toxicity. Irritation and phlebitis have been noted at the site of injection [52]. Reversible elevations of serum creatinine have occasionally developed, usually after rapid bolus injections [60]. Instances of neurotoxicity [61, 62] and marrow depression have been reported [61].

A number of studies have addressed the utility of intravenous and topical acyclovir for the treatment of mucocutaneous HSV infections in immuno-compromised cancer patients. A multicenter controlled trial of intravenous acyclovir for the treatment of mucocutaneous HSV infections in immuno-compromised patients has been performed, employing $250 \, mg/m^2$ intravenously every eight hours for seven days [52]. Of the 97 patients evaluated, 38 had lymphoma, leukemia or immunodeficiency syndromes. Acyclovir significantly reduced the period of viral shedding and lesion pain while significantly causing more rapid lesion scabbing and healing. In another study, intravenous acyclovir for 5 days exerted a beneficial effect on HSV in 6 patients with leukemia and HSV infections [54].

Topical acyclovir (five percent) has also been evaluated in a double-blind, placebo-controlled trial in 43 immunocompromised patients with progressive mucocutaneous lesions [63]. The topical use of acyclovir for 10 days significantly reduced the period of viral shedding and lesion pain.

Intravenous vidarabine has also been assessed in controlled trials for mucocutaneous HSV infections [64]. The analysis of the data showed that vidarabine significantly accelerated defervescence and loss of pain from skin lesions. 2′-Fluoro-5-iodo-1-β-D-arabinofuranosylcytosine (FIAC), a new pyrimidine nucleoside analogue, may prove effective in HSV and varicella-zoster infections [65].

While intravenous acyclovir is now the drug of choice for the prophylaxis and treatment of mucocutaneous HSV infection in cancer patients, not every patient need receive this agent. Rather, those patients with extensive lesions and whose lesions do not heal quickly would be candidates for this therapy. For prophylactic use, acyclovir may be empoyed for acute leukemia patients with HSV antibody titers of 1:16 or greater. Further evaluation of oral acyclovir in immunocompromised cancer patients is forthcoming. Oral acyclovir may play a major role in the treatment of these patients.

In disseminated cutaneous HSV infection, organ dissemination and pneumonitis, no controlled studies have been performed with acyclovir in immunocompromised cancer patients. Nevertheless, acyclovir is the most potent antiviral agent available to treat these infections.

Vidarabine is still the drug of choice for herpetic encephalitis (15 mg/kg/day) as demonstrated by controlled studies in which vidarabine reduced mortality [66, 67]. Vidarabine (Ara-A) is a purine nucleoside analogue with antiviral activity against all members of the herpesvirus group. Within cells, vidarabine is phosphorylated by cellular kinases to a triphosphate form that selectively inhibits DNA polymerase [68]. This agent is widely distributed in the body, attaining levels in cerebrospinal fluid which are one-third to one-half those in serum [68]. The agent must be administered with a large volume of fluid. Major side effects are gastrointestinal (nausea, vomiting, and diarrhea) [69] and neurologic (tremors, paresthesias, ataxia, and seizures) [70].

Evaluation of the treatment of herpetic keratitis has been conducted in well controlled trials. Topical agents such as idoxuridine, vidarabine, and trifluorothymidine have been demonstrated to be effective [71, 72]. Idoxuridine and trifluorothymidine both inhibit DNA synthesis [73]. Recently, topical acyclovir ointment has been reported to be as effective as vidarabine [74], trifluorothymidine [75], and idoxuridine [76] for the treatment of herpetic keratitis.

VARICELLA − ZOSTER VIRUS (VZV) INFECTIONS

Epidemiology

Varicella-zoster virus is a DNA virus and also a member of the herpesviruses. It is indistinguishable morphologically from other members of this group. The virus is transmitted person-to-person. Since the virus is extremely labile, it is unlikely that it can be transmitted by inanimate objects. Although it is assumed that the virus can be spread by the respiratory route, it has not been demonstrated in respiratory secretions [77]. Airborne transmission of varicella has been confirmed [78, 79]. A relationship between varicella and herpes zoster (HZ) was first suspected in the 19th century, when it was observed that susceptible children acquired varicella after contact with individuals with HZ [80]. This view was substantiated by Weller and co-workers [81]. Since the isolation of VZV, the concept that cases of HZ represent reactivation of a latent infection with VZV, has been accepted. This latent infection is manifested at a variable period of time after the primary infection with varicella. The site of latency or persistence of VZV is thought to be the dorsal root ganglia. VZV has been isolated from sensory ganglia after acute attacks of HZ [82]; but, the virus has not been detected in ganglia obtained from immune adults without histories of recent HZ [83].

Varicella (chickenpox) is usually a benign but highly contagious childhood disease. Chickenpox occurs in the late winter and early spring [84]. The course of the disease varies from mild cutaneous infection with a few lesions to extensive involvement with innumerable lesions. It is most prevalent during the first twelve years of life. The incubation period for varicella ranges from 14 to 17 days with extremes of 10 to 20 days. The typical case of varicella is infectious for 1–2 days prior to the appearance of the generalized eruption and for 4–5 days thereafter, i.e., until the last crop of vesicles has evolved to the purulent and crusted stage [80]. Among immunosuppressed cancer patients this period of infectivity is prolonged because of successive crops of cutaneous lesions.

Varicella is one of the most severe viral infections in the immunocompromised pediatric cancer patient [85–87]. Feldman et al. found a mortality rate of 7% as compared to 0.12% to 0.4% in the general population [85]. Patients in remission and off all therapy who developed varicella did not experience any mortality or visceral dissemination. In contrast, those patients who were receiving anti-cancer therapy when they developed varicella experienced a higher rate of dissemination (32%) and mortality (7%). Visceral dissemination involved the lungs, liver and central nervous system. Death from varicella dissemination occurred only in children with pneumonitis. The likelihood of dissemination was greatest in children with lymphocyte counts $<500/mm^3$. Second episodes of varicella did occur in these pediatric cancer patients. Dissemination occurred most often in the leukemia-lymphosarcoma group. Bodey also found that varicella was more likely to be severe in children with acute leukemia [87]. No large series of adults with malignancies and varicella have been reported.

HZ infection is endogenous, caused by the reactivation of VZV. The infection rate with HZ in the general population has been reported to be 5.4% [88], although it seems to rise with increasing age [83]. There is also waning of cellular immune response to VZV with age [89]. There is little information on the interval between endogenous reactivation and the appearance of symptoms. Pain in the dermatome subsequently affected may precede the skin eruption by 2–4 days [81]. (Pain is unusual in children, but is very common in the elderly.)

There is an increased frequency of HZ in both pediatric and adult patients with malignant neoplasms [86, 90–97]. Patients with Hodgkin's disease (adults and children) seem most susceptible to VZV, with infection rates ranging from 4.7% to 25% [86, 90, 93–96, 98, 99]. The incidence of HZ in lymphomas varies from 1.3% to 11.4%. HZ has been reported as a complication of solid tumors in only 0.5 to 1.8 percent of patients [93, 94, 97]. Recently, it has been reported that patients with small cell carcinoma of the lung appear to have an increased risk of developing HZ compared to those with non-small cell carcinoma of the lung [97].

Certain factors are associated with an increased incidence of HZ infections in cancer patients. Advanced stages of Hodgkin's disease (Stages III and IV) have been implicated in some studies [86, 94, 98, 100], although one large study failed to substantiate this [96]. Several studies have suggested that recent chemotherapy may be associated with zoster [95, 97, 99]; yet, no single regimen or agent has been found to be responsible.

A strong correlation of HZ infection within one year of radiation treatment has been noted by several authors [86, 90, 94, 96]. Lesions most frequently occurred in the irradiated dermatomes even though these areas were most likely to have been involved with tumor as well. Also, the combination of chemotherapy and radiation may predispose patients to HZ more than radiation alone [86, 101].

The effect of prior splenectomy is controversial. In children, prior splenectomy has not been found to be a significant predisposing factor [86, 90]. In adults, conflicting evidence exists [94–96, 101].

Not only does HZ affect patients with lymphoma more frequently than others, but it is also more severe. In immunosuppressed cancer patients, most commonly those with Hodgkin's disease, the frequency of dissemination varies from 5%–30% [86, 92, 94–96, 98, 101]. Dissemination probably results from viremia [102], and is more likely in advanced disease.

There is a low mortality associated with HZ infections even when dissemination occurs [94, 99]. Several series have reported zero mortality [94, 99], whereas others had had mortality rates less than 5% [90, 95, 96]. The morbidity of this infection as a result of dissemination and post-herpetic neuralgia are bothersome. Second cases of HZ may occur in immunosuppressed hosts, sometimes caused by exogenous sources [94].

Clinical Manifestations

Varicella usually presents as a vesicular eruption starting on the scalp or trunk, spreading centrifugally. The lesions, most commonly a few millimeters in diameter, appear in different stages of evolution. In immunocompromised cancer patients, the temperature may remain elevated beyond the usual 2–3 days as lesions continue to erupt. As the lesions subside, so does the patient's fever.

Visceral dissemination has been noted to occur in up to 32% of pediatric patients with varicella [85]. The lungs are most commonly involved, followed by the liver and brain. Varicella pneumonitis develops 3–7 days after the onset of skin lesions, and can be rapidly progressive over a few days or may linger with gradual improvement over 2–4 weeks. Death often may occur in patients with pneumonitis, who may have fulminating central nervous system varicella infection as well. Hepatitis without pneumonitis has not been fatal. The hepatitis usually resolves in 2–4 weeks. The spleen, gastrointestinal tract, lymph nodes, and bone marrow may also be involved in disseminated disease [85]. Secondary bacterial infection is common with any varicella syndrome.

HZ infection is commonly a localized vesicular eruption with dermatomal distribution. The infection is often heralded by the onset of radicular pain which may occur several days before the cutaneous lesions appear [94]. The thoracic dermatomes are most often affected, followed by cervical, lumbar, trigeminal and sacral in decreasing frequency [90]. Frequently, neuralgia follows HZ infection (18% of patients) [103].

Dissemination occurs in variable frequencies depending on the underlying malignancy, but is most common in Hodgkin's disease [86, 92, 94–96, 98, 101]. Dissemination of HZ is seen 4–11 days after the onset of localized lesions [96] and may be associated with higher mortality than localized HZ, primarily due to advanced underlying disease. Meningoencephalitis [96], pneumonitis [90], cardiac and gastrointestinal tract involvement are complications of dissemination. Atypical disseminated VZV infection has been described in patients with no antecedent localized area of zoster [94–96].

Diagnosis

The diagnosis of uncomplicated VZV infection can usually be made on clinical grounds alone. The diagnosis of varicella is based on the presence of the typical generalized vesicular eruption, often in association with a history of exposure and expected clinical features. HZ is commonly a localized infection along a dermatomal distribution. Occasionally, disseminated HSV can produce eruptions in patients with malignancy which are indistinguishable from generalized VZV eruptions. Then, viral culture of the vesicles is necessary to achieve a diagnosis. VZV grows much more poorly *in vitro* than HSV and is highly cell-associated. VZV is best isolated on human embryonic lung fibroblasts [77]. Distinctive cytopathic effects usually appear in 3–10 days. Virus can be readily isolated from vesicular fluid during the first 3 days following the onset of varicella [77]. It can be isolated for as long as 10 days in immunocompromised patients with HZ [103].

Distinguishing VZV from other vesicular non-viral eruptions can be verified by the presence of multinucleated giant cells from scrapings of the lesion base as described previously for HSV.

Immunofluorescence can be utilized to identify VZV *in vitro* [104]. Recently, counterimmunoelectrophoresis has been used to rapidly detect VZV antigen in vesicular fluid, although indirect enzyme-linked immunosorbent assay for antigen detection is 100 times more sensitive [105]. In the VZV meningoencephalitis assay, antibodies to the VZV-induced membrane antigen (FAMA) may prove a reliable means of confirming the diagnosis [106].

When visceral organs are involved, histological examination and culture of tissue may be necessary for definitive diagnosis.

Serological techniques are useful merely for the confirmation of infection. A serum specimen for complement fixation titer of VZV antibody at the onset of the illness and 2–4 weeks later is collected. A four-fold rise in titer confirms the presence of infection. The complement fixation test is being supplanted by other more sensitive procedures such as: FAMA [107], immune-adherence hemagglutination [108], the enzyme-linked immunoassay [109], the radioimmunoassay [110], and anticomplement immunofluorescence [111].

Prevention and Treatment of Varicella

Varicella infection in immunocompromised cancer patients causes serious morbidity and mortality. Progress in both preventing and treating varicella in such patients has been made.

Ross, in 1962, first showed dose-related modification or amelioration of disease after administration of gamma globulin to children exposed to varicella [112]. The most striking effect was observed in patients who received the highest doses of globulin. Since the amount of anti-VZV antibody contained in gamma globulin was presumably low and variable, zoster immune globulin (ZIG) was prepared from the sera of patients who had recently recovered from HZ. Studies performed with ZIG given to immunocompromised hosts shortly after household exposure to varicella have shown that passive immunization can protect these patients from severe or fatal varicella [113–115]. Subclinical infection did occur in these studies. Passive immunization has also been accomplished with zoster immune plasma [116, 117].

Since ZIG was in short supply, the Centers for Disease Control restricted its use to specific indications [118]. Currently, varicella-zoster immunoglobulin (VZIG) is available. It is prepared from normal plasma with high antibody titers against VZV [119]. VZIG has been demonstrated to be as effective as ZIG in a double-blind trial in cancer patients for protection against severe varicella [120]. The Centers for Disease Control have published criteria for VZIG usage when immunosuppressed children are exposed to varicella or HZ [121]. These criteria are presented in Table 2.

Another agent studied in a controlled fashion for the prevention of varicella in children with leukemia is transfer factor [122]. Children with leukemia and without VZV antibodies were randomly assigned to receive dia-

Table 2. Indications and Guidelines for the Use of Varicella-Zoster Immune Globulin (VZIG) for the Prophylaxis of Chickenpox (varicella)

1. One of the following underlying illnesses or conditions:
   a. Leukemia or lymphoma
   b. Congenital or acquired immunodeficiency
   c. Under immunosuppressive treatment
   d. Newborn of mother who had onset of chickenpox <5 days before delivery or within 48 hours after delivery
2. One of the following types of exposure to chickenpox or zoster patient(s):
   a. Household contact
   b. Playmate contact (>1 hour play indoors)
   c. Hospital contact (in same 2- to 4-bed room or adjacent beds in a large ward)
   d. Newborn contact (newborn of mother who had onset of chickenpox <5 days before delivery or within 48 hours after delivery)
3. Negative or unknown prior history of chickenpox
4. Age of <15 years, with administration to older patients on an *individual* basis
5. Time elapsed after exposure is such that VZIG can be administered within 96 hours

lyzable transfer factor from immune subjects or placebo. Varicella developed in 13 of 15 exposed patients in the placebo group, but only 1 of 16 in the transfer factor group.

Recently, live varicella vaccine was given to 23 children with lymphoreticular malignancies in remission and was effective in preventing varicella in 7 of 8 children who were exposed [123]. Live varicella vaccine has been studied in Japan [124], but latency of the virus remains a potential problem.

Both vidarabine and acyclovir have been tested in placebo-controlled trials for the therapy of varicella in immunocompromised patients with malignancies [125, 126]. Vidarabine (10 mg/kg/day for 5 days) decreased the time of new cutaneous lesion formation, daily mean lesion count, and mean duration of fever as compared with placebo [125]. Complications of visceral dissemination were reduced from 55 to 5 percent by vidarabine. Acyclovir (500 mg/m^2 every 8 hours intravenously) prevented the development of pneumonitis in immunocompromised patients; whereas, 45% of the placebo group developed this complication [126]. Acyclovir proved effective against varicella in an uncontrolled trial [54]. No controlled trial has compared vidarabine to acyclovir for the treatment of varicella.

Human leukocyte (alpha) interferon has been demonstrated in two controlled trials to be efficacious in the treatment of varicella in children with cancer [127, 128]. Arvin et al. in their first study showed that alpha interferon (4.2×10^4 to 2.5×10^5 u/kg/day) decreased the number of severe complications [127]. In their second study using higher doses of interferon, the authors showed that interferon shortened the mean number of days of new lesion formation and reduced the number of patients who had life threatening dissemination compared to the placebo. Alpha interferon is cleared from the circulation after intravenous administration with a half-life of two to three hours; after intramuscular administration, the half-life is four to six hours [129]. Toxic effects have included transient granulocyte count depression, malaise, lethargy, and fever [130]. Human interferon genes have now been cloned into bacterial and yeast clones, allowing the production of large quantities of pure interferon [131].

With the drugs currently available, it appears that an immunocompromised cancer patient with varicella should be hospitalized and treated with acyclovir.

Prevention and Treatment of HZ

HZ in cancer patients, particularly those with Hodgkin's disease, is associated with significant morbidity, but little mortality. There is an increased risk of dissemination among these patients. As a result, antiviral therapy of HZ is aimed at halting dissemination. The agents which have been proven effective are: vidarabine, acyclovir, and alpha interferon.

Two double-blind randomized studies comparing vidarabine with placebo have been performed [103, 132]. In the first study [103], the majority of patients with HZ had an underlying malignancy. Patients were randomized to receive vidarabine (10 mg/kg/day intravenously) or placebo for five days. For a second period of five days, the alternative study drug was administered. Patients receiving vidarabine for the first five days had accelerated clearing of the virus from vesicles and cessation of new vesicle formation, and a shorter time to total pustulation. Patients with reticuloendothelial neoplasia derived the greatest relative benefit.

The second study [132] enrolled patients with HZ of 72 hours duration or less. Vidarabine (10 mg/kg/day) decreased the rates of distal cutaneous dissemination from 24% to 8%, and visceral complications from 19% to 5%. Therapy also decreased the duration of post-herpetic neuralgia.

Acyclovir therapy for HZ has been studied in cancer patients in both open and controlled studies [54, 133, 134]. In a controlled trial [134], acyclovir (1500 mg/m^2/day for seven days) halted the progression of zoster as determined by development or progression of cutaneous dissemination and the development of visceral zoster, in both localized and disseminated zoster. This effect was seen whether acyclovir was started within the first three days after the onset of the exanthem or beyond three days of exanthem onset. In addition, cessation of pain occurred faster in the acyclovir treated group, although this was not statistically significant.

The efficacy of alpha interferon has been demonstrated in a placebo-controlled study [130]. The higher doses of interferon (1.7×10^5 u/kg/day and 5.1×10^5 u/kg/day) produced a significant decrease in cutaneous dissemination when used within 72 hours of the onset of lesions, and diminished severity of post-herpetic neuralgia. Only mild toxicity was seen with this schedule of interferon.

The role of antiviral therapy in the treatment of HZ is not well defined. It would seem reasonable to treat patients with advanced stage Hodgkin's disease with intravenous acyclovir due to its relatively low toxicity. As well, it is probably prudent to treat cancer patients who are severely immunocompromised to prevent dissemination. If dissemination does occur in an untreated individual, once again, intravenous acyclovir should be employed. The availability of an oral antiviral agent for HZ will facilitate the treatment of a much larger number of patients.

CYTOMEGALOVIRUS (CMV) INFECTIONS

Epidemiology

Cytomegalovirus, another member of the herpesvirus group produces unrecognized infection ubiquitously. Clinically evident disease, however, almost always is seen in those who are immunologically deficient. Like the other members of the herpesvirus family, CMV possesses the properties of latency and cell association, which play roles in the development of clinically manifested disease in the immunocompromised cancer patient. A variable time of latency after the initial infection allows the virus to reactivate at a later date, while cell association enables CMV to evade neutralizing antibodies in extracellular fluid.

Although the reactivation of latent infection is the most common cause of clinical disease, CMV disease may be transmitted via oral contact with body secretions (urine, saliva or stool) or the transfusion of blood products [135], in particular, leukocyte transfusions [136].

The prevalence of CMV antibody in the general adult population ranges from 37% in Rochester, New York to 50–60% in Nova Scotia and rises to greater than 80% in Barbados [135]. An estimate of the prevalence of CMV infections in cancer patients is more difficult since earlier estimates were from autopsy studies, while more recent studies have employed culture and serological techniques. In general, the longer patients with malignant diseases have been examined for evidence of CMV, the higher the overall rate of infection found [137].

Distinctive intranuclear inclusions due to CMV have been noted at autopsy in patients with malignancy by a number of authors. Wong and Warner reported that disseminated CMV infection occurred primarily as a terminal complication of debilitating neoplastic disease [138]. During the period from 1953 to 1963, 13 of the 394 (3%) patients at the NIH with acute leukemia who came to autopsy were found to have evidence of CMV infection [139]. In 3 patients, CMV appeared to be the cause of death. Also, in this study, the amount of time on corticosteroid therapy during the last 90 days of life was greater in CMV-infected patients than in controls. A lower prevalence of autopsy-proven CMV infections has been reported elsewhere [140].

Since CMV infection was recognized at autopsy in cancer patients and in some cases, death was attributed to the virus, investigations to assess the magnitude of the problem in living cancer patients have been undertaken. Antemortem isolation of CMV has been performed in both children and adults. Benyesh-Melnick et al. examined 515 urine specimens from 101 children and found no difference in the rate of viruria between children with leukemia (17%), those with other serious diseases (19%), and normal controls (21%) [141]. Others have reported similar findings [142]. Urinary and/or salivary excretion of virus in leukemic children can persist for months [143, 144]. Although Armstrong et al. could not detect CMV from peripheral blood cultures [143], Cox and Hughes [145] detected viremia in 11 of 36 (30.5%) children with acute lymphocytic leukemia and CMV infection by means of blood leukocyte cultures and complement-fixation antibody titers were generally $\geq 1:8$ throughout the study. The throat and stool have also been cultured effectively for CMV [144, 146].

In adults, urine and/or sputum cultures were positive for CMV in 11 of 32 (34%) patients with neoplastic disease [147]. CMV was isolated in 5 of 15 (33%) with chronic myelogenous leukemia, 2 of 6 (33%) with Hodgkin's disease, and 4 of 11 (36%) patients with other malignancies. All urine and sputum samples from 17 control subjects (composed of family members and ward personnel) were negative. An increased incidence of steroid therapy within one month of initial culture was observed in the virus-positive group compared to the virus-negative group. A single complement-fixation antibody titer was performed in the virus-positive, virus-negative and control groups, but the distribution of values for the antibody titers was essentially the same in all groups.

The use of antibody titers for the assessment of CMV prevalence has been reported for both children and adults with cancer. Sullivan et al. performed serial determinations of CMV complement-fixation (CF) titers in 41 children with a diagnosis of acute leukemia [148]. Of the 16 serum specimens obtained before or within one month of the initiation of chemotherapy, only 2 (12.5%) had antibody titers $\geq 1:4$. Of the 14 initially seronegative children, 8 (57%) underwent seroconversion 1 to 6 months after the initiation of chemotherapy, and 4 of these had clinical symptoms. In the group who were tested for CF more than a month after initiation of chemotherapy, seropositivity (48%) showed no correlation with clinical events. Armstrong et al. also found no correlation between viral isolation and CF titer [143].

In a prospective trial, 88 children receiving therapy for acute leukemia were followed for 2 to 16 (mean, 7) months [144]. Of the 88 children, 24 (27%) excreted virus: 6 in the urine, 11 in the throat, and 7 in both. Detectable antibody was more prevalent in CMV excretors: of excretors, 74% were positive by CF and 87% by indirect hemagglutination; of non-excretors, positivity was noted in 20% (CF) and 30% (indirect hemagglutination). Children who excreted virus had significantly more episodes of pneumonitis and fever with rash than non-excretors. While clinical syndromes attributed to CMV occurred during both hematologic relapse and remission, they were correlated with significant rises in CF titer only in patients in remission.

Serologic studies in adults have not been as detailed as in children. Langenhuysen et al. reported that CMV antibody titers were significantly elevated in adults with untreated Hodgkin's disease compared to healthy controls matched for age and sex [149]. However, other authors have found no difference in the prevalence or magnitude of CMV antibody titers between patients with Hodgkin's disease [150, 151], non-Hodgkin's lymphoma [150], nasopharyngeal carcinoma [151] and controls.

From the foregoing studies, it seems that CMV may be isolated as frequently or slightly more frequently from patients with malignant conditions as from controls, that the prevalence of positive serology increases with time after the initiation of chemotherapy and that CMV disease often did not correlate with seroconversion.

It has also been demonstrated that the institution isolation procedures are not helpful in decreasing the CMV infection among children with leukemia [152].

Recently, CMV infection has been associated with homosexual males who have Kaposi's sarcoma and AIDS and may actually contribute to the profound immune deficiency state present [153].

Clinical Manifestations

Although CMV infections are common in cancer, CMV disease (clinically apparent syndromes) occurs less frequently [143, 144, 148]. The clinical manifestations of CMV disease are protean. Pneumonitis [144, 148, 154], both unilateral or bilateral and fever with rubelliform rash [144], appear to be most common in the pediatric immunocompromised cancer patient. Hepatitis [144, 145], upper respiratory tract infection [145], characteristic chorioretinitis [145, 155], proctitis [145], parotitis [144], and prostatitis [144] have also been reported. Involvement of the gastrointestinal tract occurs [138, 139] and is more common in the disseminated form [146]. The gastrointestinal lesions are found with nearly equal frequency in the esophagus, stomach, small intestine and colon.

Diagnosis

Since there are many manifestations of CMV disease, the clinical diagnosis must be confirmed by: 1) isolation of the virus; 2) seroconversion or a four-fold rise in antibody titer; or 3) the presence of characteristic intranuclear inclusions in involved organs on histological examination. Viral isolation and/or seroconversion or four-fold rise in antibody titer without clinical manifestations merely denotes infection. As mentioned above, a four-fold rise in antibody titer may not appear in patients who are in hematologic relapse even though clinical manifestations are present [144].

The virus is excreted in urine [144], saliva [144], and stool [146]. CMV can also be isolated from blood leukocyte cultures. CMV can be cultured on human fibroblast monolayers [144, 146]. A major problem, however, is the length of time required before viral cytopathic effects appear, often extending beyond 2–3 weeks. The cytopathic effect can be seen as early as 5–7 days depending on the concentration of the virus in the specimen. Repeated culturing for CMV is imperative since viral excretion may be intermittent.

Several serological assays are available. The CF test has been employed in many studies and its specificity seems accepted [156]. Indirect-hemagglutination [144], enzyme-linked immunosorbent assay [157, 158] and immunofluorescence [159] techniques have also been used. The production of monoclonal antibodies to CMV to be used in immunofluorescence assays may prove to be an important immunodiagnostic tool [160].

Cytopathological examination of affected tissue can demonstrate the large intranuclear inclusions which are characteristic of CMV. Electron microscopy has been proposed for rapid diagnosis of CMV infections [161].

Recently, DNA hybridization has been utilized to rapidly detect and quantitate CMV in urine [162].

Treatment

Although numerous therapeutic trials have been undertaken in renal transplant and bone marrow transplant recipients, no prospective studies have been performed in the immunocompromised cancer patient population. Therefore, a brief review of the information in the aforementioned groups is appropriate.

Following renal transplantation, CMV causes numerous clinical syndromes [163]. Vidarabine therapy has been found to be unsatisfactory [164–166]. Acyclovir has been shown to cause more rapid improvement and faster defervescence in a placebo-controlled double-blind study [167]. Eleven of the 16 patients treated with acyclovir (1500 mg/m^2/day for seven days) were renal transplant recipients. Prophylactic alpha interferon has been demonstrated to decrease viremia [168] and CMV reactivation syndromes [169]. In a preliminary trial, a live attenuated CMV vaccine from the Towne strain has prevented the development of symptomatic CMV disease after transplantation [170].

In bone marrow transplant recipients, CMV pneumonia is a frequent and often fatal occurrence. Treatment with human leukocyte (alpha) interferon [171], recombinant leukocyte A interferon [172, 173], acyclovir [174], vidarabine and human leukocyte interferon [175], or acyclovir and human leukocyte interferon [176] has proven to be ineffective against CMV pneumonia in these patients. However, CMV immune plasma prophylaxis did significantly reduce the incidence of symptomatic infection (CMV disease), but not asymptomatic infection after marrow transplantation [177]. Also, CMV immune globulin was effective in the prevention of CMV infection when given to seronegative bone marrow transplant recipients who did not receive granulocyte transfusions [178].

As for immunocompromised cancer patients, the roles of the above-mentioned agents in both prophylaxis and treatment are unclear. Since CMV disease does pose a problem in cancer patients (although the attack rate is less than in renal and bone marrow transplants), further studies are warranted. If CMV disease is found in a cancer patient, a trial of high dose acyclovir (1500 mg/m^2/day) intravenously may be worthwhile [179].

EPSTEIN-BARR VIRUS (EBV) INFECTIONS

Epidemiology

Epstein-Barr virus is the final member of the herpesvirus group to be discussed. EBV causes heterophile-positive infectious mononucleosis, most heterophile-negative cases and occasional cases of tonsillitis and pharyngitis in childhood [180]. In addition, the virus has been associated with African Burkitt's lymphoma [181], nasopharyngeal carcinoma [182], x-linked lymphoproliferative syndrome [183], lymphoproliferative diseases accompanying immunosuppression after renal transplantation [184] and Burkitt's-like lymphoma in homosexual men [185].

As with the other members of the herpesvirus group, EBV possesses the property of latency. The virus itself infects B-lymphocytes [186] and some of these cells may persist for prolonged periods in the peripheral blood. Reactivation of EBV at a latter date under conditions of immunosuppression may then be possible.

The importance of EBV in the immunocompromised cancer population is unclear. The incidence of EBV excretion in patients with neoplastic disorders is higher than that seen in the general community. Excretion rates of EBV based on single throat samples showed that virus was recovered from 17% of healthy adults and 47% of patients with renal allografts [187]. In adult patients with solid tumors, the excretion rate was 27% whereas leukemia and lymphoma patients had a rate of 50% [188]. The same authors in a later study demonstrated EBV in the oropharyngeal secretions of 16% of healthy persons, 100% of patients with active acute lymphocytic leukemia, 16% of those with Hodgkin's disease, 74% of patients critically ill with leukemia and lymphoma, 44% of patients with myeloma and 41% of those critically ill with solid tumors, although viral excretion was not related to the duration of chemotherapy [189]. In pediatric patients with Hodgkin's disease, EBV was detected in 23% of throat washings [190].

Since EBV is prevalent in oropharyngeal secretions, it is understandable that the virus is transmitted through intimate oral contact [180]. It is unknown if EBV may be spread with the usage of blood products in immunocompromised cancer patients.

Serological evidence of EBV infection is available. Levine et al. found a higher geometric mean titer of EBV antibody in patients with Hodgkin's disease than those with other lymphoma patients and normal controls [150]. In addition, a higher viral antibody titer was present in untreated patients with more advanced Hodgkin's disease [150]. Langenhuysen et al. corroborated these findings [149]. Antibody titers rise during chemotherapy and can remain elevated for up to seven years [190]. Elevated antibody titers to EBV are also found in poorly differentiated lymphoma and chronic lymphocytic leukemia [191]. A high proportion of leukemic children have antibody titers to EBV during the first month of their illness [192].

Although EBV has been linked to lymphoproliferative disorders [183, 184, 193], there is no known cause and effect relationship between EBV and leukemia [194–196]. Immunocompromised cancer patients may be excreting EBV (be infected), but few have experienced clinically evident disease [196, 197]. Elevation of antibody titers during chemotherapy may reflect reactivation of latent virus [190].

Clinical Manifestations

In cancer patients, it appears that the incubation period of 33 to 49 days [188] seen in healthy individuals may also apply [194]. Clinical disease is uncommon, although EBV infection is quite prevalent as discussed above. Lymphadenopathy, fever, sore throat, tonsillitis, and splenomegaly have been reported as manifestations of EBV syndromes (infectious mononucleosis) when present in patients with acute lymphocytic leukemia [196]. Transient leukopenia and atypical lymphocytes have also been described in peripheral blood smears [196, 197]. (Most of the atypical lymphocytes present in peripheral blood are T-lymphocytes, although a small proportion of early atypical cells appears to be B-lymphocytes [199].)

Most often, EBV infection produces no symptoms at all. In some individuals the viral infection goes unrecognized until a lymphoproliferative disorder is diagnosed.

Diagnosis

The most useful diagnostic tests currently available are serological assays for EBV antibodies. The majority of immunosuppressed individuals infected with EBV will not demonstrate the characteristic clinical symptoms of fever, sore throat, and lymphadenopathy or the characteristic markers of atypical lymphocytosis and heterophile antibodies. Heterophile antibodies when present may be demonstrable at the onset of illness or later in the course of the illness. The detection of heterophile antibody is performed with the commercially available slide agglutination test. When heterophile antibodies are not found, IgM and IgG antibodies to EBV viral capsid antigen may be measured by immunofluorescence; IgM disappears early while IgG antibodies to viral capsid antigen persist indefinitely [180, 200]. Antibodies to Epstein-Barr nuclear antigen and complement-fixing antibodies appear 3 to 4 weeks after the onset of illness, persist indefinitely, and their detection is helpful in the diagnosis of heterophile-negative cases [180]. Early antigen antibodies are identified by immunofluorescence techniques and their presence is indicative of active or recent infection [180].

EBV may be cultured from oropharyngeal washings [188]. Unfortunately, the currently available isolation method is tedious, difficult and usually confined to research laboratories.

Treatment

EBV is sensitive *in vitro* to several antiviral agents including interferon [201], vidarabine [202], phosphonoacetic acid [203], and acyclovir [204]. EBV infections may be associated with some morbidity, but most cases are self-limited. As a result, specific treatment is rare.

Acyclovir has been tried in life-threatening EBV infections with little effect [205]. Trials are currently underway assessing the efficacy of oral acyclovir in infectious mononucleosis. Tumor regression has been seen in post-renal transplant lymphoma associated with EBV which was treated with acyclovir [193].

VIRAL HEPATITIS INFECTIONS

Epidemiology

Viral hepatitis is a major worldwide medical and public health problem. It is one of the five most frequently reported diseases in the United States [206]. The reported annual incidence from other countries varies from 10 per 100,000 in some tropical countries to 200 per 100,000 in Eastern Europe [207]. The viral agents causing this systemic infection which predominantly affects the liver are: hepatitis A virus (HAV), hepatitis B virus (HBV) and non-A, non-B virus(es) (NANB). HAV is a RNA virus, while HBV is a DNA virus. The virus(es) causing NANB hepatitis is (are) at present uncharacterized [207].

Acute viral hepatitis presents several unique clinical problems in the immunocompromised host. For instance, it is recognized that the cardinal manifestations of HBV infection may be different in patients with myeloproliferative and lymphoproliferative disorders than in other immunocompromised hosts. Viral hepatitis not only poses a hazard to cancer patients, but also poses an important occupational hazard to health care personnel [3].

As with other viral infections affecting cancer patients, serological surveys have assessed the prevalence of viral hepatitis. Since both HBV and NANB are primarily transmitted by the parenteral route, they should be more common in cancer patients who are likely to receive parenterally administered blood products. In addition, serological tests for the diagnosis of hepatitis B have been widely available since the early 1970's. A sensitive test for the diagnosis of acute hepatitis A became readily available only in the last year. At present, there are no specific laboratory tests for diagnostic or epidemiological studies of NANB hepatitis. Therefore, most of the data available involve hepatitis B.

In untreated patients with Hodgkin's disease, hepatitis B surface antigen (HB$_s$Ag) was not detected at all [149, 208]; while hepatitis B surface antibody (anti-HB$_s$) was found in four of the 25 patients in one study [149]. Sutnick et al. demonstrated a much higher frequency of HB$_s$Ag in leukemia (7.0%) and Hodgkin's disease (6.3%) than in the normal American population [2]. The frequency in acute lymphocytic, chronic lymphocytic, acute myelogenous and chronic myelogenous leukemia was 9.8%, 6.7%, 9.0% and 2.7%, respectively. HB$_s$Ag positivity was significantly associated with blood transfusions in leukemia patients and developed during the course of the leukemia. Other authors have corroborated these data, finding HB$_s$Ag in 20–50% of patients with lymphoproliferative disorders [3, 208, 209] and 17–20% [3, 209] of myeloproliferative disorders. Also, anti-HB$_s$ was present in both types of disorders [3, 209]. The high combined frequency of HB$_s$Ag and anti-HB$_s$ in myeloproliferative and lymphoproliferative disorders seemed to reflect the extensive exposure of these patients to HB$_s$Ag through multiple transfusions and hospital contacts [3, 209].

Unique characteristics of hepatitis B infection in myeloproliferative and lymphoproliferative diseases are evident from the aforementioned studies. First, serum HB$_s$Ag titers are usually much higher than in normal individuals who become infected with HBV [3]. Second, there is little evidence of ongoing hepatocellular necrosis as measured by serum aminotransferase; such patients are usually asymptomatic and anicteric. In most instances, hepatitis B infection is tolerated quite well and many patients become chronic carriers of HB_sAg, while 90–95 % of normal individuals recover and clear the virus from the blood [3, 209]. These chronic HB_sAg carriers pose a risk for transmission of HBV to other hospital personnel [3]. Third, chemotherapy had a dramatic effect on HB_sAg titers. When chemotherapy suppressed bone marrow function, HB_sAg titers increased with a decrease in titer only occurring with the recovery of marrow function [3, 209]. It would seem that the immunosuppressive effects of chemotherapy on both cellular and humoral immunity may be important in promoting HBV replication. The withdrawal of chemotherapy with subsequent recovery of immunocompetence may result in massive liver damage [210]. These observations suggest that the clinical syndrome of severe hepatitis may be related more to host defenses than to direct viral infection.

NANB hepatitis has recently been reported to be associated with chronic liver disease in children with acute lymphocytic leukemia [211, 212]. Immunofluorescence was employed to detect NANB antigen in liver tissue. Also, hepatitis due to the NANB agent(s) has been seen in adults with acute myelogenous leukemia [213, 214]. Therefore, evidence seems to be accumulating which also implicates NANB virus(es) as a cause of hepatitis in cancer patients.

Some relationship may exist between primary hepatocellular carcinoma and HBV, but the specific manner in which HBV is involved with this carcinoma is unclear [215].

Data has been reported linking hepatitis B infection to longer duration of survival in patients with acute non-lymphocytic leukemia [216] and acute lymphoblastic leukemia in children [217]. In addition, possible NANB hepatitis has been correlated with enhanced survival in acute myelogenous leukemia [213, 218]. Possibly the infection may exert a direct beneficial effect by suppressing the leukemia.

Clinical Manifestations

Patients with myeloproliferative and lymphoproliferative diseases who receive multiple blood products during chemotherapy-induced marrow suppression often become infected with HBV or NANB virus. In this situation clinically evident hepatitis is uncommon. Most patients are anicteric and asymptomatic. The prodrome of nausea, vomiting, anorexia, fatigue and malaise may not be present. Elevations in serum transaminases are common [3, 209–214]. Occasionally, transient jaundice occurs [214]. Chronic persistent hepatitis [217], chronic active hepatitis [211], chronic HB_sAg carrier states [209] and fulminant hepatitis [211] are sequelae of HBV and NANB infections.

Diagnosis

Due to the paucity of symptoms and signs, a high index of suspicion and serological methods are the mainstays of diagnosis. Radioimmunoassay tests are commercially available for HB_sAg, anti-HB_s, antibody against the core antigen, the e antigen, and the antibody against the e antigen [207]. Hepatitis A IgM and IgG antibodies may also be detected by a radioimmunoassay test [207]. No methods are readily available for NANB virus, although indirect immunofluorescence has been employed effectively [211]. Enzyme-linked immunoabsorbent assay has been used to detect HB_sAg.

Prevention and Treatment

Numerous studies have been conducted which confirm that immune globulin (IG) given before or during the incubation period of hepatitis A is protective [219, 220]. Its prophylactic value is greatest (80–90%) when given early in the incubation period and declines thereafter. Recommendations for IG prophylaxis for hepatitis A have been published by the Centers for Disease Control [221].

Studies have shown that immune globulins can prevent up to 75% of hepatitis B cases [222]. Hepatitis B immune globulin (HBIG) contains extremely high titers of anti-HB_s. Recommendations for its prophylactic use in hepatitis B have also been published [221]. There are no specific recommendations for prophylaxis with immune globulins for NANB hepatitis [221].

Inactivated HBV vaccine has been demonstrated to be efficacious in preventing HBV infection in the high risk homosexual population [223] and also medical staff of hemodialysis units [224]. It probably has a role among oncology unit staff with frequent blood exposure [225], but it is unclear if the vaccine would be helpful in cancer patients.

Neither acyclovir [226] or transfer factor [227] have been demonstrated to be effective in chronic hepatitis B infections. Steroid use in chronic active hepatitis is controversial.

INFLUENZA VIRUS INFECTIONS

Epidemiology

Influenza is a RNA virus with two antigenically distinct types. Epidemics of influenza A and influenza B recur with monotonous frequency causing thousands of deaths due to pneumonia and influenza [228]. The general behavior pattern of influenza A is such that at intervals of 10–15 years, a different family or subtype of strains appears and usually results in the occurrence of a pandemic with high attack rates in populations lacking antibodies to the emergent strain. In subsequent years, lesser outbreaks occur through recurrence of strains of the same subtype. These strains undergo minor antigenic change or drift. At the end of the time interval, a major antigenic change takes place and the cycle is repeated [229]. Less antigenic drift occurs with influenza B. The frequency of epidemics due to influenza B is less than that for influenza A and severe pandemics have not been recognized.

In patients with neoplastic disorders severe influenza epidemics influence mortality. An increase in mortality from neoplasms (2 to 3% above expected) has been reported [5]. The risk of death due to pneumonia and influenza is enhanced in people with chronic disease, including malignant neoplasms, during epidemic and non-epidemic periods [230]. It appears that in children and young adults infected with influenza A, the severity of infection is unrelated to the duration of cancer therapy, the type of therapy employed, or the status of the malignancy during infection [231]. Yet, the clinical course lasted twice as long as in the general population (1 to 2 weeks versus less than one week) and cancer therapy was interrupted.

Clinical Manifestations

The signs and symptoms of influenza in cancer patients do not differ from those seen in the general population. Signs and symptoms occur 1–4 days after exposure (average 48 hours). They include fever, cough with coryza, myalgia, malaise, headache, dizziness and pneumonia [231]. Gastrointestinal disturbances are infrequent. Pneumonia, both unilateral and bilateral, with superimposed bacterial infection, may develop [230]. Watery eyes and reddening of the nasopharyngeal membranes are frequent nonspecific findings. Reye's syndrome can be a complication of influenza infection.

Diagnosis

The clinical diagnosis of influenza can easily be made in severe cases during epidemic periods. In sporadic or isolated cases, clinical signs and symptoms are not characteristic enough to permit ready recognition of influenza virus as the cause. Laboratory diagnosis is then necessary. This is accomplished by means of isolation of the virus from the nasopharynx in rhesus-monkey-kidney-cell cultures and embryonated eggs or the demonstration of an antibody rise between acute and convalescent serum specimens. The hemagglutination-inhibition test is most commonly used to measure antibody titers [229].

Prevention and Treatment

Immunization of the population at risk with inactivated influenza vaccine is recommended to prevent infection with influenza virus. Each year new vaccines are formulated from strains that are predicted to cause infection in the upcoming influenza season. Guidelines for the use of influenza vaccine in immunocompromised hosts are published annually prior to the influenza season [232].

It has been recommended that children with malignant diseases be immunized against influenza virus [233]. Conflicting results have been reported on the efficacy of influenza vaccination in pediatric cancer patients [234–240]. Although different treatment regimens, stages of underlying disease, vaccine products and assessment of satisfactory immune response were employed in these studies, the data suggest that pediatric patients on chemotherapy do not seroconvert as frequently as normal controls or patients off chemotherapy for greater than 30 days. This pattern was seen after both a two-dose immunization schedule and a three-dose schedule [239]. Thus, patients on chemotherapy cannot be effectively vaccinated by a new antigen, and it is best to vaccinate pediatric cancer patients who have been off chemotherapy for at least one month. Studies performed in adults with malignant diseases also support the conclusion that cancer patients, in particular those receiving chemotherapy, respond to influenza immunization less frequently than normal controls [241, 242].

Amantadine is effective for the treatment of influenza A [243]. It may also be used for prophylaxis (at a dosage of 200 mg/day), but must be taken continuously throughout the duration of influenza activity.

MISCELLANEOUS INFECTIONS

An increased incidence of viral warts has been reported in patients with Hodgkin's disease, malignant lymphoma, and chronic lymphocytic leukemia compared to control subjects [4]. In addition, the average number of warts in these patients as compared to controls was increased and the appearance of the warts preceded the onset of symptoms from the underlying disease. Patients with multiple myeloma and other solid tumors demonstrated no increased incidence of viral wart infections. It was hypothesized that the higher incidence of viral warts appeared in patients with Hodgkin's disease and lymphoma due to the defect in cell-mediated immunity present in these diseases. The reason for the increased presence in chronic lymphocytic leukemia is unclear.

Measles (rubeola) can be a severe and fulminating infection in patients with hematological malignancies, although the course is not invariably fatal and may be similar to that in the normal population [244]. Bacterial pneumonia, a common complication of measles, and encephalitis can pose serious problems to the immunocompromised host [245]. Currently, a live attenuated vaccine is usually given as part of routine immunization in early childhood, thus protecting most of the population. Efforts are underway to eradicate measles. Live attenuated vaccine is not indicated in the immunosuppressed cancer patient. In event of exposure to the infection, a susceptible patient should receive immune serum globulin.

Rubella is not associated with a severe clinical course. A live attenuated vaccine for rubella is now administered in early childhood as well, but is contraindicated in the immunocompromised patient.

Mumps virus rarely causes infections in cancer patients [246]. Immunization with an attenuated vaccine is routinely performed in early childhood. Once again, this vaccine should not be administered to the immunosuppressed.

SUMMARY

Viral infections cause significant morbidity and mortality in patients with neoplastic disorders. The susceptibility of these individuals to viruses results from the interaction of the organism, the environment and the host. The cell-mediated immunity of the host which provides most of the protection against viruses may be altered due to the neoplastic disease itself, or chemotherapy used to treat the malignancy, leaving the host vulnerable to viral infection. Some viruses such as the herpesvirus group produce a state of latent infection which allows them to reactivate and cause disease at the time of host immunosuppression. At times, viruses themselves may be oncogenic.

With the recent advances in the prevention and treatment of viral diseases with vaccines, immune globulin and antiviral agents, more effective supportive care can be offered by physicians caring for cancer patients. Further breakthroughs are necessary, but the management of viral infections in cancer patients should evolve rapidly in the future.

ACKNOWLEDGEMENTS

I wish to thank Dr. Wendy Wolfman and Corrine Cesari for assistance in the preparation of this manuscript.

REFERENCES

1. Evans AS: Epidemiological concepts and methods. In: Viral infections of humans: epidemiology and control (Second edition), Evans AS (ed), New York, Plenum Medical, 1982, p 3–42.
2. Sutnick AI, London WT, Blumberg BS, Yankee RA, Gerstley BJS, Millman I: Australia antigen (a hepatitis-associated antigen) in leukemia. J Natl Cancer Inst 44:1241–1249,1970.
3. Wands JR, Walker JA, Davis TT, Waterbury LA, Owens AH, Carpenter CJ: Hepatitis B in an oncology unit. N Engl J Med 291:1371–1375, 1974.
4. Morrison WL: Viral warts, herpes simplex and herpes zoster in patients with secondary immune deficiencies and neoplasms. Brit J Dermatol 92:625–630, 1975.
5. Housworth J, Langmuir A: Excess mortality from epidemic influenza 1957–1966. Am J Epidemiol 100:40–48, 1974.
6. Stevens DA, Merigan TC: Interferon antibody and other host factors in herpes zoster. J Clin Invest 51:1170–1178, 1972.
7. Notkins AL: Immune mechanisms by which the spread of viral infections is stopped. Cell Immunol 11:478–483, 1974.
8. Merigan TC: Host defenses against viral disease. N Engl J Med 290:323–329, 1974.
9. Root RK: Humoral immunity and complement. In: Principles and practice of infectious diseases, Mandell GL, Douglas RG, Bennett JE (eds), New York, John Wiley and Sons, 1979, p 21–63.
10. Oleske JM, Minnefor AB: Viral and chlamydial infections. In: Infections in the abnormal host, Grieco MH (editor), New York, Yorke Medical Books, 1980, p 382–405.
11. Stewart WE II: Purification and characterization of interferons. In: Interferons and their actions, Stewart WE II (ed), Cleveland, CRC Press, 1977, p 49–72.
12. Young RC, Corder MD, Haynes HA, DeVita VT: Delayed hypersensitivity in Hodgkin's disease. A study of 103 untreated patients. Am J Med 52:63–72, 1972.
13. Eltringham JR, Kaplan HS: Impaired delayed hypersentitivity responses in 154 patients with untreated Hodgkin's disease. Natl Cancer Inst Monogr 36, International Symposium on Hodgkin's Disease, 1973, p 107–115.
14. Burdick JF, Wells SA, Herbeman RB: Immunologic evaluation of patients with cancer by delayed hypersensitivity reactions. Surg Gynecol Obstet 141:779–792, 1975.
15. Bodey GP, Hersh EM, Valdivesco M, Feld R, Rodriguez V: Effects of cytotoxic and immunosuppressive agents on the immune system. Postgrad Med 67(7):67–74, 1975.
16. Hersh EM: Immunosuppressive agents. In: Antineoplastics and immunosuppressive agents, Satorelli AC, Joans DJ (eds), New York, Springer-Verlag, Inc, 1974, p 577–617.
17. Markoe AM, Saluk PH: The effects of radiation on the immune response: A review. Appl Radiol 6:63–72, 1977.
18. Rafla S, Yang SJ, Meleka F: Changes in cell-mediated immunity in patients undergoing radiotherapy. Cancer 41:1076–1086, 1978.
19. Slater JM, Ngo E, Lau BHS: Effect of therapeutic irradiation on the immune responses. Am J Roentgenol 126:313–320, 1976.
20. Fauci AS, Dale DC, Balow JE: Glucocorticosteroid therapy: Mechanisms of action and clinical considerations. Ann Intern Med 84:304–315, 1976.
21. Fauci AS: Mechanisms of the immunosuppressive and anti-inflammatory effects of glucocorticosteroids. J Immunopharmacol 1:1–25, 1978.
22. Fauci AS, Dale DC: The effect of in vivo hydrocortisone on subpopulations of human lymphocytes. J Clin Invest 53:240–246, 1974.
23. Hirsch MS: Herpes simplex virus. In: Principles and practice of infectious diseases, Mandell GL, Douglas RG, Bennett JE (eds), New York, John Wiley and Sons, 1979, p 1283–

1294.

24. Douglas RG, Couch RB: A prospective study of chronic herpes simplex virus infection and recurrent herpes labialis in humans. J Immunol 104:289–295, 1970.

25. Nahmias AJ, Josey WE, Naib AM, Luce CF, Duffey A: Antibodies to herpes virus hominis types 1 and 2 in humans. 1. Patients with genital herpetic infections. Am J Epidemiol 91:539–546, 1970.

26. Rawls WE, Gardner HL, Flanders RW, Lowry SP, Kaufman RH, Melnick JL: Genital herpes in two social groups. Am J Obstet Gynecol 110:682–689, 1971.

27. Embil JA, Stephens RG, Manuel FR: Prevalence of recurrent herpes labialis and aphthous ulcers among young adults on six continents. Can Med Assoc J 113:627–630, 1975.

28. Muller SA, Herrmann EC, Winkelmann RK: Herpes simplex infections in hematologic malignancies. Am J Med 52:102–114, 1972.

29. Ramsey PG, Fife KH, Hackman RC, Meyers JD, Corey L: Herpes simplex pneumonia. Ann Intern Med 97:813–820, 1982.

30. Nash G, Ross JS: Herpetic esophagitis. A common cause of esophageal ulceration. Hum Pathol 5:339–345, 1974.

31. Weiden PL, Schuffler MD: Herpetic esophagitis complicating Hodgkin's disease. Cancer 33:1100–1102, 1974.

32. Lightdale CJ, Wolf DJ, Marcucci RA, Salyer WR: Herpetic esophagitis in patients with cancer. Antemortem diagnosis by brush cytology. Cancer 39:223–226, 1977.

33. Sperling HV, Reed WG: Herpetic gastritis. Digest Dis 22:1033–1034, 1977.

34. Rosen P, Hajdu SI: Visceral herpes virus infections in patients with cancer. Am J Clin Path 56:459–465, 1971.

35. Faden HS, Bybee BL, Overall JC, Lahey ME: Disseminated herpes virus hominis infection in a child with acute leukemia. J Pediatr 90:951–953, 1977.

36. O'Donoghue S, Miller KJ, Weinberg PB, Rose RC: Herpes simplex virus type II meningoencephalitis in an immunocompromised adult. South Med J 76:538–539, 1983.

37. Vonderheid EC, Milstein HJ, Thompson KD, Wu BC: Chronic herpes simplex infection in cutaneous T-cell lymphomas. Arch Dermatol 116:1018–1022, 1980.

38. Boulton AJ, Slater DN, Hancock BW: Herpes virus colitis: A new cause of diarrhea in a patient with Hodgkin's disease. Gut 23:247–249, 1982.

39. Segal FP, Lopez C, Hammer GS, Brown AE, Kornfeld SJ, Gold J, Hassett J, Hirschman S, Cunningham-Rundles C, Adelsberg BR, Parham DM, Siegel M, Cunningham-Rundles S, Armstrong D: Severe acquired immunodeficiency in homosexuals manifested by chronic perianal ulcerative herpes simplex lesions. N Engl J Med 305:1439–1444, 1981.

40. Aston DL, Cohen A, Spindler MA: Herpes virus hominis infection in patients with myeloproliferative and lymphoproliferative disorders. Brit Med J 4:462–465, 1972.

41. Lam MT, Pazin GJ, Armstrong JA, Ho M: Herpes simplex infection in acute myelogenous leukemia and other hematologic malignancies: A prospective study, Cancer 48:2168–2171, 1981.

42. Buss D, Scharyj M: Herpes virus infection of the esophagus and other visceral organs in adults. Am J Med 66:457–462, 1977.

43. Spruance SL, Overall JC, Kern ER, Kreuger GG, Pliam V, Miller W: The natural history of recurrent herpes simplex labialis — Implications for antiviral therapy. N Engl J Med 297:69–75, 1977.

44. Nahmias AJ, Josey WE: Epidemiology of herpes simplex viruses 1 and 2, In: Viral infections of humans: epidemiology and control (Second edition), Evans AS (ed), New York, Plenum Medical, 1982, p 351–372.

45. Nahmias AJ, Shore SL, DelBuono I: Diagnosis By immunofluorescence of human viral infections with emphasis on herpes simplex viruses. In: Viral immunodiagnosis, Kurstak E, Morisset R (eds), New York, Academic Press, 1974, p 157–172.

46. Nahmias AJ, Roizman B: Infection with herpes-simplex viruses 1 and 2. N Engl J Med 289:781–789, 1973.
47. Redfield DC, Richman DD, Cleveland PH, Albanil S, Oxman MN: Detection and typing of herpes simplex virus by DNA hybridization. Abstract, 23rd Interscience Conference on Antimicrobial Agents and Chemotherapy, October 24–26, 1983, Las Vegas, Nevada.
48. McIntosh K, Wilfert C, Chernesuy M, Plotkin S, Matthesis M: Summary of a workshop on new and useful techniques in rapid viral diagnosis. J Infect Dis 142:793–802, 1980.
49. Saral R, Burns WH, Laskin OL, Santos GW, Lietman PS: Acyclovir prophylaxis of herpes simplex virus infections: A randomized, double-blind controlled trial in bone marrow transplant recipients. N Engl J Med 305:63–67, 1981.
50. Gluckman E, Lotsberg J, Devergie A, Zhao XM, Melo R, Gomez-Morales M, Niebout T, Mazeron MC: Prophylaxis of herpes infections after bone marrow transplantation by oral acyclovir. Lancet 2:706–708, 1983.
51. Saral R, Ambinder RF, Burns WH, Angelopulos CM, Griffin DE, Burke PJ, Leitman PS: Acyclovir prophylaxis against herpes simplex virus infection in patients with leukemia: a rendomized double-blind placebo-controlled study. Ann Intern Med 99:773–776, 1983.
52. Meyers JD, Wade JC, Mitchell CD, Saral R, Lietman PS, Durack DT, Levin MJ, Segretti AC, Balfour HH: Multicenter collaborative trial of intravenous acyclovir for treatment of mucocutaneous herpes simplex virus infection in the immunocompromised host. Am J Med 73(1A):229-235, 1982.
53. Mitchell CD, Bean B, Gentry SR, Groth KE, Boen JR, Balfour HH: Acyclovir therapy for mucocutaneous herpes simplex infections in immunocompromised patients. Lancet 1:1389–1392, 1981.
54. Van der Meer JWM, Versteeg J: Acyclovir in severe herpes virus infections. Am J Med 73(1A):271-274, 1982.
55. Elion GB: Mechanism of action and selectivity of acyclovir. Am J Med 73(1A):7-13, 1982.
56. McGuirt PV, Furman PA: Acyclovir inhibition of viral DNA chain elongation in herpes simplex virus-infected cells. Am J Med 73(1A):67-71, 1982.
57. Schaeffer HJ: Acyclovir chemistry and spectrum of activity. Am J Med 73(1A):4-6, 1982.
58. Field HJ, Larder BA, Darby G: Isolation and characterization of acyclovir resistant strains of herpes simplex virus. Am J Med 73(1A):369-371, 1982.
59. Burns WH, Saral R, Santos GW, Laskin OL, Leitman PS, McClaren C, Barry DW: Isolation and characterization of resistant herpes simplex virus after acyclovir therapy. Lancet 1:421-424, 1982.
60. Peterslund NA, Black PFT, Tauris P: Impaired renal function after bolus injections of acyclovir. Lancet 1:243-244, 1983.
61. Wade JC, Hintz M, McGuffin RW, Springmeyer SC, Connor JD, Meyers JD: Treatment of cytomegalovirus pneumonia with high dose acyclovir. Am J Med 73(1A):249-256, 1982.
62. Wade JC, Meyers JD: Neurologic symptoms associated with parenteral acyclovir treatment after marrow transplantation. Ann Intern Med 98:921-925, 1983.
63. Whitley R, Barton N, Collins E, Whelchel J, Diethelm AG: Mucocutaneous herpes simplex virus infections in immunocompromised patients: A model for evaluation of topical antiviral agents. Am J Med 73(1A):236-239, 1982.
64. Whitley RJ, Spruance S, Hayden FG, Overall J, Alford CA, Jr, Gwaltney JM, Soong S-J and The NIAID Collaborative Antiviral Study Group: Vidarabine therapy for mucocutaneous herpes simplex virus infections in the immunocompromised host. J Infect Dis 149:1-8, 1984.
65. Young CW, Schneider R, Leyland-Jones B, Armstrong D, Tan CTC, Lopez C, Watanabe

KA, Fox JJ, Philips FS: Phase I evaluation of 2′-Fluoro-5-iodo-1-β-D-arabinofuranosylcytosine in immunosuppressed patients with herpesvirus infection. Cancer Res 43:5006–5009, 1983.

66. Whitley RJ, Soong S-J, Dolin R, Galasso CJ, Chien LT, Alford CA and the Collaborative Study Group: Adenine arabinoside therapy of biopsy proved herpes simplex encephalitis: National Institute of Allergy and Infectious Diseases collaborative antiviral study. N Engl J Med 297:289–294, 1977.

67. Whitley RJ, Soong S-J, Hirsch MS, Karchmer AN, Dolin R, Galasso G, Dunnick JK, Alford CA and the NIAID Collaborative Antiviral Study Group: Herpes simplex encephalitis: Vidarabine therapy and diagnostic problems. N Engl J Med 304:313–318, 1981.

68. Whitley R, Alford C, Hess F, Buchanan R: Vidarabine: A preliminary review of its pharmacological properties and therapeutic use. Drugs 20:267–282, 1980.

69. Sacks SL, Smith JL, Pollard RB, Sawhney V, Mahol AS, Gregory P, Merigan TC, Robinson WS: Toxicity of vidarabine. JAMA 241:28–29, 1979.

70. Ross AH, Julia A, Balakrishnan C: Toxicity of adenine arabinoside in humans. J Infect Dis 133 (Suppl A):192–198, 1976.

71. Coster DJ, McKinnon JR, McGill JI, Jones BR, Fraunfelder FT: Clinical evaluation of adenine arabinoside and trifluorothymidine in the treatment of corneal ulcers caused by herpes simplex virus. J Infect Dis 133 (Suppl A):173–177, 1976.

72. Chin GN: Treatment of herpes simplex keratitis with idoxuridine and vidarabine: A double-blind study. Ann Ophthalmol 10:1171–1174, 1978.

73. Hirsch MS, Schooley RT: Treatment of herpes virus infections. N Engl J Med 309:963–970, 1034–1039, 1983.

74. Laibson PR, Pavan-Langston D, Yearkley WR, Lass J: Acyclovir and vidarabine for the treatment of herpes simplex keratitis. Am J Med 73(1A):281–285, 1982.

75. Lalau C, Oosterhuis JA, Versteeg J, van Rij G, Renardel De, Lavalette JO, Craandijk A, Lamers WR, Mierlobensteyn TH: Multicenter trial of acyclovir and trifluorothymidine in herpetic keratitis. Am J Med 73(1A):305–306, 1982.

76. Collum LMT, Logan P, Hillary IB, Ravenscroft T: Acyclovir in herpes keratitis. Am J Med 73(1A):290–293, 1982.

77. Brunell PA: Varicella-zoster virus. In: Principles and practice of infectious diseases, Mandell GL, Douglas RG, Bennett JE (eds), New York, John Wiley and Sons, 1979, p 1295–1306.

78. LeClair JM, Zaia JA, Levin MJ, Congdon RG, Goldmann DA: Airborne transmission of chickenpox in a hospital. N Engl J Med 302:450–453, 1980.

79. Gustafson TL, Lavely GB, Brawner ER, Jr, Hutcheson RH, Jr, Wright PF, Schaffner W: An outbreak of airborne nosocomial varicella. Pediatrics 70:550–556, 1982.

80. Weller TH: Varicella – herpes zoster virus. In: Viral infections of humans (Second edition), Evans AS (ed), New York, Plenum Medical, 1982, p 569–595.

81. Weller TH, Witton HM: The etiologic agents of varicella and herpes zoster: Serologic studies with the viruses as propagated in vitro. J Exp Med 108:869–890, 1958.

82. Bastian FO, Rabson AS, Yee CL, Tralka TS: Herpes virus varicellae: Isolated from human dorsal root ganglia. Arch Pathol 97:331–333, 1974.

83. Dolin R, Reichman RC, Mazur MH, Whitley RJ: Herpes zoster – varicella infection in immunosuppressed patients. Ann Intern Med 89:375–388, 1978.

84. Gordon JE, Ingalls TH: Chickenpox: An epidemiological review. Am J Med Sci 244:362–389, 1962.

85. Feldman S, Hughes WT, Daniel CB: Varicella in children with cancer: Seventy-seven cases. Pediatrics 56:385–397, 1975.

86. Reboul F, Donaldson SS, Kaplan HS: Herpes zoster and varicella infections in children

with Hodgkin's disease. Cancer 41:95–99, 1978.

87. Bodey G, McKelvey E, Karon M: Chickenpox in leukemic patients. Pediatrics 34:562–564, 1974.
88. Hope-Simpson RE: The nature of herpes zoster. A long-term study and a new hypothesis. Proc R Soc Med 58:9–20, 1965.
89. Burke BL, Steele RW, Beard OW, Wood JS, Cain TD, Marmer DJ: Immune responses to varicella-zoster in the aged. Arch Intern Med 142:291–293, 1982.
90. Feldman S, Hughes WT, Kim HY: Herpes zoster in children with cancer. Am J Dis Child 126:178–184, 1973.
91. Pancoast HK, Pendergrass EP: The occurrence of herpes zoster in Hodgkin's disease. Am J Med Sci 196:326–334, 1924.
92. Shanbrom E, Miller S, Haar H: Herpes zoster in hematologic neoplasms: Some unusual manifestations. Ann Intern Med 53:523–533, 1960.
93. Wright ET, Winer LH: Herpes zoster and malignancy. Arch Dermatol 84:242–244, 1961.
94. Schimpff S, Serpick A, Stoler B, Rumack B, Mellin H, Joseph JM, Block J: Varicella-zoster infection in patients with cancer. Ann Intern Med 76:241–254, 1972.
95. Goffinet DR, Glatstein EJ, Merigan TC: Herpes zoster-varicella infections and lymphoma. Ann Intern Med 76:235–240, 1972.
96. Mazur MH, Dolin R: Herpes zoster at the NIH: A 20 year experience. Am J Med 65:738–744, 1978.
97. Feld R, Evans WK, DeBoer G: Herpes zoster in patients with carcinoma of the lung. Am J Med 73:795–801, 1982.
98. Sokal JE, Firat D: Varicella-zoster infection in patients with cancer. Am J Med 39:452–463, 1965.
99. Feld R, Bodey GP: Infections in patients with malignant lymphoma treated with combination chemotherapy. Cancer 39:1018–1025, 1977.
100. Wilson JF, Marsa GW, Johnson RE: Herpes zoster in Hodgkin's disease. Clinical, histologic, and immunologic correlations. Cancer 29:461–465, 1972.
101. Schimpff SC, O'Connell MJ, Greene WH, Wiernik P: Infections in splenectomized patients with Hodgkin's disease. Am J Med 59:695–701, 1975.
102. Feldman S, Chaudary S, Ossi M, Epp E: A viremic phase for herpes zoster in children with cancer. J Pediatr 91:597–600, 1977.
103. Whitley RJ, Chien LT, Dolin R, Galasso GJ, Alford CA and the Collaborative Study Group: Adenine arabinoside therapy of herpes zoster in the immunosuppressed. N Engl J Med 294:1193–1199, 1976.
104. Weller TH, Coons AH: Fluorescent antibody studies with agents of varicella and herpes zoster propagated in vitro. Proc Soc Exp Biol Med 86:789–794, 1954.
105. Frey HM, Steinberg SP, Gershon AA: Rapid diagnosis of varicella-zoster virus infections by countercurrent immunoelectrophoresis. J Infect Dis 143:274–280, 1981.
106. Andiman WA, White-Greenwald M, Tinghitella T: Zoster encephalitis: Isolation of virus and measurement of varicella-zoster specific antibodies in cerebrospinal fluid. Am J Med 73:769–772, 1982.
107. Williams V, Gershon A, Brunell PA: Serologic response to varicella-zoster membrane antigens measured by indirect immunofluorescence. J Infect Dis 130:669–672, 1974.
108. Gershon AA, Kalter ZG, Steinberg S: Detection of antibody to varicella-zoster virus by immune adherence hemagglutination. Proc Soc Exp Biol Med 152:762–765, 1976.
109. Forghani B, Schmidt NJ, Dennis J: Antibody assays for varicella-zoster virus: Comparison of enzyme immunoassay with neutralization immune adherence agglutination and complement fixation. J Clin Microbiol 8:545–552, 1978.
110. Forghani B, Schmidt NJ, Lennette EH: Sensitivity of a radioimmunoassay method for

detection of certain viral antibodies in sera and cerebrospinal fluids. J Clin Microbiol 4:470–478, 1976.

111. Gallo D, Schmidt NJ: Comparison of anticomplement immunofluorescence and fluorescent antibody-to-membrane antigen tests for determination of immunity status to varicella-zoster virus and for serodifferentiation of varicella-zoster and herpes simplex virus infections. J Clin Microbiol 14:539–543, 1981.

112. Ross AH: Modification of chickenpox in family contacts by administration of gamma globulin. N Engl J Med 267:369–376, 1962.

113. Gershon AA, Steinberg S, Brunell PA: Zoster immune globulin: A further assessment. New Engl J Med 290:243–245, 1974.

114. Orenstein WA, Heymann D, Ellis RJ, Rosenberg RL, Nakano J, Halsey NA, Overturf GD, Hayden GF, Witte JJ: Prophylaxis of varicella in high risk children: Dose-responsive effect of zoster immune globulin. J Pediatr 98:368–373, 1981.

115. Meyers JD, Witte JJ: Zoster immune globulin in high risk children. J Infect Dis 129:616–618, 1974.

116. Geiser CF, Bishop Y, Myers M, Jaffe N, Yankee R: Prophylaxis of varicella in children with neoplastic diseases: Comparative results with zoster immune plasma and gamma globulin. Cancer 35:1027–1030, 1975.

117. Balfour HH, Groth KE, McCullough J, Kalis JM, Marker SC, Nesbit ME, Simmons RL, Najarian JS: Prevention or modification of varicella using zoster immune plasma. Am J Dis Child 131:693–696, 1977.

118. Centers for Disease Control: Zoster immune globulin and varicella zoster immune globulin. Morbid Mortal Weekly Rep 26:359–360, 1977.

119. Zaia JA, Levin MJ, Wright GG, Grady GF: A practical method for preparation of varicella-zoster immune globulin. J Infect Dis 137:601–604, 1978.

120. Zaia JA, Levin MJ, Preblud SR, Leszczynski J, Wright GG, Ellis RJ, Curtis AC, Valerio MA, LeGore J: Evaluation of varicella-zoster immunosuppressed children after household exposure to varicella. J Infect Dis 147:737–743, 1983.

121. Centers for Disease Control: Varicella-zoster immune globulin – United States. Morbid Mortal Weekly Rep 30:15–23, 1981.

122. Steele RW, Myers MG, Vincent MM: Transfer factor for the prevention of varicella-zoster infection in childhood leukemia. N Engl J Med 303:355–359, 1980.

123. Brunell PA, Geiser C, Shehab Z, Waugh JE: Administration of live varicella vaccine to children with leukemia. Lancet 2:1069–1072, 1982.

124. Izawa T, Ihara T, Hattori A, Iwasa T: Application of live varicella vaccine in children with acute leukemia or other malignant diseases. Pediatrics 60:805–809, 1977.

125. Whitley R, Hilty M, Haynes R, Bryson Y, Connor JD, Soong S-J, Alford CA: Vidarabine therapy of varicella in immunosuppressed patients. J Pediatr 101:125–131, 1982.

126. Prober CG, Kirk LE, Keeney RE: Acyclovir therapy of chickenpox in immunosuppressed children – A collaborative study. J Pediatr 101:622–625, 1982.

127. Arvin AM, Feldman S, Merigan TC: Human leukocyte interferon in the treatment of varicella in children with cancer: A preliminary controlled trial. Antimicrob Agents Chemother 13:605–607, 1978.

128. Arvin AM, Kushner JH, Feldman S, Baehner RL, Hammond D, Merigan TC: Human leukocyte interferon for the treatment of varicella in children with cancer. N Engl J Med 306:761–765, 1982.

129. Jordan GW, Fried RP, Merigan TC: Administration of human leukocyte interferon in herpes zoster. I. Safety, circulating antiviral activity, and host responses to infection. J Infect Dis 130:56–62, 1974.

130. Merigan TC, Rand KH, Pollard RB, Abdallah PS, Jordan GW, Fried RP: Human leukocyte interferon for the treatment of herpes zoster in patients with cancer. N Engl J Med

298:981–987, 1978.

131. Horning SJ, Levine JF, Miller RA, Rosenberg SA, Merigan TC: Clinical and immunologic effects of recombinant leukocyte A interferon in eight patients with advanced cancer. JAMA 247:1718–1722, 1982.

132. Whitley RJ, Soong S-J, Dolin R, Betts R, Linnemann C, Alford CA, and NIAID Collaborative Antiviral Study Group: Early vidarabine therapy to control the complications of herpes zoster in immunosuppressed patients. N Engl J Med 307:971–975, 1982.

133. Spectro SA, Hintz M, Wyborny C, Connor JD, Keeney RE, Liao S: Treatment of herpesvirus infections in immunocompromised patients with acyclovir by continuous intravenous infusion. Am J Med 73(1A):275-280, 1982.

134. Balfour HH, Bean B, Laskin OL, Ambinder RF, Meyers JD, Wade JC, Zaia JA, Aeppli D, Kirk LE, Segreti AC, Keeney RE: Acyclovir halts progression of herpes zoster in immunocompromised patients. N Engl J Med 308:1448–1453, 1983.

135. Gold E, Nankervis GA: Cytomegalovirus. In: Viral infections of humans: epidemiology and control (Second edition), Evans AS (ed), New York, Plenum Medical, 1983, p 167–186.

136. Winston DJ, Ho WG, Howell CL, Miller MJ, Mickey R, Martin WJ, Lin C-H, Gale RP: Cytomegalovirus infections associated with leukocyte transfusions. Ann Intern Med 93:671–675, 1980.

137. Ho M, Dowling JN: Cytomegalovirus infection in transplant and cancer patients. In: Current clinical topics in infectious diseases (Vol. 1), Remington JS, Swartz MN (eds), New York, McGraw-Hill, 1980, p 45–67.

138. Wong TW, Warner NE: Cytomegalic inclusion disease in adults. Reports of 14 cases with review of literature. Arch Pathol 74:403–422, 1962.

139. Bodey GP, Wertlake PT, Douglas G, Levin RH: Cytomegalic inclusion disease in patients with acute leukemia. Ann Intern Med 62:899–906, 1965.

140. Rosen P, Hajdu S: Cytomegalovirus inclusion disease at autopsy of patients with cancer. Am J Clin Pathol 55:749–756, 1971.

141. Benyesh-Melnick M, Dessy SI, Fernback DJ: Cytomegaloviruria in children with acute leukemia and in other children. Proc Soc Exp Biol Med 117:624–630, 1974.

142. Dyment PG, Orlando SJ, Isaacs H, Jr, Wright HT, Jr: The incidence of cytomegaloviruria and post-mortem cytomegalic inclusions in children with acute leukemia. J Pediatr 72:533–536, 1968.

143. Armstrong D, Haghbin M, Balakrishnan SL, Murphy ML: Asymptomatic cytomegalovirus infection in children with leukemia. Am J Dis Child 122:404-407, 1971.

144. Henson D, Siegel SE, Fuccillo DA, Matthew E, Levine AS: Cytomegalovirus infections during acute childhood leukemia. J Infect Dis 126:469–481, 1972.

145. Cox F, Hughes WT: Cytomegaloviremia in children with acute lymphocytic leukemia. J Pediatr 87:190–194, 1975.

146. Cox F, Hughes WT: Fecal excretion of cytomegalovirus in disseminated cytomegalic inclusion disease. J Infect Dis 129:732–736, 1974.

147. Duvall CP, Casazza AR, Grimley PM, Carbone PP, Rowe WP: Recovery of cytomegalovirus from adults with neoplastic disease. Ann Intern Med 64:531–541, 1966.

148. Sullivan MP, Hanshaw JB, Cangir A, Butler JJ: Cytomegalovirus complement-fixation antibody levels of leukemic children: Results of a longitudinal study. JAMA 206:569–574, 1968.

149. Langenhuysen MMAC, Cazemier T, Houwen B, Brouwers TM, Halie MR, The JH, Nieweg HO: Antibodies to Epstein-Barr virus, cytomegalovirus and Australia antigen in Hodgkin's disease. Cancer 34:262–267, 1974.

150. Levine PH, Ablashi DV, Berard CW, Carbone PP, Waggoner DE, Malan L: Elevated antibody titers to Epstein-Barr virus in Hodgkin's disease. Cancer 27:416–421, 1971.

151. Hilgers F, Hilgers J: An immunofluorescence technique with counterstain on fixed cells for the detection of antibodies to human herpesviruses: Antibody patterns in patient with Hodgkin's disease and nasopharyngeal carcinoma. Intervirology 7:309–327, 1976.

152. Cox F, Hughes WT: The value of isolation procedures for cytomegalovirus infections in children with leukemia. Cancer 36:1158–1161, 1975.

153. Urmacher C, Myskowski P, Ochoa M, Jr, Kris M, Safai B: Outbreak of Kaposi's sarcoma with cytomegalovirus infection in young homosexual men. Am J Med 72:569–575, 1982.

154. Abdallah PS, Mark JBD, Merigan TC: Diagnosis of cytomegalovirus pneumonia in compromised hosts. Am J Med 61:326–332, 1976.

155. Cox F, Meyer D, Hughes WT: Cytomegalovirus in tears from patients with normal eyes and with acute cytomegalovirus chorioretinitis. Am J Ophthamol 80:817–824, 1975.

156. Wentworth BB, Alexander ER: Seroepidemiology of infections due to members of the herpesvirus group. Am J Epidemiol 94:496–507, 1971.

157. Castellano GA, Hazzard GT, Madden DL, Sever JL: Comparison of the enzyme-linked immunosorbent assay and the indirect hemagglutination test for detection of antibody to cytomegalovirus. J Infect Dis 136(Suppl):337–340, 1977.

158. Cappel R, DeCuyper F, DeBraekeleer J: Rapid detection of IgG and IgM antibodies for cytomegalovirus by enzyme-linked immunosorbent assay (ELISA). Arch Virol 58:253–258, 1978.

159. Rubin RH, Russell PS, Levin M, Cohen C: Summary of a workshop on cytomegalovirus infections during organ transplantation. J Infect Dis 139:728–734, 1979.

160. Goldstein LC, McDougall J, Hackman R, Meyers JD, Thomas ED, Nowinski RC: Monoclonal antibodies to cytomegalovirus: Rapid identification of clinical isolates and preliminary use in diagnosis of cytomegalovirus pneumonia. Infect Immun 38:273–281, 1982.

161. Lee FK, Nahmias AJ, Stagno S: Rapid diagnosis of cytomegalovirus infection in infants by electron microscopy. N Engl J Med 299:1266–1270, 1978.

162. Chou S, Merigan TC: Rapid detection and quantitation of human cytomegalovirus in urine through DNA hybridization. N Engl J Med 308:921–925, 1983.

163. Glenn J: Cytomegalovirus infections following renal transplantation. Rev Infect Dis 3:1151–1178, 1981.

164. Rytel MV, Kauffman HM: Clinical efficacy of adenine arabinoside in therapy of cytomegalovirus infections in renal allograft recipients. J Infect Dis 133:202–205, 1976.

165. Marker SC, Howard RJ, Groth KE, Mastri AR, Simmons RL, Balfour HH, Jr: A trial of vidarabine for cytomegalovirus infection in renal transplant patients. Arch Intern Med 140:1441–1444, 1980.

166. Ch'ien LT, Cannon NJ, Whitley RJ, Diethelm AG, Dismukes WE, Scott CW, Buchanan RA, Alford CA, Jr: Effect of adenine arabinoside on cytomegalovirus infections. J Infect Dis 130:32–39, 1974.

167. Balfour HH, Jr, Bean B, Mitchell CD, Sachs GW, Boen JR, Edelman CK: Acyclovir in immunocompromised patients: A controlled trial in one institution. Am J Med 73(1A):241–248, 1982.

168. Cheeseman SH, Rubin RH, Stewart JA, Tolkoff-Rubin NE, Cosimi AB, Cantell K, Gilbert J, Winkle S, Herrin JT, Black PH, Russell PS, Hirsch MS: Controlled clinical trial of prophylactic human leukocyte interferon in renal transplantation: Effects on cytomegalovirus and herpes simplex virus infections. N Engl J Med 300:1345–1349, 1979.

169. Hirsch MS, Schooley RT, Cosimi AB, Russell PS, Delmonico FL, Tolkoff-Rubin NE, Herrin JT, Cantell K, Farrell ML, Rota TR, Rubin RH: Effects of interferon-alpha on cytomegalovirus reactivation syndromes in renal transplant recipients. N Engl J Med 308:1489–1493, 1983.

170. Glazer JP, Friedman HM, Grossman RA, Starr SE, Barker CF, Perloff LJ, Huang ES,

Plotkin SA: Live cytomegalovirus vaccination of renal transplant candidates: Preliminary trial. Ann Intern Med 91:676–683, 1979.

171. Meyers JD, McGuffin RW, Neiman PE, Singer JW, Thomas ED: Toxicity and efficacy of human leukocyte interferon for treatment of cytomegalovirus pneumonia after marrow transplantation. J Infect Dis 141:555–562, 1980.

172. Winston DJ, Ho WG, Schroff RW, Champlin RE, Gale RP: Safety and tolerance of recombinant leukocyte A interferon in bone marrow transplant recipients. Antimicrob Agents Chemother 23:846–851, 1983.

173. Meyers JD, Day LM, Lum LG, Sullivan KM: Recombinant leukocyte a interferon for the treatment of serious viral infections after marrow transplant: A phase I study. J Infect Dis 148:551–556, 1983.

174. Wade JC, Hintz M, McGuffin RW, Springmeyer SC, Connor JD, Meyers JD: Treatment of cytomegalovirus pneumonia with high dose acyclovir. Am J Med 73(1A):249–256, 1982.

175. Meyers JD, McGuffin RW, Bryson YJ, Cantell K, Thomas ED: Treatment of cytomegalovirus pneumonia after marrow transplant with combined vidarabine and human leukocyte interferon. J Infect Dis 146:80–84, 1982.

176. Wade JC, McGuffin RW, Springmeyer SC, Newton B, Singer JW, Meyers JD: Treatment of cytomegaloviral pneumonia with high dose acyclovir and human leukocyte interferon. J Infect Dis 148:557–562, 1983.

177. Winston DJ, Pollard RB, Ho WG, Gallagher JG, Rasmussen LE, Huang SN, Lin C, Gossett TG, Merigan TC, Gale RP: Cytomegalovirus immune plasma in bone marrow transplant recipients. Ann Intern Med 97:11–18, 1982.

178. Meyers JD, Leszczynski J, Zaia JA, Flournoy N, Newton B, Snydman DR, Wright GG, Levin MJ, Thomas ED: Prevention of cytomegalovirus infection by cytomegalovirus immune globulin after marrow transplantation. Ann Intern Med 98:442–446, 1983.

179. Tyms AS, Seamans EM, Naim HM: The in vitro activity of acyclovir and related compounds against cytomegalovirus infections. J Antimicrob Chemother 8:65–72, 1981.

180. Evans AS, Niederman JC: Epstein-Barr virus. In: Viral infections of humans: epidemiology and control (Second edition), Evans AS (ed), New York, Plenum Medical, 1982, p 3–42.

181. Epstein MA, Achong BG, Barr YM: Virus particles in cultured lymphoblasts from Burkitt's lymphoma. Lancet 1:702–703, 1964.

182. Klein G: The relationship of the virus to nasopharyngeal carcinoma. In: The Epstein-Barr virus, Epstein MA, Achong BG (eds), Berlin, Springer-Verlag, 1979, p 339–350.

183. Purtilo DT, Sakamoto K, Barnabei V, Seeley J, Bechtold T, Rogers G, Yetz J, Harada S: Epstein-Barr virus-induced diseases in boys with the x-linked lymphoproliferative syndrome. Am J Med 73:49–56, 1982.

184. Hanto DW, Frizzera G, Purtilo DT, Sakamoto K, Sullivan JL, Saemundsen AK, Klein G, Simmons RL, Najarian JS: Clinical spectrum of lymphoproliferative disorders in renal transplant recipients and evidence of the role of Epstein-Barr virus. Cancer Res 41:4253–4261, 1981.

185. Ziegler JL, Drew WL, Miner RC, Mintz L, Rosenbaum E, Gershow J, Lennette ET, Greenspan J, Shillitoe E, Beckstead J, Casavant C, Yamamoto K: Outbreak of Burkitt's-like lymphoma in homosexual men. Lancet 2:631–633, 1982.

186. Jondal M, Klein G: Surface markers on human B and T lymphocytes. II. Presence of Epstein-Barr virus receptors on B lymphocytes. J Exp Med 138:1365–1378, 1973.

187. Strauch B, Siegel N, Andrews LL, Miller G: Oropharyngeal excretion of Epstein-Barr virus by renal transplant recipients and other patients treated with immunosuppressive drugs. Lancet 1:234–237, 1974.

188. Chang RS, Lewis JP, Abildgaard CF: Prevalence of oropharyngeal excretors of leukocyte

transforming agents among a human population. N Engl J Med 289:1325–1329, 1973.

189. Chang RS, Lewis JP, Reynolds RD, Sullivan MJ, Neuman J: Oropharyngeal excretion of Epstein-Barr virus by patients with lymphoproliferative disorders and by recipients of renal homografts. Ann Intern Med 88:34–40, 1978.

190. Lange B, Arbeter A, Hewetson J, Henle W: Longitudinal study of Epstein-Barr virus antibody titers and excretion in pediatric patients with Hodgkin's disease. Int J Cancer 22:521–527, 1978.

191. Johansson B, Klein G, Henle W, Henle G: Epstein-Barr virus (EBV)-associated antibody pattern in malignant lymphoma and leukemia. II. Chronic lymphocytic leukemia and lymphocytic lymphoma. Int J Cancer 8:475–486, 1971.

192. Sutton RNP, Marston SD, Pullen HJM, Darby CW, Evans DIK, Emond RTD: Antibodies to Epstein-Barr and other viruses in children with acute lymphoblastic leukemia. Arch Dis Child 49:540–544, 1974.

193. Hanto DW, Frizzera G, Gajl-Peczalska KJ, Sakamoto K, Purtilo DT, Balfour HH, Jr, Simmons RL, Najarian JS: Epstein-Barr virus-induced B-cell lymphoma after renal transplantation: Acyclovir therapy and transition from polyclonal to monoclonal B-cell proliferation. N Eng J Med 306:913–918, 1982.

194. Levine PH, Stevens DA, Coccia PF, Dabich L, Roland A: Infectious mononucleosis prior to acute leukemia: A possible role for the Epstein-Barr virus. Cancer 30:875–880, 1972.

195. Rosner F, Grunwald HW: Infectious mononucleosis and acute leukemia. JAMA 246:1783–1784, 1981.

196. Stevens DA, Levine PH, Lee SK, Sonley MJ, Waggoner DE: Concurrent infectious mononucleosis and acute leukemia: Case reports. Review of the literature and serologic studies with the herpes-type virus (EB virus). Am J Med 50:208–217, 1971.

197. Langenhuysen NMAC: Concurrent infectious mononucleosis and acute myelocytic leukemia. Acta Hemat 51:121–127, 1974.

198. Hoagland RJ: The incubation period of infectious mononucleosis. Am J Public Health 54:1699–1705, 1964.

199. Pattengale PK, Smith RW, Perlin E: Atypical lymphocytes in acute infectious mononucleosis. N Eng J Med 291:1145–1148, 1974.

200. Edwards JMB, McSwiggan DA: Studies on the diagnostic value of an immunofluorescence test for EB virus specific IgM. Clin Pathol 27:647–651, 1974.

201. Adams A, Strander H, Cantell K: Sensitivity of Epstein-Barr virus transformed human lymphoid cell lines to interferon. J Gen Virol 28:207–217, 1975.

202. Coker-Vann M, Dolin R: Effect of adenine arabinoside on Epstein-Barr virus *in vitro*. J Infect Dis 135:447–453, 1977.

203. Summers WC, Klein G: Inhibition of Epstein-Barr virus DNA synthesis and late gene expression by phosphonoacetic acid. J Virol 18:151–155, 1976.

204. Colby BM, Shaw JE, Datta AK, Pagano JS: Replication of Epstein-Barr virus DNA in lymphoblastoid cells treated for extended periods with acyclovir. Am J Med 73(1A):77–81, 1982.

205. Sullivan JL, Byron KS, Brewster FE, Sakamoto K, Shaw JE, Pagano JS: Treatment of life-threatening Epstein-Barr virus infections with acyclovir. Am J Med 73(1A):262–266, 1982.

206. Centers for Disease Control: Summary – Cases specified. Notifiable diseases, United States. Morbid Mortal Weekly Rep 32:654, 1983.

207. McCollum RW: Viral hepatitis. In: Viral infections of humans: epidemiology and control (Second edition), Evans AS (ed), New York, Plenum Medical, 1983, p 327–350.

208. Grange MJ, Erlinger S, Teillet F, Schlegel N, Barge J, Degott C: A possible relationship between hepatitis-associated antigen and chronic persistent hepatitis in Hodgkin's disease. Gut 14:433–437, 1973.

209. Wands JR, Chura CM, Roll FJ, Maddrey WC: Serial studies of hepatitis-associated antigen and antibody in patients receiving antitumor chemotherapy for myeloproliferative and lymphoproliferative disorders. Gastroenterology 68:105–112, 1975.

210. Galbraith RM, Eddleston ALWF, Williams R, Zuckerman AJ, Bagshawe KD: Fulminant hepatic failure in leukemia and choriocarcinoma related to withdrawal of cytotoxic drug therapy. Lancet 2:528–530, 1975.

211. Locasciulli A, Alberti A, Barbieri R, Realdi G, Uderzo C, Portmann B, Masera G: Evidence of non-A, non-B hepatitis in children with acute leukemia and chronic liver disease. Am J Dis Child 137:354–356, 1983.

212. Vergani D, Locasciulli A, Masera G, Alberti A, Moroni G, Tee DEH, Portmann B, Mieli Vergani G, Eddleston ALWF: Histological evidence of hepatitis-B virus infection with negative serology in children with acute leukemia who develop chronic liver disease. Lancet 1:361–364, 1982.

213. Barton JC, Conrad ME: Beneficial effects of hepatitis in patients with acute myelogenous leukemia. Ann Intern Med 90:188–190, 1979.

214. Armitage JO, Burns CP, Kent TH: Liver disease complicating the management of acute leukemia during remission. Cancer 41:737–742, 1978.

215. Szmuness W: Hepatocellular carcinoma and the hepatitis B virus: Evidence for a causal association. Prog Med Virol 24:40–49, 1978.

216. Rotoli B, Formisano S, Martinelli V, Nigro M: Long-term survival in acute myelogenous leukemia complicated by chronic active hepatitis. N Eng J Med 307:1712–1713, 1982.

217. Masera G, Locasciulli A, Jean G, Jankovic M, Rossi MR, Recchia M, Uderzo C: Hepatitis B and childhood acute lymphoblastic leukemia. J Pediatr 99:98–100, 1981.

218. Foon KA, Yale C, Clodfelter K, Gale RP: Post-transfusion hepatitis in acute myelogenous leukemia. JAMA 244:1806–1807, 1980.

219. Kluge T: Gamma globulin in the prevention of viral hepatitis: A study of the effect of medium size doses. Acta Med Scand 174:469–477, 1963.

220. Mosly JW, Reisler DM, Brachott D, Roth D, Weiser J: Comparison of two lots of immune serum globulin for prophylaxis of infectious hepatitis. Am J Epidemiol 87:539–550, 1968.

221. Centers for Disease Control: Immune globulins for protection against viral hepatitis. Morbid Mortal Weekly Rep 30:423–435, 1981.

222. Maynard JE: Passive immunization against hepatitis B: A review of recent studies and comment on current aspects of control. Am J Epidemiol 107:77–86, 1978.

223. Francis DP, Hadler SC, Thompson SE, Maynard JE, Ostrow DG, Altman N, Braff EH, O'Malley P, Hawkins D, Judson FN, Penley K, Nylund T, Christie G, Meyers F, Moore JN, Jr, Gardner A, Doto IL, Miller JH, Reynolds GH, Murphy BL, Schable CA, Clark BT, Curran JW, Redeker AG: The prevention of hepatitis B with vaccine: Report of the Centers for Disease Control multi-center efficacy trial among homosexual men. Ann Intern Med 97:362–366, 1982.

224. Szmuness W, Stevens CE, Harley EJ, Zang EA, Alter HJ, Taylor PE, Devera A, Chen GTS, Kellner A, and the Dialysis Vaccine Trial Study Group: Hepatitis B vaccine in medical staff of hemodialysis units: Efficacy and subtype cross-protection. N Engl J Med 307:1481–1486, 1982.

225. Centers for Disease Control: Inactivated hepatitis B virus vaccine. Morbid Mortal Weekly Rep 31:317–328, 1982.

226. Smith CI, Scullard GH, Gregory PB, Robinson WS, Merigan TC: Preliminary studies of acyclovir in chronic hepatitis B. Am J Med 73(1A):267–270, 1982.

227. Jain S, Thomas HC, Sherlock S: Transfer factor in the attempted treatment of patients with HB$_s$Ag-positive chronic liver disease. Clin Exp Immunol 30:10–15, 1977.

228. Serfling RE, Sherman IL, Housworth WJ: Excess pneumonia-influenza by age and sex in three major influenza A2 epidemics, United States, 1957–58, 1960, and 1963. Am J Epidemiol 86:433–441, 1967.

229. Davenport FM: Influenza viruses. In: Viral infections of humans: epidemiology and control (Second edition), Evans AS (ed), New York, Plenum Medical, 1983, p 373–396.

230. Barker WH, Mullooly JP: Pneumonia and influenza deaths during epidemics: Implications for prevention. Arch Intern Med 142:85–89, 1982.

231. Feldman S, Webster RG, Sugg M: Influenza in children and young adults with cancer: 20 cases. Cancer 39:350–353, 1977.

232. Centers for Disease Control: Influenza vaccines, 1983–84. Morbid Mortal Weekly Rep 32:333–337, 1983.

233. Committee on Infectious Diseases of the American Academy of Pediatrics: Immunization of children at high risk from influenza infection. Morbid Mortal Weekly Rep 25:285–286, 1976.

234. Sumaya CV, Williams TE, Brunell PA: Bivalent influenza vaccine in children with cancer. J Infect Dis 136(Suppl):656–660, 1977.

235. Lange B, Shapiro SA, Waldman MTG, Proctor E, Arbeter A: Antibody responses to influenza immunization of children with acute lymphoblastic leukemia. J Infect Dis 140:402–406, 1979.

236. Smithson WA, Siem RA, Ritts RE, Jr, Gilchrist GS, Burgert EO, Ilstrup DM, Smith TF: Response to influenza virus vaccine in children receiving chemotherapy for malignancy. J Pediatr 96:632–634, 1978.

237. Gross PA, Lee H, Wolff JA, Hall CB, Minnefore AB, Lazicki ME: Influenza immunization in immunosuppressed children. J Pediatr 92:30–35, 1978.

238. Steinherz PG, Brown AE, Gross PA, Braun D, Ghavimi F, Wollner N, Rosen G, Armstrong D, Miller DR: Influenza immunization of children with neoplastic diseases. Cancer 45:750–756, 1980.

239. Brown AE, Steinherz PG, Miller DR, Armstrong D, Kellick MG: Immunization against influenza in children with cancer: Results of a three dose trial. J Infect Dis 145:126, 1982.

240. Borella L, Webster RG: The immunosuppressive effects of long-term combination chemotherapy in children with acute leukemia in remission. Cancer Res 31:420–426, 1971.

241. Ortbals DW, Liebhaber H, Presant CA, van Amburg AL, III, Lee JY: Influenza immunization of adult patients with malignant diseases. Ann Intern Med 87:552–557, 1977.

242. Silver RT, Utz JP, Fahey J, Frei E: Antibody response in patients with acute leukemia. J Lab Clin Med 56:634–643, 1960.

243. Amantadine: Does it have a role in the prevention and treatment of Influenza? A National Institutes of Health Consensus Development Conference. Ann Intern Med 92:256–258, 1980.

244. Jones HE: Immunosuppression and fatal measles. Lancet 2:1255–1256, 1969.

245. Breitfeld V, Hashida Y, Sherman FE, Odagiri K, Yunis EJ: Fatal measles infection in children with leukemia. Lab Invest 28:279–291, 1973.

246. Robertson MG: Mumps with orchitis and lymphosarcoma. JAMA 215:1827, 1971.

4. Infection Prophylaxis in Granulocytopenic Patients with Antimicrobial Drugs Selected for Their Indifferent Activity to Resident (Anaerobic) Protective Flora

D. VAN DER WAAIJ and H. G. DE VRIES-HOSPERS

INTRODUCTION

A growing body of information is being focused on the infection hazard of special care areas in hospitals. The sources of infection appear to be both endogenous and exogenous in origin. The sources of nosocomial exogenous infection are no longer a mystery. The bacteria, yeasts and molds associated with these infections can be traced to other patients in the unit, to intravenous and urinary catheters and to wash sinks and utility areas. It is generally agreed that prime factors in their transmission are the personnel who work in these units. Consequently, for practical and financial reasons, more emphasis is in general given to handwashing than to strict isolation and architectural design of special care units.

A considerable proportion of special care patients are those with hematological malignancies who are hospitalized to receive chemotherapy. These patients are extremely susceptible to infections because they are granulocytopenic ($<1,000$ granulocytes/mm^3 blood) for several weeks. In addition to profound granulocytopenia, in patients under aggressive chemotherapy, the mucosa of the various tracts suffers greatly. This increases the likelihood that potentially pathogenic bacteria and fungi will colonize, invade, and ultimately infect.

The decreased host defense to infections renders the patient apparently almost equally susceptible to endogenous potentially pathogenic microbes as to those of nosocomial origin. This is based on the observation that even under conditions of effective strict reverse isolation, infections are frequently seen in granulocytopenic patients [1]. The bacteria involved in infections are mostly gram-negative bacilli, i.e., *Enterobacteriaceae* and *Pseudomonadaceae* species [2–4]. Apart from the fact that strict reverse isolation in laminar flow isolators [5–8] or in so-called patient bed-isolators [9–11] is extremely difficult and expensive, the net result appears limited. Infections in

Higby, DJ (ed), The Cancer Patient and Supportive Care. ISBN 0-89838-690-X.
© *1985, Martinus Nijhoff Publishers, Boston. Printed in The Netherlands.*

perfectly isolated patients are obviously caused by organisms which had colonized the patient prior to isolation. Isolation alone, however, is not of much use [12, 13]. If a patient is admitted from another hospital, or even if there has been an intervening period at home, his/her flora may harbor resistant hospital-acquired strains which may cause infection during a granulocytopenic period.

In a study of the Gnotobiotic Project Group of the EORTC in 54 patients with acute leukemia, 36% of 32 patients treated under ward conditions experienced no bacteriologically documented infection, while not many more (41%) of 22 strictly isolated patients had no such infection. Other groups have reported similar experiences [14, 15].

The mixed (endogenous and exogenous) origin of microbial infections in granulocytopenic patients has lead to attempts to prevent these infections by 'gut sterilization' [12–16]. Briefly, patients have been treated orally with combinations of broad spectrum non-absorbable antibiotics in such doses that the gastrointestinal (GI) tract flora should disappear. Several factors, such as bacterial resistance to the antibiotics used, as well as inactivation of these antibiotics by gastrointestinal contents, however, negatively influenced the results [17]. The occurrence of overgrowth with multiply resistant organisms during total antibiotic decontamination (sterilization) of the digestive tract has been reported. As in experimental animals [18], total decontamination of the digestive tract appears to render patients extremely susceptible to colonization by resistant organisms [19–21].

Since this is the case, total gut sterilization as a clinically useful goal must include strict isolation of the patient to prevent severe infections from resistant organisms; or else, regimens need to be designed to which resistance cannot develop. Neither is a very feasible possibility at this time.

COLONIZATION RESISTANCE

Studies in experimental animals have revealed that both chemotherapy and X-irradiation as well as complete decontamination (sterilization) of the digestive tract with non-absorbable antibiotics strongly enhances overgrowth by antibiotic-resistant microbes. The mechanisms which control the colonization pattern of potentially pathogenic microorganisms in the digestive tract are thus related to cytotoxic injury to host defenses (especially those related to the mucosal barrier of the tract) and to effects of the antibiotics on the normal flora in the digestive tract. Mechanisms related to cytotoxic agents are largely, if not completely, dependent on host factors (e.g., pre-existing mucosal integrity, age, bowel transit time, etc.), whereas those mechanisms related to antibiotics are largely associated with the anaerobic bacterial flora of the digestive tract. The mechanisms related to alteration in anaerobic flora account for most of the colonization-controlling factors, collectively termed 'Colonization Resistance' (CRes) [18]. Anaerobic bacteria live in close association with the mucosa of the colon and in that way may block adherence of potentially pathogenic bacteria and yeasts; colonization of bacteria and yeasts requires that they adhere, or live otherwise in intimate association with the mucosa [21].

HOST-RELATED ASPECTS OF COLONIZATION RESISTANCE

The adherence of potentially pathogenic microorganisms to mucosal surfaces *in vivo* is a complex process which depends on many host and microbial variables. During good health, the mucosal surfaces appear to provide excellent protection against bacterial invasion. The mucous membranes are virtually impervious to colonization by pathogenic bacteria because of highly effective defense barriers. The surfaces are continuously 'bathed' by saliva and mucus, which contain a variety of active chemical agents such as glycoproteins, fibronectin, antibacterial enzymes and antibodies, all of which coat or damage bacteria. Antibodies which only coat bacteria in the digestive tract are of IgA class. These antibodies appear to prevent microorganisms from making contact with binding sites on mucosal cells [22–25]. Several different glycoproteins also limit adhesion of pathogens to mucosal cells of the host by blocking receptor sites [26]. The removal of secretions, the generation of factors blocking receptors for bacteria, the normal fluid flow of secretions, and the desquamation of mucosal cells, all occur more rapidly than the multiplication of most potentially pathogenic microorganisms. Thus, new bacteria are eliminated by mechanical means before they can begin to colonize (although these normal mechanisms can be overcome by mass effects (e.g., exposure to very large numbers of organisms).

FLORA-RELATED ASPECTS OF COLONIZATION RESISTANCE

Blocking of receptor sites occurs also by resident bacteria. Many, if not all resident bacteria, appear to have the capacity to complement host-related mechanisms in the control of bacterial colonization. The resident bacteria live in close association with the mucosa, particularly in the lower part of the digestive tract. Since the great majority (more than 99%) of the bacteria in the digestive tract are anaerobic, it appears that the anaerobic fraction of the flora has the predominant protective effect in preventing colonization by pathogens. Sprunt and co-authors, however, have provided evidence that aerobic streptococci may also have a colonization-controlling effect, especially in the oropharynx, namely where viridans streptococci may share activity with anaerobes in minimizing colonization by gram-negative bacilli [27, 28]. Flora-related CRes is also subject to mass effects.

Colonization and Infection

Colonization implies that the organisms adhere to and multiply on the surface of the mucosa, from which they can penetrate the mucous membrane in sufficient numbers to cause clinical infection. When cellular and humoral defense mechanisms are compromised, serious infections may be caused by organisms of relatively low intrinsic pathogenicity and by smaller inocula of organisms than would be required in the normal individual. The major defense against infection (as opposed to adherence or colonization) is the level of criculating granulocytes.

Epidemiological Consequences

Maintenance of a strong CRes is of importance for the patient, but also has great epidemiological consequences. The higher the CRes, the smaller the chance that contamination of the patient with small numbers of potentially pathogenic microbes will occur. In turn, the chance of colonization and infection of the host and subsequent contamination of the hospital environment, is lessened.

SCREENING OF ANTIBIOTICS

With the discovery that there was a causal relationship between impairment of CRes and acquisition of infection, it seemed possible that strengthening of impaired CRes during intensive cytotoxic therapy (e.g., the remission induction of acute leukemia) might have clinical utility. Since the host mechanisms contributing to CRes could not be easily altered, attention was directed to the mechanisms related to endogenous flora. Could the protective microorganism population be maintained, and if so, would this reduce the likelihood of colonization and infection with potentially pathogenic organisms? Studies were performed in mice, in which a variety of antimicrobial agents were screened for their effects on the flora thought responsible for CRes. The agents were administered orally several times a day for several weeks [29–33]. Some of the more promising agents were screened in man [34, 35]. These tests showed that the majority of available antibiotics do adversely affect the CRes-responsible flora. Poorly absorbed antibiotics which are significantly toxic to gram-positive organisms, tend to have the greatest effect on flora related to CRes, whereas those antibiotics which are almost completely absorbed or those whose spectrum is largely limited to gram-negative organisms (polymyxin, nalidixic acid) or to yeasts (nystatin, amphotericin B), were found to have little effect on CRes. In fact, these latter agents appear to enhance the CRes, specifically for those organisms against which they have activity. With sufficient doses, these agents not only prevent colonization by susceptible nosocomial strains, but also suppress endogenous gram-negative flora selectively. This technique of selectively suppressing potentially pathogenic organisms was termed 'Selective Decontamination of the Digestive Tract' (SDD) [29, 36].

When SDD was applied in granulocytopenic patients, stool cultures were generally negative for gram-negative bacilli within one week of treatment [36, 37]; selective decontamination of the oropharynx usually takes longer and is rarely as successful as that applied to the intestines. Later in this chapter, more detailed information will be provided about the clinical results of SDD.

Some drugs with significant broad spectrum activity, which include gram-negative bacteria and which are not completely absorbed (e.g., oral cephalosporins), do not follow the general rule that activity against gram-positive bacteria is contraindicated if one aims to maintain the CRes. This includes both antimicrobial drugs chemically bound to an ester (bacampicillin, pivmecillinam) which renders them biologically inactive in the intestinal lumen, and drugs like co-trimoxazole which have activity against only some gram-positive cocci. Co-trimoxazole therefore can be given in rather high doses before it becomes detrimental to the CRes. In the literature, a suppressive effect of co-trimoxazole to gram-negative bacilli has been described following relatively low daily doses (one regular tablet) [38]. A higher proportion of patients has been found freed of susceptible *Enterobacteriaceae* species during treatment with four tablets per day. However, higher doses of four to six regular co-trimoxazole tablets appear to give optimal success in studies of others [36, 39, 40]. An even higher dose has been applied by Hughes and co-authors [41] to prevent *Pneumocystis carinii* [41]. This group also reported the high incidence of stool cultures negative for gram-negative bacilli. However, in addition they noticed an increase of colonization by *Candida albicans*. The latter could indicate that the flora-related part of the CRes had suffered from the dose used in these patients [21].

DETERMINATION OF THE COLONIZATION RESISTANCE IN PATIENTS

In the foregoing, a rationale has been advanced regarding the importance of maintaining the flora-associated part of the CRes of the digestive tract in

granulocytopenic patients. This may even be more important in patients undergoing chemotherapy, which may affect their mucosal linings and therewith the host-related part of the CRes. Maintenance of a good protective microflora in these patients is necessary for two reasons:
1) to keep the patient optimally resistant to colonization following oral contamination
2) because an intact anaerobic flora will prevent overgrowth by already colonizing potentially pathogenic bacteria, which could lead to infection and septicemia

Thus, the preservation of an intact flora-related part of the CRes forms the basis for SDD.

The most direct way of investigating the CRes-responsible microflora is the comprehensive anaerobic culturing of the feces in order to inventory the presence and number of the various anaerobic bacterial species. This is, however, extremely laborious and costly, not to speak of the technical difficulties involved in proper sampling and transportation of fecal samples to the anaerobic laboratory. The next best direct method may be microscopic counting of anaerobes according to the method described by Holdeman and co-authors [42]. A relatively simple indirect way of investigating the CRes, which has in our hands a good correlation with the quality of the CRes of the digestive tract, is based on the fact that anaerobes associated with the CRes produce an enzyme which cleaves β-aspartyl-glycine [43–45]. β-Aspartyl-glycine is a normal end-product of protein metabolism and is excreted into the urine as well as the digestive tract. Mammals lack the enzyme which further degrades the molecule. Thus, in individuals (man and animals) in whom the CRes-responsible part of the flora is significantly affected by an antibiotic that reaches the intestinal contents in suppressing concentrations, β-aspartyl-glycine is excreted with the feces. The concentration of β-aspartyl-glycine thus inversely correlates with the mass of anaerobic flora, and therefore, the integrity of the CRes. In antibiotic-decontaminated patients with no anaerobic flora left, the concentration of β-aspartyl-glycine is high, whereas in individuals with a normal flora, the molecule is not detectable in the feces.

The technique by which β-aspartyl-glycine concentrations can be determined is simple and inexpensive. Briefly, fecal supernatants are subjected to high voltage paper electrophoresis. The papers are then stained with ninhydrin. After subsequent heating for ten minutes at 150 °C, β-aspartyl-glycine stains blue. The intensity of the color of the spot reflects the concentration of β-aspartyl-glycine semi-quantitatively.

CLINICAL APPROACH

As mentioned in the first part of this chapter, infection is still a leading cause of death in the neutropenic patient. Gram-negative bacilli belonging to the families of the *Enterobacteriaceae* and *Pseudomonadaceae* species account for the majority of the infectious episodes. *S. aureus,* yeasts, and fungi are next. Many of these microorganisms are normal residents of the GI tract. When the mucosal barrier is affected, as with leukemia remission induction chemotherapy, these bacteria may easily become invasive. This is complicated further by the fact that the patient is then in general also severely granulocytopenic. Infection prevention in these patients is therefore indicated. This is done by applying SDD [36, 37], aiming at selective elimination of potentially pathogenic microorganisms from the gut.

The ability of SDD to attenuate and prevent infection has been determined in a prospectively randomized clinical trial [36]. Briefly, patients with hematological malignancies, mainly acute leukemia and idiopathic granulocytopenia, were randomized to either SDD or to a control group. In the control group (52 patients), 46% developed a severe infection. In the SDD group (53 patients), 20% developed such infections. Of all infections in this study, about 60% could be documented bacteriologically. When only infections were included which were caused by gram-negative bacilli and yeasts – the 'target group' of microorganisms most suppressed by our SDD regimen at that time – these figures were 23% and 4%, respectively. In SDD patients, reduction was also seen in the number of clinically documented infections in comparison with the control group. One of the two SDD 'target group' infections in the SDD group was preceded by gastrointestinal colonization. In a period during which the patient refused to take oral amphotericin B, massive *Candida* colonization occurred, followed by septicemia. The other severe microbiologically documented infection in the SDD group may have originated from outside the GI tract. This patient experienced a secondary infected thrombophlebitis. Severe acquired infections due to gram-negative bacilli or yeasts in the control group occurred 12 times. In many of these cases, the causative bacterium had been isolated beforehand from the fecal samples and/or the throat swabs. This confirms that the gastrointestinal tract is an important port of entry for infections in these kinds of patients.

Oral administration of the SDD regimen resulted in a significant decrease in the number of fecal and throat swab cultures positive for gram-negative bacilli and/or yeasts. In the oropharynx, SDD appeared much more difficult to achieve than in the lower part of the digestive tract (feces), especially as far as yeasts were concerned. It appeared even more difficult when there were foreign bodies involved, such as dentures or a nasogastric tube. Dentures could be removed, but removal of a nasogastric tube could not usually be done, since this was required for tube-feeding in patients who had severe problems with emesis and for anorexia. The tube was also often used for administration of the SDD drugs. In this situation, however, the oral cavity was bypassed, i.e., not exposed to the SDD drugs. *Candida* species which colonize the oropharynx of about half of the severely compromised patients are a particular problem in this situation. To reduce the risk of dense growth and thereby of infection, lozenges each containing 10 mg of amphotericin B [46] were given to these patients 4 times per day for suppression of yeasts in the mouth. Although it is very difficult to eradicate yeasts completely from the oropharynx, suppression of growth can in this way successfully be accomplished [47]. Gram-negative colonization in the oropharynx seems to be controlled by co-trimoxazole, probably because this causes effective anti gram-negative concentrations in the saliva [48]. Kurrle et al. also noted the absence of gram-negative bacilli in the oral washings of co-trimoxazole-treated patients [49].

Colonization of *S. aureus* in the oropharynx is seen in only a small percentage of leukemic patients. In such cases, we add cefradin to the SDD regimen. In general, this results in prompt disappearance of *S. aureus*. Although *S. aureus* is *in vitro* often susceptible to co-trimoxazole, the suppressive effect is not always as prompt and complete as that of cefradin.

ISOLATION CONDITIONS

SDD can be applied on the open hematological ward without substantial isolation procedures. This is possible because the CRes-responsible flora is maintained. During SDD, the CRes is even artificially increased by the concentration of the SDD drugs in the intestines. Contaminations of the patients with high numbers of potentially pathogenic bacteria, however, must be avoided since they may be resistant to the drugs used for SDD. Therefore, one should be aware of the major environmental sources of potentially pathogenic microorganisms. Raw meat and vegetables as well as freshly prepared fruit salads, for example, can be heavily contaminated by gram-negative bacilli [50]. It is therefore necessary to avoid this kind of food. The necessity of minimally contaminated food is illustrated by our experience with tube feeding. At the time we started to use tube feeding, the food was prepared and handled without special precautions on the ward, and was therefore not sterile at the onset. After several hours of storage on the ward, bacterial multiplication (which was to be expected) did occur. We soon experienced an outbreak of *Pseudomonas* septicemia among the tube fed leukemic patients. At that time, *Pseudomonas aeruginosa* was isolated from tube feeding in concentrations as high as 10^6/ml. When we switched to ready-for-use sterile tube feeding, food-born septicemia no longer was noted.

Another important effective measure to control transmission of gram-negative bacilli is handwashing[62]. This simple precaution is too easily forgotten, especially when more than one patient occupies a room and the medical staff is going from patient to patient.

PRACTICAL APPROACH

Ideally, from every patient, the results of recently obtained baseline cultures should be available before the start of SDD. When these indicate gram-negative flora susceptible to polymyxin, the patient should be selectively decontaminated with this drug. After oral intake, usually 2–3 days elapse before susceptible gram-negative bacilli have disappeared from the gut, provided the bowel function is normal. This rapid disappearance of gram-negative bacilli is important; the shorter this period, the less the chance that a resistant strain will emerge.

However, in cases where one cannot wait for the results of baseline cultures, a combination of polymyxin or colistin and one of the absorbable drugs (whether co-trimoxazole or nalidixic acid is used, or newer derivatives, depends on the patient's history of allergies and his/her condition) should then be started empirically after throat swabs and fecal samples are obtained and sent to the microbiology laboratory. When SDD is started 'blindly', *Proteus sp.* and related species which are essentially resistant to polymyxin should be included in the spectrum of activity of the empiric drug combinations. Both co-trimoxazole and nalidixic acid meet this requirement. When the fecal flora is free of gram-negative bacilli, we usually discontinue one of the two drugs; which one is discontinued is determined by the results of the inventory cultures. Both the detection of potentially pathogenic organisms as well as their sensitivity patterns play a role.

For elimination of yeasts, we prefer amphotericin B because of its higher activity and better palatability. Nystatin, however, remains a good alternative, although higher doses are required [21]. Ketoconazole, on the other hand, may have no place in the control of *Candida* colonization and prevention of mycotic infections in the neutropenic patient. After oral administration, the drug is partially absorbed. Its subsequent excretion with the saliva could be of advantage in the control of yeast proliferation in the oropharyngeal area. However, absorption of ketoconazole in the gut depends on the pH in the stomach and the condition of the mucosa, both of which are affected by chemotherapy. There is also clinical evidence indicating that ketoconazole is not the drug of choice for elimination of yeasts [51]. Cefradin is included only when the patient is colonized by *S. aureus* [52], in which case it is continued for at least three weeks.

SDD for gram-negative bacilli and yeasts is applied as long as the patient is severely granulocytopenic, i.e., granulocyte counts less than $500/mm^3$. Thereafter, all drugs for SDD are stopped.

SURVEILLANCE CULTURES

Bacteriological monitoring of the neutropenic patient during SDD should include, at least, cultures of fresh throat swabs or oral washings and fecal samples. Inventory cultures should also include a urine sample, a swab from the anterior nares and if skin or mucosal infections are in sight, material from these lesions. Cultures from feces and throat should be repeated at least twice a week. This is necessary because the flora of the environment, although maintained in as low a concentration as possible with standard hygienic measures, and microbes in food and beverages, both may contaminate the patient to a variable degree.

The finding of resistant bacteria in two sonsecutive fecal samples, with the concentration of the bacterium rising, is an indication for adjustment of the decontamination regimen according to its sensitivity spectrum for SDD drugs [37]. The mere presence of *Pseudomonas aeruginosa* in a throat or fecal culture, however, is potentially more dangerous. This requires immediate adjustment of the SDD drug combination. In our experience, a change in the SDD regimen because of the isolation of resistant bacteria in rising concentration or the finding of serious pathogens is necessary in about 30–40% of the decontamination periods.

COMPARISON WITH OTHER PROPHYLACTIC REGIMENS

Infection prevention by SDD or similar CRes-preserving regimens have been shown to be efficacious. There is a decrease in the infection frequency in comparison with control patients who are not prophylactically treated [36, 53, 54]. There is, however, only one trial in which SDD is compared with total decontamination in strict reverse isolation. Both methods of infection prevention appeared to be equally effective [55, 56]. This study also contrasted different SDD regimens. There was a slight advantage for the regimen in which co-trimoxazole was included.

Other investigators are inconclusive about the prophylactic effect of co-trimoxazole [57]. In a number of studies in which co-trimoxazole was applied for infection prophylaxis, the drug was given in combination with a CRes-decreasing drug [58–60]. Based on our hypothesis, this would be counter-productive and may result in resistant microorganisms colonizing the patient. The dose of the SDD agents is also crucial; those investigators who used a daily dose of 6 tablets co-trimoxazole (480 mg trimethoprim and 2400 mg sulfamethoxazole) in patients with less than 500 granulocytes per mm^3 found clinical benefit. The administration of 4 regular tablets of co-trimoxazole will eliminate gram-negative bacilli within ten days in 50–60% of the patients [61], whereas this figure approached 100% in our study in patients who received six regular tablets [37].

Another important difference in reported studies is in the management of the results of the surveillance cultures. Three approaches have been reported:

1. Oral administration of antimicrobial agents for selective decontamination without monitoring the effect on the fecal flora, so that it is unknown whether patients are really decontaminated or not.
2. Oral administration of antibiotics for prophylaxis, with the performance of surveillance cultures, so that while it was known which bacteria were eliminated and which ones were not, no adjustment in the regimen was made.
3. Studies in which the aim was elimination of all potentially pathogenic bacteria from the GI tract. Surveillance cultures were used to indicate whether SDD was successful or not. If not, the drugs were adjusted when possible.

We prefer the last approach in which the finding of positive cultures dictates the alteration and adjustments of the SDD regimen. Our purpose is not to study the effect of administration of certain fixed combinations of antimicrobial agents, but to eliminate potential pathogens from the digestive tract flora. In the hands of an experienced team, one SDD drug at the time can be sufficient to achieve this goal. However, since treatment must usually be started blindly, a fixed combination (for example, co-trimoxazole and polymyxin) is to be recommended. These drugs cover a broad spectrum of potential pathogens which reduces the need for readjustment [40].

INFECTION PREVENTION IN PATIENTS UNDERGOING AUTOLOGOUS BONE MARROW TRANSPLANTATION FOR SOLID TUMORS: PRELIMINARY DATA

Seventeen patients with solid tumors (small cell lung cancer, non-seminomatous testicular cancer, ovarian cancer) received aggressive ablative chemotherapy with increasing doses of cyclophosphamide (4.5 g/m^2–7 g/m^2) and VP-16-213 (0.6 g/m^2–2.5 g/m^2). Four days after the end of chemotherapy, previously frozen autologous bone marrow was infused. Since it requires about two weeks for the bone marrow to 'take' and because the mucous membranes are heavily affected by this chemotherapy, these patients temporarily have strongly enhanced susceptibility to infection. For this reason, all patients were selectively decontaminated. Because of the possible risk of bone marrow suppression, only non-absorbable drugs were used for SDD; the use of co-trimoxazole was avoided. The SDD regimen in these patients consisted of oral treatment with polymyxin (800 mg/day) and neomycin (1000 mg/day), together with antimycotic drugs. Neomycin was included in the combination to cover polymyxin-resistant bacteria such as *Providencia* and *Proteus* species. Elimination of the gram-negative bacilli form the GI tract was successful in these patients except in one who was colonized with a *Serratia* species resistant to all antimicrobial agents at that time available for SDD. The non-absorbable regimen was not very successful with regard to infection prevention in the eight patients who were treated in this way [63]. All patients developed fever which was most likely due to infection in seven. Microbiological documentation of the infection was possible in four patients, revealing *Serratia, H. influenzae* + *S. pneumoniae, Pseudomonas fluorescens* and *Candida.*

Because of the ineffectiveness of our standard SDD regimen, we have searched for alternative drugs. In a study in volunteers, it appeared that twice daily administration of 250 mg temocillin intramuscularly resulted in disappearance of gram-negative bacilli from the intestines after 2–3 days [64]. There were no signs of disturbance of the CRes. Temocillin is active against most members of the family of the *Enterobacteriaceae* species, inclusive of *Proteus* species. *Pseudomonas* species as well as staphylococci and streptococci are resistant. Temocillin was subsequently used in nine autologous bone marrow transplantation patients. They were treated intravenously with 250 mg temocillin twice daily. In most patients, temocillin administration occurred via a Hickman catheter. In addition, polymyxin and amphotericin B were given orally in the usual dose regimen. In two patients, temocillin administration had to be stopped because of allergic reactions. In the remaining seven patients, elimination of the intestinal gram-negative bacilli was successful. All patients developed fever due to bacteriologically documented infections. Two infections were only documented at autopsy. In one of these patients, *Candida* was seen microscopically in the wall of the appendix. This patient previously experienced septicemia with *S. epidermidis* and viridans streptococci. The other patient showed bacteria in multiple organs microscopically. The infections in the remaining five patients were all caused by gram-positive cocci. Three septicemias were caused by viridans streptococci, most probably originating from the oropharynx. Mucositis of the oropharyngeal area may have contributed to these infections. Catheter-related infections were found in two patients: one *S. aureus* and one *S. epidermidis*. One patient had a sinusitis maxillaris from which *S. epidermidis* was isolated.

The results of our recent experiments with patients undergoing autologous bone marrow procedures demonstrate: 1) that despite the disappointing clinical results of our studies, there did seem to be a correlation between the organisms causing the infections and those found in surveillance cultures; and 2) that the regimens used were effective in eliminating those organisms against which they were targeted. Obviously, further investigations should allow for more clinically useful regimens.

It may also be that the degree of injury to the host components of CRes might have been substantially greater with the kinds of regimens used in the autologous marrow transplantation experiments, so that protection of CRes by maintaining the microbial aspects of this defense was not enough to make a difference in the clinical end result.

CONCLUSION

Selective decontamination of the digestive tract as described above has proven effective in reducing the frequency and severity of infection in neutropenic individuals by potentially pathogenic host flora during the remission induction phase of the treatment of acute myelogenous leukemia. Obviously, as this new approach is studied further and as additional selective antibiotics are developed, the success of this approach should increase.

Similar principles may be applied eventually to the external sites of infection by normally benign host organisms, although the role of flora in the protection of the host from organisms such as *Staphylococcus epidermidis,* which is a growing problem as the use of indwelling central venous catheters rises, is as yet unknown.

Finally, further profit may come from attempting to manipulate the host aspects of CRes. Can mucosal damage from cytotoxic agents be selectively limited? Can artificial products be used to substitute for the natural barriers associated with mucus and saliva? Can host factors such as transit time be manipulated so as to reduce the number of organisms residing in the digestive tract without causing serious other difficulties to the host?

Obviously, the principles of eliminating access to the host by all potential pathogens is an area of great promise for improved supportive care during the treatment of many malignancies, especially those which seem to have the potential for cure with more aggressive cytotoxic therapy.

REFERENCES

1. EORTC Gnotobiotic Project Group Writing Committee – Dankert J, Gaus W, Krieger D, Linzenmeier G, van der Waaij D: Protective isolation and antimicrobial decontamination in patients with high susceptibility to infection. A prospective study of gnotobiotic care in acute leukemia patients. III. The quality of isolation and decontamination. Infection 6:3-19, 1978.

2. Levine AS, Schimpff SC, Graw RG: Hematologic malignancies and marrow failure states: Progress in the management of complicating infections. Semin Hematol 11:141-202, 1974.

3. Mortenstein N, Mortenstein BT, Nissen NI: Bacteremia in patients with leukemia and allied neoplastic diseases. Scand J Infect Dis 8:145-149, 1976.

4. Van der Waaij D, Tielemans-Speltie TM, De Roeck-Houben AMJ: Infection by and distribution of biotypes of Enterobacteriacea species in leukemic patients treated under ward conditions and in units for protective isolation in seven hospitals in Europe. Infection 5:188-194, 1977.

5. Solberg CO, Matsen JM, Vesley D, Wheeler DJ, Good RA, Meuwissen HJ: Laminar airflow protection in bone marrow transplantation. Appl Microbiol 21:209-216, 1971.

6. Van der Waaij D, Vossen JM, Korthals Altes C: Patient isolators designed in the Netherlands. In: Germ-free Research Biological Effect of Gnotobiotic Environments, Heneghan JB (ed), New York, Academic Press, 1973, pp 31-36.

7. Schimpff SC: Laminar airflow room reverse isolation and microbial suppressio suppression to prevent infection in patients with cancer. Cancer Chem Ther 59:1055-1060, 1975.

8. Pederson PD, Penland WZ, Ufford KA: Laminar flow patient isolation systems in cancer treatment – Current status. Proc Internatl Symp Contam Control Ed Black, SICCLS, 1974, pp 149-154.

9. Schwartz SA, Perry S: Patient protection in cancer chemotherapy. JAMA 197:623-627, 1966.

10. Dietrich M, Fliedner TM: Gnotobiotic care of patients with immunologic deficiency diseases. Transplant Proc 5:1271-1277, 1973.

11. Trexler PC, Spiers ASD, Gaya H: Plastic isolators for treatment of acute leukemia patients under 'germ-free' conditions. Brit Med J 4:549-553, 1975.

12. Yates JW, Holland JF: A controlled study of isolation and endogenous microbial suppression in acute myelocytic leukemia patients. Cancer 32:1490-1498, 1973.

13. EORTC Writing Committee – Dietrich M, Gaus W, Vossen J, Van der Waaij D, Wendt F: Protective isolation and antimicrobial decontamination in patients with high susceptibility to infection. A prospective cooperative study of gnotobiotic care in acute leukemia patients. I. clinical results. Infection 5:107-114, 1977.

14. Levine AS, Siegel SE, Schreiber AD, Hauser J, Preisler HD, Goldstein IM, Seidler F, Simon R, Perry S, Bennett JE, Henderson ES: Protective environments and prophylactic antibiotics. A prospective controlled study of their utility in the therapy of acute leukemia. N Engl J Med 288:477-483, 1973.

15. Schimpff SC, Greene WH, Young VM, Fortner CL, Jepsen L, Cusack N, Block JB, Wiernik PH: Infection prevention in acute non-lymphocytic leukemia. Ann Intern Med 82:351-358, 1975.

16. EORTC Writing Committee – Gaus W, Kurrle E, Linzenmeier G, Nowrousian R, de Vries-Hospers HG, Van der Waaij D: A prospective cooperative study of antimicrobial decontamination in granulocytopenic patients. Comparison of two different methods. Infection 10:131-138, 1982.

17. Hazenberg MP, van de Boom M, Bakker M, van de Merwe JP: Binding to faeces and influence on human anaerobes of antimicrobial agents used for selective decontamination.

Antonie van Leeuwenhoek 49:111–117, 1983.

18. van der Waaij D, de Vries JM, Lekkerkerk JEC: Colonization resistance of the digestive tract in conventional and antibiotic treated mice. J Hygiene 69:405–410, 1971.

19. Schimpff SC, Greene WH, Young VM, Fortner CL, Jepsen L, Cusack N, Block J, Wiernik PH: Infection prevention in acute non-lymphocytic leukemia. Laminar air flow room reverse isolation with oral, non-absorbable antibiotic prophylaxis. Ann Intern Med 82:351–358, 1975.

20. Hanhn DM, Schimpff SC, Fortner CL, Smyth AC, Young VM, Wiernik PH: Infection in acute leukemia patients receiving oral nonabsorbable antibiotics. Antimicrob Agents Chemother 13:958–964, 1978.

21. van der Waaij D: Gut resistance to colonization: Clinical usefulness of selective use of orally administered antimicrobial and antifungal drugs. In: Infections in Cancer Patients, Klastersky J (ed), New York, Raven Press, 1982, pp 73–85.

22. Reed W, Williams RC: Bacterial adherence: First step in pathogenesis of certain infections. J Chron Dis 31:67–72, 1978.

23. Brinton CC: Contribution of pili to the specificity of bacterial surface. In: The Specificity of Cell Surface, Davis BD (ed), Englewood Cliffs, New York, Prentice-Hall, 1967, pp 37–70.

24. Ofek I, Mirelman D, Sharon N: Adherence of E. coli to human mucosal cells mediated by mannose receptors. Nature 265:623–625, 1977.

25. Johanson WG, Woods DE, Chandhuri T: Association of respiratory tract colonization with adherence of gram-negative bacilli to epithelial cells. J Infect Dis 139:667–673, 1979.

26. Beachy EH: Bacterial adherence: Adhesion-receptor interactions mediating the attachment of bacteria to mucosal surfaces. J Infect Dis 143:325–345, 1981.

27. Sprunt K, Redman W: Evidence suggesting importance of role of interbacterial inhibition in maintaining balance of normal flora. Ann Intern Med 68:579–590, 1968.

28. Sprunt K, Leidy GA, Redman W: Prevention of bacterial overgrowth. J Infect Dis 123:1–10, 1971.

29. van der Waaij D, Berghuis-de Vries JM: Selective elimination of Enterobacteriaceae species from the digestive tract in mice and monkeys. J Hygiene 72:205–211, 1974.

30. Emmelot CH, van der Waaij D: The dose at which neomycin and polymyxin B can be applied for selective decontamination of the digestive tract in mice. J Hygiene 84:331–340, 1980.

31. van der Waaij D, Aberson J, Thijm HA, Welling GW: The screening of four aminoglycosides in the selective decontamintion of the digestive tract in mice. Infection 10:35–40, 1982.

32. van der Waaij D, Hofstra W, Wiegersma N: Effect of beta-lactam antibiotics on the resistance of the digestive tract of mice to colonization. J Infect Dis 146:417–422, 1982.

33. Wiegersma N, Jansen G, van der Waaij D: Effect of twelve antimicrobial drugs on the colonization resistance of the digestive tract of mice and on endogenous potentially pathogenic bacteria. J Hygiene 88:221–230, 1982.

34. van der Waaij D, de Vries-Hospers HG, Welling GW: Selective decontamination of the digestive tract with aztreonam: A study in ten human volunteers. In: Proc 13th Internatl Congress Chemotherapy, Vienna, Austria (8/28–9/2/83), Spitzy KH, Karrer KP (eds), 1983.

35. Mulder JG, Wiersma WE, Welling GW, van der Waaij D: Low dose tobramycin treatment for selective decontamination of the digestive tract: A study in human volunteers. J Antimicrob Ther, 13:495–504, 1984.

36. Sleijfer DT, Mulder NH, de Vries-Hospers HG, Fidler V, Nieweg HO, van der Waaij D, van Saene HKF: Infection prevention in granulocytopenic patients by selective decontamination of the digestive tract. Eur J Cancer 16:859–869, 1980.

37. de Vries-Hospers HG, Sleijfer DT, Mulder NH, van der Waaij D, Nieweg HO, van Saene

HKF: Bacteriological aspects of selective decontamination of the digestive tract as a method of infection prevention in granulocytopenic patients. Antimicrob Agents Chemother 19:813–820, 1981.

38. Knothe H: The effect of a combined preparation of trimthoprim and sulfamethoxazole following short-term and long-term administration on the flora of the human gut. Chemotherapy 18:285–296, 1973.

39. Wade JC, de Jongh CA, Newman KA, Crowley J, Wiernik PH, Schimpff SC: Selective antimicrobial modulation as prophylaxis against infection during granulocytopenia: Trimethoprim-sulfamethoxazole versus nalidixic acid. J Infect Dis 147:624–634, 1983.

40. Rozenberg-Arska M, Dekker AW, Verhoef J: Colistin and trimethoprimsulfamethoxazole for the prevention of infection in patients with acute non-lymphocytic leukemia. Decrease in the emergence of resistant bacteria. Infection 11:167–169, 1983.

41. Hughes WT, Kuhn S, Chandhary S, Feldman S, Verzosa M, Aur RJA, Pratt CH, George SL: Successful chemoprophylaxis for pneumocystis carinii pneumonitis. N Engl J Med 297:1419–1426, 1977.

42. Holdeman LV, Cato EP, Moore WEC: Quantitative estimates of anaerobes: Direct microscopic and cultural counts. In: *Anaerobic Laboratory Manual* (4th edition), Holdeman LV, Moore WEC (eds), Virginia Polytechnique Institute and State University Anaerobe Laboratory, 1978, p 124.

43. Welling GW, Groen G: Beta-aspartylglycine, A substance unique to faecal contents of germ-free and antibiotic treated mice. Biochem J 175:807–812, 1978.

44. Welling GW: Beta-aspartylglycine, An indicator of decreased colonization resistance? In: New Criteria for Antimicrobial Therapy, van der Waaij D, verhoef J (eds), Amsterdam-Oxford, Excerpta Medica, 1979, pp 65–71.

45. Welling GW: Comparison of methods for the determination of beta-aspartylglycine in fecal supernatants of leukemic patients treated with antimicrobial agents. J Chrom 232:55–62, 1982.

46. de Vries-Hospers HG, van der Waaij D: Salivary concentrations of amphotericin B following its use as an oral lozenge. Infection 8:63–65, 1980.

47. de Vries-Hospers HG, Mulder NH, Sleijfer DT, van Saene HKF: The effect of amphotericin B on the presence and number of candida cells in oropharynx of neutropenic leukemia patients. Infection 8:63–65, 1983.

48. Hansen I, Nielsen ML, Bertelsen S: Trimethoprim in human saliva, bronchial secretions, and lung tissue. Acta Pharmac Tox 32:337–344, 1973.

49. Kurrle E, Bhaduri S, Krieger D, Pflieger H, Heimpel H: Antimicrobial prophylaxis in acute leukemia: Prospective randomized study comparing two methods of selective decontamination. Klin Wochenschr 61:691–698, 1983.

50. Remmington JS, Schimpff SC: Please don't eat the salads. N Engl J Med 304:433–435, 1981.

51. Meunier-Carpentier F, Snoeck R, Ceuppens AM, Klastersky J: Treatment of oropharyngeal candidiasis in cancer patients. In: Proceedings of 13th International Congress of Chemotherapy (Vienna, Austria), Spitzy KH, Karrer K (eds), 1983, p 40, 14–17.

52. van Saene HKF, Driessen LHHM: Importance of the treatment Staphylococcus aureus carriership in the prevention and therapy of Staphylococcus aureus infections. In: New Criteria for Antimicrobial Therapy, van der Waaij D, Verhoef J (eds), Amsterdam-Oxford, Excerpta Medica, 1979, pp 197–207.

53. Dekker AW, Rozenberg-Arska M, Sixma JJ, Verhoef J: Prevention of infection by trimethoprim-sulfamethoxazole plus amphotericin B in patients with acute non-lymphocytic leukemia. Ann Intern Med 95:555–559, 1981.

54. Guiot HFL, van den Broek PJ, van der Meer JWM, van Furth R: Selective antimicrobial modulation of the intestinal flora of patients with acute non-lymphocytic leukemia: A dou-

ble-blind, placebo-controlled study. J Infect Dis 147:615–623, 1983.

55. Bhaduri S, Kurrle E, Krieger D, Pflieger H, Arnold R, Kubanek B, Heimpel H: Infection prophylaxis in acute leukemia patients. Comparison of selective and total antimicrobial decontamination of gastrointestinal tract. Folia Haematol 109:377–389, 1982.

56. Krieger D, Vanek E, Strekke R: Influence of total and selective decontamination on the aerobic and anaerobic gastrointestinal flora in patients with acute leukemia. In: Recent Advances in Germ-free Research, Sasaki S, Ozawa A, Hashimoto K (eds), Tokyo, Tokai University Press, 1981, pp 715–718.

57. Wilson JM, Huiney DG: Failure of oral trimethoprim-sulfamethoxazole prophylaxis in acute leukemia. N Engl J Med 306:16–20, 1982.

58. Enno A, Darrell J, Hows J, Lank BA, Harding GKM, Ronald AR: Cotrimoxazole for prevention of infection in acute leukemia. Lancet ii:395–397, 1978.

59. Watson JG, Powels RL, Lawson DN, Morgenstern GR, Jameson B, McElwain TJ, Judson D, Lumley H, Kay MEM: Co-trimoxazole versus nonabsorbable antibiotics in acute leukemia. Lancet i:6–9, 1982.

60. Pizzo PA, Robichaud KJ, Edwards BK, Schumaker C, Kramer BS, Johnson A: Oral antibiotic prophylaxis in patients with cancer: A double-blind randomized placebo-controlled trial. J Pediatr 102:125–133, 1983.

61. Weiser B, Lange M, Fialk MA, Singer C, Szatrowski TH, Armstrong D: Prophylactic trimethoprim-sulfamethoxazole during consolidation chemotherapy for acute leukemia: A controlled trial. Ann Intern Med 95:436–438, 1981.

62. Nauseef WM, Maki DG: A study of the value of simple protective isolation in patients with acute granulocytopenia. N Engl J Med 304:448–453, 1981.

63. Postmus PE, de Vries-Hospers HG, Sleijfer DT, van Imhoff GW, Meinesz AF, Vriesendorp R, Mulder NH, de Vries EGE: Failure of selective decontamination of the digestive tract with non-absorbable antibiotics in preventing infections in patients treated with high dose chemotherapy and autologous bone marrow transplantation. In: EORTC Monograph: Autologous Bone Marrow Transplantation in Solid Tumors, McVie JG, Dalesio O, Smith IE, New York, Raven Press, 1984.

64. de Vries-Hospers HG, Hofstra W, Welling GW: The influence of BRL 17421 on the intestinal flora of mice and man: Usefulness for selective decontamination? Abstracts of the 1982 ICAAC Meetings, Number 771, 1982, p 201.

5. Cancer in the Elderly

MONICA B. SPAULDING

INTRODUCTION

Figures obtained in the most recent census indicated that there are approximately 25.5 million people over the age of 65 in United States [1]. With improvements in nutrition, better sanitation, antibiotics, newer drugs and general health care, the average American is living longer: the average life expectancy for a person at age 70 is over 13 years, and at age 80 is 8.2 years. There is every reason to believe that the numbers of 'elderly' individuals in this country will continue to increase as will their requirements for health care. Cancer is an important cause of this need for health care, as 50% of the malignancies in the United States are diagnosed in those over age of 65, (Table 1) [2] a number estimated as over 500,000 in 1982 [3].

Many authors have speculated on the causes for the increased incidence of cancer with age, citing decreased immune surveillance [4], cumulative exposure to carcinogens [5], dietary habits including both an absence of such protection as offered by Vitamin A [6] or selenium [7] and an increase

Table 1.

Types of Cancer	Incidence 1983	Age at Greatest Risk
Leukemia	23,000	More than half over age 60
Breast	114,900	> age 50
Uterine	55,000	Peak age 50–64
Stomach	24,500	> age 50
Colorectal	126,000	> age 50
Prostate	75,000	> age 50
Oral Cavity	27,100	Peak age 60–70
Lung	135,000	Peak age 50–64

From Cancer Facts and Figures 1983, ACS and Cancer: Principles and Practice DeVita.

Higby, DJ (ed), The Cancer Patient and Supportive Care. ISBN 0-89838-690-X.
© 1985, Martinus Nijhoff Publishers, Boston. Printed in The Netherlands.

in dietary fats [8] and finally hormonal changes [9] as being reasons for this increased susceptibility. It is, of course, unlikely that there is a single explanation for the high incidence but rather a complex set of factors which result in the cellular changes necessary for the development of neoplasia. Separate from their possible etiologic importance, factors such as the status of the immune system, the quality of nutrition, and hormonal status become important when an elderly person develops cancer and therapeutic decisions must be made. A cancer developing in an older patient raises therapeutic social and moral issues that differ from issues raised in the young. For many reasons adequate consideration may not be given to appropriate cancer management.

The types of cancer seen in the elderly are frequently those which are surgically curable if detected at an early stage. Early detection is difficult in the elderly, possibly because the available screening programs are limited [10] and certainly because the multiple medical problems of the older individual may mask and confuse symptomatology. Moreover, diagnostic tests are more difficult to perform in the elderly who become less mobile and have more discomfort lying on hard surfaces. Even though associated medical problems of the elderly do increase the risks of major surgery, increasing the patient's life span by successful tumor resection must still be weighed against the pain, discomfort, and shortened life span associated with the untreated tumor. In those tumors which are not surgically treatable, there is concern that chemotherapeutic agents, although offering potential cure in some tumor types and significant palliation in others, offer such toxicity to the elderly that this treatment is not tolerable. Because many large-scale chemotherapy studies exclude patients on the basis of age alone, there is relatively little objective data to support the common suspicion of increased toxicity due to age alone.

Decisions concerning cancer treatment in the elderly can only be made with a knowledge of the natural history of the tumor in question, of its stage when diagnosed and with an appreciation for the treatment and its associated morbidity.

This chapter consists of two parts. Part 1 considers the three modalities of therapy (surgery, radiation therapy, and chemotherapy) with specific reference to whether the elderly tolerates them less well than the younger population. Part II discusses some specific tumors common in the older population, the special problems they present, some of the options in management and their results.

PART I: TREATMENT MODALITIES IN THE ELDERLY

The modalities of surgery, radiation, and chemotherapy may be used individually or in combination, in the treatment of malignant disease. Combined modality therapy, the planned use of chemotherapy plus surgery or surgery plus radiation or a similar combination is a new concept. While it holds promise for the management of many tumors, the majority of data concerning the morbidity of treatment in the elderly concerns a single modality.

Surgery
The most common modality used in the treatment of cancer is surgery. Although some cancers are not amenable to surgical cure by their nature, such as leukemias and most lymphomas, and many are not curable because they are detected at a late stage when curative resection is not possible, more tumors are cured by the appropriate utilization of surgical resection than by any of the other modalities. Whether the surgery is done in an attempt for cure or whether it is done for palliation, the ability of the elderly patient to tolerate the procedure is of overwhelming importance. In general, surgery in the elderly must be performed with caution [11]. Mortality rates increase directly with age, being approximately 11.3% in those between ages 60–70 and rising to 15.1% between age 70–89. In those over age 90, mortality rates are over 20%. These numbers were determined by Linn et al. who reviewed 108 papers written about surgical mortality in the aged [12]. It is important to note that the risk of an elective procedure is generally one third or less than the risk of an emergency operation.

The major risk associated with emergency procedures in the elderly is not surprising. Renal, cardiovascular, and pulmonary disease are common; the devastation caused by a sudden hemorrhage or perforated viscus to an already compromised system can be overwhelming. Various authors have shown that there is a significant reduction in mortality, if the patient can be prepared for surgery [13, 14, 15]. Preparation involves transfusions, rehydration, and frequently, hyperalimentation to improve the patient's physical condition before he goes to the operating room. Although this approach may delay surgery by even several weeks, the reduction in peri-operative complications, sepsis and death in properly prepared patients is well worth the time [13].

In reviewing the outcome of surgery in the elderly, it is clear that each patient must be evaluated in terms of his physiologic and functional state rather than simply using age per se in estimating operative risk. The preoperative evaluation scale used by anesthetists is useful in that regard [16]. Djokovic looked at the outcome of 500 patients over age 80 who underwent major surgery. Those patients who were class 2 i.e. mild to moderate systemic disturbance caused either by the condition to be treated surgically or by other pathophysiologic processes, had a mortality rate less than 1%. The rate increased progressively to 25% of those judged to be class 4, i.e. a patient with severe systemic disorder that is already life threatening and not always correctable by the operative procedure. Several other conclusions could be drawn from the report. Intra-arterial pressure monitoring was important as it afforded early recognition of problems such as hypotension or reduction in blood volume. The authors also recommended prolonged constant volume ventilation postoperatively and continued monitoring of arterial blood gases for several days after surgery to reduce problems associated with the postoperative period.

A major pitfall in the management of elderly patients with cancer is the failure to consider treatment options. Age alone should not be a deterrent to the performance of a curative procedure. Surgery can also significantly palliate many patients with cancer. Proper preparation and patient monitoring both during and after the procedure can make surgery a viable treatment option to prolong life and improve its quality.

Radiation Therapy

Radiation therapy is the second modality useful in the treatment of cancer. It is curative for certain well defined tumors such as small laryngeal carcinomas and localized Hodgkin's Disease, but its greatest usefulness in the elderly population is palliation. Radiation therapy is almost always a locally directed modality, non-invasive, and free from those risks associated with surgery. It does not have the systemic effects associated with chemotherapy but it does cause a certain amount of toxicity to normal tissues. With careful localization of the target to be radiated and a policy of treating as small a volume as possible, the risk to normal tissues is reduced. While there is no suggestion that the tolerance of normal tissues to radiation therapy decreases with age, there are some recognizable radiation reactions that may be more difficult to manage in the elderly. A realization that these might occur, allows the physician to be better prepared to manage them. For example, radiation treatment of prostatic carcinoma or advanced carcinoma of the cervix results in damage to the normal intestine. The more common reactions are tenesmus, diarrhea and bleeding but rarely there may be such serious narrowing of the bowel lumen that a colostomy is necessary. Radiation of lung cancer can cause radiation pneumonitis which may disastrously affect pulmonary status in a patient with already compromised lung function. An awareness of these complications should influence the planning of radiation therapy, whether for cure or palliation.

In many settings, radiation therapy has great usefulness. It gives relief of bone pain secondary to metastatic cancer. It may be used to stop bleeding from unresectable lesions of the lung or the rectum. Ulcerative unresectable lesions of the breast may be treated with radiation therapy to control growth, pain, bleeding and even a foul-smelling discharge.

Because it is relatively free of systemic toxicity and is noninvasive, there is a tendency to propose palliative radiation therapy to the elderly rather than to consider curative approaches. The expediency of this approach must be consciously avoided when weighing therapeutic risks and benefits.

Chemotherapy

The third and most recently developed modality in the treatment of cancer is chemotherapy; many, however question its use in the elderly. The upper age limit in most formal chemotherapy protocols restricts participation to those under age 65 or age 70, or dose modifications solely on age may be mandated, e.g., the Milan adjuvant study for breast cancer[17]. Pharmacologic studies of the action and metabolism of many drugs have shown changes in distribution[18], alterations in rates of drug clearance[19] and enhancement of drug binding to receptors[20], in the older patient. Although similar studies have not been done with cancer drugs, there is concern that drug disposition and metabolism might differ in the elderly as compared to younger individuals. The illnesses associated with aging and the multiplicity of other drugs which the older patient may be taking also increase the concern about the use of chemotherapeutic agents in the elderly. Despite such concern, there are relatively few studies, which specifically address the above issues.

Some single agent drug trials have suggested age-related toxicity. Bleomycin-induced pulmonary toxicity was initially reported to occur with greater frequency in the older individual: Haas et al. reported that the incidence of pulmonary fibrosis was twice as frequent in those over the age of 70 versus those less than 70[21]. However those over 70 are more likely to have significant pre-existing pulmonary damage, and whether there is an increased risk to the elderly for bleomycin when pulmonary function is normal is not presently known.

Doxorubicin is cardiotoxic and the risk of developing drug related congestive heart failure increases with age[22]. Previous cardiac disease and hypertension are known to be factors which increase the risk. Pre-existent but undiagnosed cardiac disease cannot be excluded as causing the age related sensitivity to doxorubicin. Following dose guidelines as well as monitoring left venticular function by measuring the systolic time interval or the cardiac ejection fraction are reasonable ways to minimize the risk with administration of this or other cardiotoxic drugs.

Neurotoxicity is a significant side effect associated with procarbazine[23], vindesine [24] and, in particular, vincristine [25]. The neurotoxicity of vincristine has been studied in greatest detail and appears to be due to a direct effect on peripheral nerve fibers with loss of myelin and axonal degeneration. These have been anecdotal reports of severe neurotoxicity developing in patients with pre-existing neuropathies, suggesting that the drug should be used with caution in such patients. The drug has, however, been used without significant problem in diabetics and alcoholics with peripheral neuropathy and there is no data to support restricting its use solely based on age.

Most tumors are treated with combination chemotherapy, which generally yields higher response rates than single agent therapy but also gives more reason for concern about drug toxicity. The Eastern Cooperative Oncology Group reviewed the incidence of drug toxicity in elderly patients who were receiving drugs for metastatic lung, colorectal or breast cancer [26]. The patients reviewed were over age 70 in the case of the lung and colorectal cancer and over 60 in those cases of breast cancer. There were 2981 patients analyzed and there was no difference in the incidence or severity of toxicity in comparison of the 'elderly' patients to younger patients. These 'elderly' had not been selected in a way that would favor them and a comparison of performance status, previous therapy and extent of disease showed no difference between the two groups. Furthermore there was no evidence that dose modification in the elderly patients occurred more frequently. These findings are summarized in Table 2.

Although there is widespread belief that age alone increases the risk of prohibitive toxicity from chemotherapy, there is little evidence to support that belief. When a patient with cancer is a candidate for chemotherapy, the same physiologic guidelines used in younger individuals should be used. These patients with a history of congestive heart failure or evidence of poor left ventricular function are at risk when given doxorubicin no matter what age. Similarly those with obstructive pulmonary disease are at increased

Table 2. Percent with severe or worse toxicity from chemotherapy

	Hematologic		Comiting		Infection		Neurologic	
Lung	<70	>70	<70	>70	<70	>70	<70	>70
Patient	14.5	11.5	7.2	6.8	1.2	2.0		
Colorectal								
Patient	19.6	23.1	7.2	6.9	1.2	0.6	1.5	2.3
Breast	<60	>60	<60	>60	<60	>60	<60	>60
Patient	28.3	36.7	10.2	8.5	3.8	5.6	4.4	2.8

From *Cancer: Principles and Practice* (DeVita)

risk when given bleomycin, as are patients with renal insufficiency when given platinol. As with all patients the risks associated with chemotherapy must be balanced against potential benefit, particularily the likelihood of cure or significant palliation.

PART II: SPECIFIC TUMORS IN WHICH AGE APPEARS TO PLAY A ROLE IN ETIOLOGY OR TREATMENT

Based on natural history, the tumors seen in the elderly can be grouped into three classes. The first, the epithelial tumors, include tumors of the lung, gastro-intestinal tract, and head and neck region and show a steady increase in incidence with age substitute semi-colon; this may be due to cumulative carcinogen exposure.

Lung tumors as well as tumors arising from the head and neck area are known to be carcinogen-induced: the risk of developing a lung tumor is directly related to duration of tobacco exposure [27], and a similar association can be shown for tobacco and alcohol together in the case of head and neck tumors [28]. The etiology of gastro-intestinal cancer is not as clear but there is suggestion that high fat intake [29], caffeine [30] and nitrites [31] may play a role in the development of colon, pancreatic and gastric cancer respectively. In general, the best chance for cure in these tumors is if they are recognized early, when surgical management is feasible. Curative surgery may offer greater risks for the elderly than for the younger individual but the risks, although real, have sometimes been exaggerated. Furthermore palliative treatments are particularly important for these tumors.

The second group is those tumors in whom hormonal factors are important not only in their etiology but in their management. Most important in this group are breast cancer and prostatic cancer. Surgery, radiation therapy, and hormonal agents as well as the usual chemotherapeutic agents may all be useful in these patients. Age becomes a factor in choosing the modality used in these tumors.

Lastly there are a variety of tumor types which occur in all age groups but which appear to be different in their clinical behavior when seen in the older individual. These include Hodgkin's Disease, thyroid carcinoma, and the acute leukemias. Although the management of these tumors in the older individual does not differ from the management in the younger, the clinical course may be so different as to suggest a different etiology; there may also be enhanced toxicity from the treatment for the previously mentioned reasons.

The following section reviews the information available on the management of the specific types of tumors in the elderly.

EPITHELIAL TUMORS

1. *Cancer of the Lung*

Bronchogenic carcinoma is a leading cause of cancer deaths in males in the U.S. and second only to breast cancer in females as the cause of cancer deaths [2]. The incidence rises with age in this tumor, as might be expected in a cancer in whom prolonged and repeated exposure to a known carcinogen is the common cause. Lung tumors may be classified histologically as either small cell, in which surgery is generally contra-indicated and the treatment of choice is radiation therapy and chemotherapy, and non-small cell carcinomas, in which surgery is the only modality offering curative potential.

Three-fourths of all lung cancers are non-small cell in type and the guidelines for surgical resection are well established. The tumor's extent in the chest must be such that a pneumonectomy or less can remove all the tumor and the patient must not have metastatic disease. The intrathoracic stage of lung cancer is determined by tumor size and nodal spread as indicated by chest X-ray, tomography, mediastinoscopy and occasionally gallium scanning. In general, patients with Stage I and II disease are considered resectable. The limits of staging are such, however, that approximately half of the patients believed to be resectable on the basis of preoperative evaluation will be found to be unresectable at the time of surgery because of bulky mediastinal spread of tumor or tumor invastion of the chest wall, great vessels or pericardium.

When resectability has been established, consideration must be given to the patient's ability to tolerate surgery. At any age and with any tumor, other medical problems, such as cardiac disease, markedly increase the risk of surgery and problems with anesthesia. The major problem in patients with lung cancer, however, is concern about their postoperative pulmonary reserve. Virtually all patients with lung cancer have diminished pulmonary function before surgery due to the effects of years of cigarette smoking on lung parenchyma. Hypoxemia ($PO_2 < 50$) at rest or with exercise, hypercapnea ($PCO' > 45$ mm Hg) at rest or with exercise or a predicted postresection FEV-1 of < 800 cc have been accepted as criteria for unresectability [32]. In the minds of many however, age by itself is also important and a thoracotomy for lung cancer may be performed reluctantly in those over age 70.

Kirsch et al. reported the results of major pulmonary resection in 75 patients over the age of 70 performed at their institution from 1959 to 1969 [33]. The patients had been staged by standard chest X-rays, tomograms, and bronchoscopy and were felt to have Stage I or II disease. Of these 75, 17 could not have surgery because of associated medical problems and received radiation therapy alone. The median survival of the group receiving radiation therapy was only 7.7 months, with all but one dying of uncontrolled lung cancer. The remaining 58 went to surgery. Fifty-five were resected, 49 undergoing a lobectomy, the remaining six a pneumonectomy. Their overall surgical mortality was 14%. This is somewhat higher than the expected surgical mortality in pulmonary resection of lung cancer but the five-year survival of 30% was quite satisfactory, even when compared to younger patients with lung cancer.

The higher operative mortality rate observed in older individuals has also been substantiated by Weiss, who reported a large retrospective review of surgical results in patients with lung cancer, examining the date of surgery, age at the time of surgery, date of death, and other followup information on 1076 cases operated on in 12 teaching hospitals in the Philadelphia area between 1956 to 1965 [34]. He concluded that the operative mortality increased with age, reaching a high of 19% in males over the age of 70. The five-year survival in this age group of only 11% do not support the results of Kirsch and suggest that resection of lung cancer is not indicated in males over the age of 70. The causes of the high postoperative mortality in the latter study included a variety of factors including peri-operative myocardial infarction, cerebrovascular accidents and pulmonary emboli, but the most frequent was respiratory insufficiency.

There have been two improvements in surgical management which are particularly important in selecting elderly patients for thoracotomy, and which make less applicable the findings of Weiss. The first is the refinement in the pre-operative evaluation of pulmonary function using combined radio-nucleotide perfusion scans [35]. In this evaluation, a patient under-goes routine pulmonary function tests with the spirometer. A perfusion lung scan is then performed, using technetium tetroxide to determine the blood flow to each lung. The post operative pulmonary function can then be pre-dicted by calculating the fraction of radioactivity contributed by the lung contralateral to that containing the tumor. Boysen et al., used this technique to select for thoracotomy 38 high risk patients whose surgery would not have been performed based on the results of routine testing. During the first postoperative year, there was only one death attributable to pulmonary insufficiency, indicating the utility of this type of evaluation [36].

The second important change in operative management concerns the type of surgery done in those patients. The first successful operations for lung cancer were pneumonectomies and many believed that lesser operations were insufficient for cancer. However the loss of functional pulmonary par-enchyma with a pneumonectomy may be prohibitive in the older patient. Jensik et al. have reported their results with a segmental resection of lung cancer [37]. In this procedure, a peripherally located tumor in which there is no hilar or lobar adenopathy is 'wedged' out from the parenchyma. This operation was performed in 118 patients with Stage I lung cancer who were not candidates for bigger operations because of cardiovascular disease, renal disease, previous malignancies or severe chronic obstructive pulmonary disease. The postoperative mortality and morbidity was acceptable and the five-year survival rate was 54%, with the majority of deaths being due to medical illness rather than carcinoma. The other tissue-sparing operation useful in those with pulmonary insufficiency is the sleeve lobectomy, in which a pneumonectomy is avoided in certain patients with proximal lesions of the right bronchus by an anastomosis of the lower lobe to the main stem bronchus. In 1981, Breyer et al. confirmed the usefulness of the operation in the elderly, when they published the results of thoracotomy in 150 patients over the age of 70 [38]. The postoperative mortality rate in this series was only 4% and there was a five-year survival rate of 27% which is comparable to that reported by Kirsh et al. [33]. The major factor contributing to the reduced mortality in their series was the performance of lung-sparing operations whenever possible. Fifty of their patients were treated with a segmental or wedge resection. Thirteen had a sleeve resection only. Only 18 patients required a pneumonectomy. Mortality in those with the pneumonectomy or lobectomy was 5%, whereas it was only 2% of patients undergoing a segmental or subsegmental resection.

The conclusion that can be reached from these studies is that no patient should be denied an attempt at curative surgery on the basis of age alone. Surgically resectable lung lesions in the elderly should be viewed with the same criteria used in the younger patient. When metastases are ruled out, staging with bronchoscopy and mediastinoscopy is necessary to identify those with Stage I and II disease who are then candidates for surgery. With resonable pulmonary functions, a thoracotomy can be performed even in the elderly without undue risk. Furthermore a conservative approach to surgery with a segmental or wedge resection is adequate for many tumors. Finally in situations where a pneumonectomy might seem to be required, the possibility of a lobectomy with a sleeve resection, to maximize residual functioning lung tissue, should be considered. At the present time chemotherapy remains experimental for patients with non-small cell carcinoma. Its use in the older patient depends upon the patient's physiologic condition as well as his and his family's philosophy about cancer treatment.

Small cell carcinoma of the lung is treated primarily by chemotherapy and there are patients with the disease who have been cured by its appropriate and aggressive use. Precisely because of the 'aggressiveness' of chemotherapeutic regimens used effectively in this disease, there is reluctance to use them in the older patient. Clamon et al., however, reported their experience with chemotherapy for small cell carcinoma in 24 patients over the age of

70 [39]. All but two of the patients had other major medical problems including cardiac disease [14]. obstructive lung disease [10], renal insufficiency [4], hypertension [8] and seven had other malignant disorders. The patients received standard chemotherapy with 67% requiring dosage reductions during the course of therapy for various reasons, generally leukopenia. There was one treatment-related death. Treatment results showed a median survival of eight months in those with limited disease, and ten months in those with extensive disease. Placebo-treated patients with small cell carcinoma have a survival of only 3–5 months. The number of patients on this study was small but the minimal toxicity observed and the associated improvement in survival suggests that an upper age limit on protocols should not be accepted *a priori.*

2. *Carcinomas of the Head and Neck*

Cancers of the head and neck, like lung cancers, show a rising incidence with age. The median age for patients with tumors arising in the mouth, pharynx and larynx is 58 years [40], thus about half of the patients with this disease are over the age of 60. Although small lesions are frequently manageable by radiation therapy, more than half require surgery, frequently extensive procedures necessitating reconstruction and radical neck dissections. The patient with head and neck cancer generally is a heavy smoker as well as drinker and not only has reduced pulmonary reserves, but may also have hepatic damage, as well as the other accompaniments of old age, i.e. cardiovascular, cerebrovascular and renal disease. The question arises as to whether these features lead to such an increased risk that curative surgery may not be possible, and less extensive palliative procedures should be the rule.

In 1966, Loewy and Huttner compared the medical problems seen in a group of patients with head and neck over the age of 70 to a similar group between the ages of 55–69 [41]. The number of older patients with cardiovascular and metabolic disease was approximately twice that of the younger group. Pulmonary disease was extremely common in both, although more frequent in the older population. When the incidence of postoperative complications was reviewed, it was not suprising to note that these were more common in the older patients. The peri-operative mortality rate however, was much less than that in comparable patients of the same age group undergoing other types of major surgery. Because of the nature of head and neck surgery, many of the complications associated with surgery on other parts of the body are not seen. Since the abdominal cavity is not entered, nasogastric feeding tubes can be inserted at the time of surgery and enteral fluid and protein repletion can be started within the first 24 hours of surgery.

A tracheostomy is a necessary part of laryngectomy, but a prophylactic tracheostomy is extremely important in the surgical management of the older patient undergoing any major head and neck surgery. The tracheostomy allows for frequent catheter suctioning and assists in clearing the bronchi of secretions. As long ago as 1938, Hayes Martin noted that the most frequent cause of postoperative deaths in older patients with head and neck cancer was pneumonia [42]. He recommended not only doing a prophylactic tracheostomy but leaving the tube in place for one to two weeks after surgery to reduce the likelihood of this complication.

Fifteen years after the review by Loewry and Huttner, Morgan et al. reviewed their experience with head and neck surgery in the elderly [40]. The peri-operative mortality in this study was only 3.5% reflecting a significant advances in medical care. Nevertheless pneumonia remained the chief cause of death, with half of their patients dying from this or other pulmonary complications.

It would appear that major head and neck surgery in the elderly carries an acceptable risk with fewer potential complications than in surgery done in the thoracic or abdominal cavity. A full medical workup prior to surgery is essential to identify medical problems, and these should be corrected as well as possible before surgery. If the medical problem is stable and unlikely to improve with time, it is reasonable to proceed with surgery if that would result in cure or significant palliation. Untreated or inadequately palliated head and neck cancer leads to starvation or asphyxiation as a cause of death and the risk of surgery will generally be the lesser evil.

3. Carcinoma of the Stomach

Although gastric carcinoma has been decreasing in incidence in this country, it remains the seventh leading cause of cancer death (fifth in men and eighth in women) [2]. At any rate, gastric carcinoma is extremely lethal, with five-year survivals of less than 10% [44].

The problem with gastric carcinoma is the fact that symptoms are rarely noted until the tumor is large enough to be felt or there is enough local extension to cause pain or symptoms of obstruction. Of 201 patients seen at the Massachusetts General Hospital with gastric carcinoma, three-fourths had lymph node spread at the time of diagnosis and one third had peritoneal implants [45]. One fourth had presented with a palpable abdominal mass. Ninety-two of the patients underwent operations that were felt to be potentially curable, but only 22 of these survived five years. No patient who underwent a less than curative operation survived five years. The authors concluded that any patient fit for surgery should be explored. Distal gastrectomies done for lesions in the distal stomach had the best prognosis, with a 47% five-year survival. Total gastrectomies frequently required removal of the spleen, pancreatic tail and mesentery. This operation had a 10% mortality and only a 16% five-year survival.

Bittner recently reviewed the results of surgery for carcinoma of the stomach in a series of 88 patients over the age of 70 [46]. Twenty-four required a total gastrectomy, with an operative mortality of 28%. Those patients who could be treated with a distal gastrectomy fared better, with an operative mortality of 16%. The major cause of postoperative mortality was pneumonia (a complication that might be lessened with aggressive attention to pulmonary care including tracheostomy for management of secretions, if necessary (*vide supra*). Forty-one percent of their patients were alive at two years.

In spite of the high operative mortality in gastric carcinoma, there should be an attempt to relieve symptoms even if only by palliative surgery. Stern et al. showed that by doing a subtotal or total gastrectomy in those with advanced carcinoma, survival was improved from 7 months to 19.4 months in patients with nodal spread at the time of surgery (Stage III disease) [47]. In 89 Stage IV patients (distant metastases present) survival was improved from 5.6 to 15.5 months. Doing a major palliative resection did not add to operative mortality or morbidity but certainly improved the quality of life. Presumably the prolongation of survival in the resected group was due to the removal of potential sites of hemorrhage, obstruction and perforation.

4. *Carcinoma of the Colon and Rectum*

Unlike gastric carcinoma, colon carcinoma continues to increase in frequency in this country and is presently the second leading cause of cancer deaths, second to lung in males and breast in females [2].

The mean age of incidence of colon carcinoma is 65; clinical studies show that the incidence of carcinoma in those under the age of 40 is 5 per 100,000 whereas it is 300 per 100,000 in those over 80 [48].

The presenting symptoms of colon carcinoma in the elderly are similar to those in the younger population. Unfortunately however, the symptoms, such as fatigue, change in bowel habits, or weakness may easily be attributed to age and associated illness. Adam et al. noted that the average delay between the onset of symptoms and diagnosis was nine months in patients over the age of 80 with colorectal carcinoma [49]. A similar sutdy showed that the average delay in seeking medical care and diagnosis in younger patients with colorectal carcinoma was only 3 months [49].

Particularly in the elderly, the diagnosis may not be made until a catastrophic event such as hemorrhage, obstruction or perforation occurs. Emergency surgery done in these patients is particularly hazardous. They may have anemia, hypovolemia, or septicemia in addition to their long-standing co-existing medical problems. Boyd reviewed the pre-existing conditions which might increase the risk of colorectal surgery in the elderly and found that the presence of two or more medical problems doubled the mortality rate for emergency operations as opposed to elective procedures [14]. The pre-operative conditions examined included cardiovascular disease, pulmonary factors such as previous lung resection, chronic obstructive pulmonary disease or pneumonia, renal disease manifested by an increased serum creatinine, metabolic abnormalities, hepatic dysfunction, and nutritional deficiencies. Twenty-five percent of the patients between the age of 60–69, and 41% of those over 80, had two or more major pre-existing medical problems. Thus the decline in survival time in older patients with colon carcinoma is due to both a delay in diagnosis and the increased surgical risk associated primarily with emergency operations.

In spite of these figures, all authors agree that every attempt should be made to do curative operations in older patients with this diagnosis. Careful pre-operative evaluation accompanied by correction of existing problems can be shown to reduce operative mortality as seen in the difference between elective and emergency surgery. Kragelung et al. reviewed the mortality and morbidity occurring in the elderly patients in two different time periods, 1950 to 1964 and 1965 to 1975, to determine whether improvements in medical care would mean an improvement in the results of an elective resection. They found that operative mortality decreased significantly in carcinoma of the rectum from 36% to 15% in those over age 75. There was no significant change, however, in those with carcinoma of the colon [50].

There is a role for conservative management of colorectal carcinoma for those patients who cannot immediately tolerate a colectomy. In the case of colon carcinoma, a palliative diversion or bypass improves the quality of remaining life and prevents catastrophic complications such as obstruction or perforation. It is simpler to do a diversion than a total colectomy. In high risk patients with rectal carcinoma however, the rectal lesion may continue to be a source of blood loss or foul-smelling mocous discharge, as well as a cause of obstructive symptoms. Electrocoagulation as a means of treating these symptoms yields good results [51]. Gingold has used this method as the sole treatment for elderly patients with rectal carcinoma who could not medically tolerate conventional surgery or who were felt to be unable to manage a colostomy. Although his report involved a relatively small number of patients, the results were quite good [52].

5. Carcinoma of the Pancreas

There are fewer age-related decisions to be made in pancreatic carcinoma because the overall results of treatment are poor at any age. Sixty to eighty percent of these tumors are unresectable at the time of diagnosis. The diagnosis tends to be made late because of the nonspecific symptoms and the inadequacy of diagnostic techniques for detection of small lesions. The procedure of choice in resectable carcinoma of the pancreas is probably a radical pancreatoduodenectomy (Whipple procedure) which has a high morbidity and a mortality ranging from 5–30% [52b]. The risk of such surgery is higher in the elderly with their associated medical problems and its use must be weighed with caution. Out of 64 patients with pancreatic carcinoma who underwent such surgery, only 15% were alive at three years and less than 5% at five years [53]. Because of these poor surgical results, palliation is important.

Jaundice and severe pruritis secondary to obstruction of the biliary tree from pancreatic cancer was a symptom which was formerly relieved by operative bypass. The risk of bypass in an elderly patient who is sick and frequently malnourished is significant. Endoscopic placement of catheters for decompression has lessened if not eliminated the need for this operation.

Radiation therapy has been recommended for palliation but when delivered to the upper abdomen, there are many radiation-sensitive organs (the small intestine, stomach, kidney, liver and spinal cord) in the radiation port. The dose necessary (4000–6000 R) is unlikely to be delivered without side effects. This should be considered in planning treatment for the older patient.

HORMONE DEPENDENT TUMORS

The next group of tumors in the elderly are the adenocarcinomas which arise in hormone-responsive tissues, (the prostate, breast and corpus uteri). Each of these tumor types is much more common in those over the age of 50 and each has the potential of excellent palliation with the proper use of hormonal agents. An understanding of the of these tumors is important in the decision as to when to apply the less toxic hormonal therapy as opposed to therapeutic modalities which despite higher toxicity, may be indicated in some situations.

1. *Carcinoma of the Prostate*
Carcinoma of the prostate is presently the second most common malignancy in males in the United States and is particularly common in those over the age of 60. It is increasing in frequency in the United States primarily because the age to which the average American survives is increasing. Just as this tumor increases in frequency with each decade, the prognosis also appears to change with succeeding decades.

Halbert and Schmalhorst performed careful sections on the prostates of

100 consecutive deceased veterans between the ages of 70 and 79. Only two of these patients had known carcinoma before death but 39 additional tumors were found [54]. In a similar study, Hirst and Bergman performed serial sections on the prostates of 39 males who died after the age of 80 [55]. Twenty-one were found to contain tumors, an incidence of 53.8%. Interestingly, if one divided the patients according to age groups, prostatic cancer was found in 42% of the patients between age 80 and 84; 71% of these between 85 and 89, and 80% of the patients over age 90. The incidence in patients under age 50 is less than 4% [56]. Despite the high incidence in older males, it has been estimated that of 100 patients with carcinoma of the prostate, only seven will die of it; thus it seems that there is a tendency to latency (benignity) which increases with age. Although the prognosis of prostatic cancer is poor for the patient under the age of 60, it is quite good for those over the age of 70. In those over 80, is similar to that general population [57].

Besides age, the stage of the disease is the most important factor determining prognosis and management. Stage A is the clinically inapparent prostatic lesion which is found incidently at the time of a transurethral prostatectomy or at the time of autopsy. In the older patient, who is without symptoms, no therapy other than repeated observation is necessary.

Although rectal examinations detect prostate carcinoma (Stage B) in asymptomatic patients, few cases are actually identified in this way. The majority of patients present with symptoms either of local disease with obstruction, hematuria, or dysuria or of disseminated disease with metastases. In fact, few patients who present with local symptoms truly have local disease. Stage B carcinoma (e.g. localized to the prostate) accounts for less than 10% of newly diagnosed cases. Most patients with local symptoms have Stage C carcinoma with local extension of tumor through the capsule of the prostate into the surrounding periprostatic fat, bladder, or seminal vesicles, or asymptomatic distant spread. Stage D carcinoma includes those with lymphatic spread (D1) and those (D2) with spread to the bone and other tissues. The spread of prostatic cancer to pelvic, iliac and para-aortic nodes often causes no symptoms. Although bone scans and bone marrow aspirates are effective ways of identifying patients with Stage D2 disease, there is no easy way to define Stage D1 disease short of exploratory laparotomy. Lymphangiography has been used but a high rate of false negatives makes this test less than ideal [58]. Unfortunately the majority of patients who are felt clinically to have Stage B and C disease and thus to be treatable by locally directed surgery or radiation therapy, actually have metastases to the lymph nodes, and are thus not curable. This fact plus the apparently less aggressive nature of prostatic cancer in the elderly may affects decisions regarding therapy.

There is no question that the presence of symptoms due to prostatic carcinoma requires therapy. Patients with Stage D2 carcinoma at the time of diagnosis generally come to a physician's attention because of pain due to bony involvement. The mainstay for systemic therapy of metastatic prostatic carcinoma is withdrawal of androgens either by an orchiectomy or by administration of estrogens which results in inhibition of release of luteinizing hormone, in turn reducing testosterone production. Such therapy results in relief of bone pain, shrinkage of the primary tumor and its metastases, improvement in the hemoglobin level and a generally increased sense of well being.

There appears to be no difference in the degree of response obtained by either estrogen therapy or orchiectomy, and estrogen therapy, being less invasive, is generally preferred. Diethyl stilbesterol (DES) (1 mgm/day) has been shown to result in a tumor response equivalent to that obtained by larger doses and causes few side effects. Although obtaining a response does not appear to depend on absolute suppression of testosterone secretion, many investigators prefer to use 3 mgm/day which lowers serum testosterone to castrate levels, yet spares the patient the cardiovascular side-effects associated with larger doses [59].

If the patient has severe obstructive symptoms associated with the primary tumor as well as systemic spread, an orchiectomy may be preferred to oral estrogen therapy because the response is more rapid. Patients who have such severe cardiovascular disease that they cannot tolerate even minimal fluid retention associated with the estrogen administration, as well as unreliable patients who may not take their daily oral medication, are also candidates for orchiectomy.

In the patients with apparently localized carcinoma of the prostate (no evidence of spread to bones by X-rays, scans or the bone marrow aspiration and biopsy) management at any age is less than satisfactory, as suggested by the many approaches to treatment of local tumor, including radical prostatectomy, brachy radiotherapy with 125 iodine implantation, and external radiotherapy to a total prostatic dose of 7000 R. Kagan and Hinty concluded 'it is apparent that many different therapies are dispensed to reasonably comparable clinical states with what seemingly are not very disparate results in terms of life span' [60]. It is important to treat patients with whatever therapy best maintains a good quality of life.

A radical prostatectomy has been used most often for patients with Stage B and C disease (less than 10–20 percent of all). The operation has a mortality rate of less than 1%. All patients are impotent following the operation, although an effective penile prosthesis can lessen the seriousness of this complication. Another serious complication however is incontinence, occurring in up to 20% of the patients. Boxer et al. reported a five-year cure rate of 82% for Stage A and B tumors and 67% for Stage C tumors following radical prostatectomy [61]. Less than 30% of his patients were over 65 and only 10% were over 70. The high complication rate, however, makes the procedure of questionable benefit in older patients who may have a biologically less active tumor.

Radiation therapy appears to be very useful in controlling symptoms of locally invasive prostatic carcinoma and survival statistics are comparable to those achieved with surgery. Bagshaw et al. reported a 70% five-year survival in patients with Stage B disease treated with external beam radiation therapy to the prostate [62]. The radiation dose of 7000 to 7600 rads took seven and a half weeks to deliver and was also associated with side effects such as diarrhea, rectal urgency, dysuria, and frequency. Persistence of symptoms beyond the course of treatment was frequent, although the majority resolved within one year. Radiation therapy plays a most important role in the management of localized painful bone lesions. Doses of 3500 to 4000 rads will achieve significant, if not absolute, pain relief with few side effects.

In summary, retrospective and autopsy studies show that prostatic carcinoma is extremely common in elderly males but rarely symptomatic. When diagnosed because of symptoms, attention should be directed towards relieving symptoms in the method most free of unpleasant side effects. Systemic therapy directed at reducing testosterone levels is extremely effective in relieving bone pain and reducing tumor masses. Surgery and radiation therapy are effective in relieving symptoms of obstructive uropathy but both are associated with side effects which may be significant in the older patient. Since both surgery and radiation therapy results in similar survival, the decision as to which modality to employ in the older patient must be based on consideration of side effects.

2. Carcinoma of the Breast

Carcinoma of the breast shows a steady increase in incidence with age. For several reasons, it does not create as many problems in management as do other tumors arising in the elderly. A mastectomy is done without entering body cavities and thus does not result in the type of operative morbidity seen with abdominal or thoracic operations. The surgical mortality in this operation is that of the anesthetic, which is quite small, and the complications are generally only those related to wound healing.

The radical mastectomy was once considered the operation of choice for localized, breast cancer. However, although definitive studies are still in progress, current thinking is that less radical procedures, e.g. lumpectomy, simple mastectomy, are quite suitable in many cases. Older women have been shown to tolerate radical mastectomy [63, 64, 65] so there is no question as to their ability to tolerate less extensive procedures.

One of the major problems in dealing with breast cancer is that recurrence may be delayed for many years after the original mastectomy. The likelihood of recurrence can be predicted by the size of the primary tumor and the status of the axillary nodes [66]. In the post-menopausal female, this likelihood of recurrence brings up two questions of management. The first is what to do if and when metastatic disease develops.

Like prostatic carcinoma, breast carcinoma may respond to hormonal manipulation. The presence and quantity of estrogen and progesterone receptors in the breast tumor allows the physician to determine whether hormonal therapy is likely to be effective. Unlike prostatic carcinoma, there are many options for hormonal manipulation including the use of anti-estrogens, progesterone, estrogens, androgens and amino glutethimide. Although the patient with prostatic cancer is unlikely to have further response to hormonal manipulation after failing on estrogen therapy, patients with breast cancer are very likely to respond to second and even subsequent hormonal manipulations. This ability to have repeated responses is of significant benefit in the elderly patient, as the side effects of hormonal manipulation tend to be minimal and not age-related. These drugs can also reproduce the effect of surgical ablating procedures such as oophrectomy and adrenalectomy, avoiding the morbidity associated with those more formidable operations.

In the case of the elderly patient with metastatic disease who either fails to respond to hormonal manipulation, is refractory after an initial response, or whose tumor has absent estrogen or progesterone receptors, other therapeutic decisions must be made. When there is localized, symptomatic disease, such as painful bone lesion, radiation therapy generally brings prompt relief without undue toxicity.

If the patient has widespread metastases, she is a candidate for chemotherapy. Objective responses can be achieved in 45–60% of patients using regimens such as methotrexate, 5-fluorouracil (CMF) or cyclophosphamide, adriamycin, and 5-fluorouracil (CAF), or cyclophosphamide, 5-fluorouracil methotrexate, vincristine, and prednisone (CMFVP) [67]. The decision to use chemotherapeutic agents in the older patient with metastatic disease must take into account the need to relieve symptoms and the toxicity of the chemotherapy. Survival of patients with metastatic breast cancer has not changed significantly since the introduction of combination chemotherapy [68]. In the period before combination chemotherapy was available, the percent alive one year following recurrence was 63.3% and 6.6% at one and five years respectively. Following the introduction of combination chemotherapy, the percent alive at one and five years respectively was only 69.5%

and 7.9%. Thus it is probably only useful to treat symptomatic patients with metastatic breast carcinoma with chemotherapy, and then to treat only if the toxicity from the chemotherapy warrants the benefit.

The second important question in the management of patients with breast cancer pertains to the use of adjuvant chemotherapy. The rationale for post-mastectomy chemotherapy is based on the data previously mentioned. Patients with involved axillary nodes have a high incidence of relapse: effective combination chemotherapy is available for patients with known metastatic disease. There have been a multitude of studies of adjuvant therapy in both pre and postmenopausal patients. The present studies indicate now that the administration of adjuvant chemotherapy to postmenopausal women has no advantage. Studies continue however, and enrollment of an older patient in such a study requires a judgment regarding benefit and toxicity, a decision which can only be made on the basis of other health problems faced by the patient, her life expectancy, tumor status, and the toxicity of the drug regimen involved.

TUMORS WITH A DIFFERENT BEHAVIOR IN THE ELDERLY

The third group of tumors are those which appear to have a somewhat different pattern of behavior in the elderly than in the younger patient. Chief among these are Hodgkin's Disease, thyroid carcinoma and, to some extent, acute leukemia, which presents in many older patients with a long prodrome or pre-leukemic state.

1. *Hodgkin's Disease*

In 1963, MacMahon observed that Hodgkin's Disease occured in a bimodal age distribution with an initial peak occurring between the years of 15 to 35 and a second peak occured after age 50 [69]. This suggested to him that there might be a different etiology in the different age groups. Whether this is true or not, several distinctions may be made between the disease as seen in the younger group and the elderly. Lokich et al. reviewed the course of 47 patients over the age of 60 who presented with Hodgkin's Disease and found that the older patient was more likely to present with constitutional symptoms, Stage III and IV disease, and intra-abdominal involvement, including invasion of the gastro-intestinal tract [70]. Although adenopathy as a presenting complaint was more common in the elderly, cervical and mediastinal adenopathy was unusual. Most important, the older patient had a distinctly shorter survival, which Lokich attributed to different therapeutic approaches used in the elderly. Peterson et al., however, reviewed data collected by Cancer and Acute Leukemia Group B and found that those over

60 had both a low frequency of response to standard chemotherapy and a brief duration of response when compared to younger patients [71]. This poor response rate did not appear to be due to differences in drug dosage, (reduction due to increased toxicity) or to other complications.

2. *Leukemia*

The chronic leukemias, myelocytic and lymphocytic, present few controversies in management in the older patient. These tend to run a relatively predictable course and usually respond readily to non-toxic methods of management.

Acute leukemia is generally a disease with a dramatic onset, and a short duration of symptoms prior to diagnosis, resulting in rapid demise if untreated. The peripheral blood and bone marrow examination are diagnostic. In the elderly, however, more than half the patients present with rather non-specific symptoms, including fatigue, anorexia and weakness. The peripheral blood may show cytopenia but on bone marrow examination, there is an increased number of blasts, a picture frequently referred to as 'smoldering' leukemia. Other elderly patients present with a long prodrome, labeled as a 'refractory' anemia or myelodysplastic syndrome. This prodrome may be very stable, and be present for a number of years before evolving into a picture more characteristic of acute leukemia.

Because of the variabilities in presentation in the elderly, treatment decisions may be different, particularly in the patient with multiple other medical problems. The patient with indolent disease should probably receive supportive care including transfusions as necessary. The elderly patient with overt acute leukemia presents a different therapeutic decision. The therapy of acute leukemia requires ablation of functioning marrow, and many have felt that the resulting period of complete marrow aplasia was more than the elderly patient could tolerate. Several recent studies, however, have shown that intensive chemotherapeutic regimens can be tolerated by some elderly patients and such treatment can yield results that are comparable to those achieved in younger patients [72, 73, 74]. Exceptions to this finding include those patients whose acute leukemia evolved from a pre-leukemic syndrome, who have a particularly poor response to induction chemotherapy and a shorter survival [75], and those patients who cannot physiologically tolerate the chemotherapy.

3. *Carcinomas of the Thyroid Gland*

Thyroid carcinoma is a disease which also has two peaks of incidence and a more malignant clinical course in the elderly patient. Papillary and follilcular carcinoma account for 95% of the thyroid tumors seen in the younger age group. These tumors are curable by surgery if detected while confined to the thyroid, are slowly progressive, and when metastatic respond to therapy with radioactive iodine. Carcinoma of the thyroid in the elderly is quite different, being usually of undifferentiated histology, and rapidly progressive. Rarely are these tumors resectable [71] and they do not usually respond to radio-active iodine. Although there are some reports of tumor shrinkage from external radiation, these are unusual.

CONCLUSION

Cancer in the older patient involves a number of issues which are not of major importance in the management of younger patients. The presumption that the life span of the older individual is necessarily limited and aggressive therapy is not indicated is clearly not based on fact. Many studies have already been done to show that the elderly patient, however defined, can tolerate much of the same treatment as the younger patient. More studies need to be done to further define selection criteria for various treatments and more drug studies need to be done on the use of chemotherapeutic agents in the elderly to determine the limiting side effects. Further understanding of the natural history of common malignant disease in the elderly is necessary so that the physician can make better judgements as to exactly when therapeutic intervention is called for.

REFERENCES

1. Siegel JS, Taeuber CM: The 1980 census and the elderly: new data available to planners and practitioners. Gerontologist 22:144–145, 1982.
2. Cancer facts and figures 1983. American Cancer Society, 1982.
3. Cancer facts and figures 1982. Your patient and cancer, April 1983.
4. Hersh EM, Mavligit GM, Gutterman JU: Immunodeficiency in cancer and the importance of immune evaluation of the cancer patient. Med Clin N Amer 60:623–639, 1976.
5. Miller DG: On the nature of susceptibility to cancer. The presidential address. Cancer 46:1307–1318, 1980.
6. DeCosse JJ: Potential for chemoprevention. Cancer 50:2550–2553, 1982.
7. Griffin AC: Role of selenium in the chemoprevention of cancer. Adv Cancer Res 29:419–442, 1979.
8. Weisburger JH, Wynder EL, Horn CL: Nutritional factors and etiologic mechanisms in the causation of gastrointestinal cancers. Cancer 50:2541–2549, 1982.
9. Lipsett MB: Hormones, medications and cancer. Cancer 51:2426–2429, 1983.
10. Holmes FF, Hearne E: Cancer stage-to-age relationship: implications for cancer screening in the elderly. J Am Geriatr Soc 20:55–57, 1981.
11. Santos AL, Gelperin A: Surgical mortality in the elderly. J Am Geriatr Soc 23:42–46, 1975.
12. Linn BS, Linn MW, Wallen N: Evalution of results of surgical procedures in the elderly, Ann Surg 195:90–96, 1982.

13. Smale BF, Mullen JL, Buzby GP, et al: The efficacy of nutritional assessment and support in cancer surgery. Cancer 47:2375–2381, 1981.
14. Boyd JB, Bradford B, Watne AL: Operative risk factors of colon resection in the elderly. Ann Surg 192:735–746, 1980.
15. Nagasaki F, Flehinger BJ, Martini N: Complications of surgery in the treatment of carcinoma of the lung. Chest 82:25–29, 1982.
16. Djokovic JL, Hedley-Whyte J: Prediction of outcome of surgery and anesthesia in patients over 80. JAMA 242:2301–2306, 1979.
17. Bonadonna G, Brusamolino E, Valagussa P, et al: Combination chemotherapy as an adjuvant treatment in operable breast cancer. N Engl J Med 294:405–410, 1976.
18. Vestal RE: Drug use in the elderly. Drugs 16:358–382, 1978.
19. Crooks J, O'Malley K, Stephenson IH: Pharmacokinetics in the elderly. Clin Pharmacokin 1:280–296, 1976.
20. Wallace S, Whiting D, Runcie J: Factors affecting drug finding in plasma of elderly patients. Br J Clin Pharmacol 3:327–330, 1976.
21. Haas CD, Coltman CA, Gottlieb JA, et al: Phase II evaluation of bleomycin: A Southwest Oncology Group Study. Cancer 38:8–12, 1976.
22. Von Hoff D, Layard MW, Basa P, et al: Risk factors for doxorubicin-induced congestive heart failure. Ann Int Med 91:710–717, 1979.
23. Brunner KW, Young CW: A methylhydrazine derivative in Hodgkin's disease and other malignant neoplasms. Ann Int Med 63:69–86, 1965.
24. Hande K, Gay J, Gober J, et al: Toxicity and pharmacology of bolus vindesine injection and prolonged vindesine infusion. Cancer Treat Rep 7:25–30.
25. Weiss HD, Walker MD, Wiernak PH: Neurotoxicity of commonly used antineopalstic agents (second of two parts). N Engl J Med 291:127–133, 1972.
26. Begg CB, Cohen JL, Ellerton J: Are the elderly predisposed to toxicity from cancer chemotherapy. Cancer Clin Trials 3:369–374, 1980.
27. Wynder EL: Etiology of lung cancer. Reflection on two decades of research. Cancer 30:1332–1339, 1972.
28. Wynder EL, Bross IJ, Feldman RM: A study of the etiologic factors in cancer of the mouth. Cancer 10:1300, 1957.
29. Weisburger JH, Wynder EL, Horn CL: Nutritional factors and etiologic mechanisms in the causation of gastrointestinal cancers. Cancer 50:2541–2549, 1982.
30. MacMahon B, Yen S, Trichopolous D, et al: Coffee and cancer of the pancreas. N Engl J Med 304:630–633, 1981.
31. Weisburger JH, Marquardt H, Mower HF, et al: Inhibition of carcinogenesis: Vitamin C and the prevention of gastric cancer. Prev Med 9:352–361, 1980.
32. Mountain CF: Surgical therapy in lung cancer: biologic, physiologic, and technical determinants. Sem Onc 1:253–258, 1974.
33. Kirsh MM, Rotman H, Bove E, et al: Major pulmonary resection for bronchogenic carcinoma in the elderly. Ann Thor Surg 22:369–373, 1976.
34. Weiss W: Operative mortality and five year survival rates in patients with bronchogenic carcinoma. Am J Surg 128:799–804, 1974.
35. Olsen GN, Block AJ, Tobias JA: Prediction of postpneumonectomy pulmonary function using quantitative macroaggregate lung scanning. Chest 66:13–16, 1974.
36. Boysen PG, Harris JO, Block AJ, et al: Prospective evaluation for pneumonectomy using perfusion scanning followup beyond one year. Chest 80:163–166, 1981.
37. Jensik RJ, Faber LP, Kittle CF: Segmental resection for bronchogenic carcinoma. Ann Thor Surg 28:475–483, 1979.
38. Breyer RH, Zippe C, Pharr WF, et al: Thoracotomy in patients over age 70 years. J Thorac Cardiovasc Surg 81:187–193, 1981.

140

39. Clamon GH, Audeh MW, Pinnick S: Small cell lung carcinoma in the elderly. J Am Geriatr Soc 30:299–302, 1981.
40. Cancer of the head and neck. Ed. Suen JY, Meyers EN. Churchill Livingstone, New York, 1981.
41. Loery A, Huttner DJ: Head and neck surgery in patients just past 70. Arch Otolaryngol 84:523–526, 1966.
42. Martin H, Rasmussen LH, Perras C: Head and neck surgery in patients of the older age group. Cancer 8:707–711, 1955.
43. Morgan RF, Hirata RM, Jaques DA, et al: Head and neck surgery in the aged. Am J Surg 144:449, 1982.
44. Lundt G, Burn JI, Kolig G, et al: A cooperative international study of gastric cancer. Ann R Coll Surg 54:219, 1974.
45. Buchholtz TW, Welch CE, Malt RA: Clinical correlates of resectabilty and survival in gastric carcinoma. Ann Surg 188:711–714, 1978.
46. Bittner R, Berger HG, Krass E, et al: Should we operate on patients with gastric carcinoma who are 70 years old and older. Langenbecks Arch Chir 344:293, 1978.
47. Stern JL, Denman S, Elias EG, et al: Evaluation of palliative resection in advanced carcinoma of the stomach. Surg 77:291–298, 1975.
48. Gardner B, Dotan J, Shaikh L, et al: The influence of age upon the survival of adult patients with carcinoma of the colon. Surg Gynecol Obstet 153:366–368, 1981.
49. Adam YG, Calabrese C, Volk H: Colorectal cancer in patients over 80 years of age. Surg Clin N A 52:883–889, 1972.
50. Kragellung E, Balslev I, Bardram L, et al: Resectability, operative moratality, and survival of patients in old age with carcinoma of the colon and rectum. Dis Col and Rect 17:617–621, 1974.
51. Salvati EP, Rubin RJ: Electrocoagulation as primary therapy for rectal carcinoma. Am J Surg 132:583–586, 1976.
52a. Gingold BS: Local treatment (electrocoagulation) for carcinoma of the rectum in the elderly. J Am Ger Soc 29:10–13, 1981.
52b. MacDonald JS, Gunderson LL, Cohl I: Cancer of the pancreas in Cancer: Principles and Practice of Oncology editor DeVita VT, Hellmen S, Rosenberg SA. J.B. Lippincott, Philadelphia, 1982, pp 575–576.
52. Warren KW, Christophi C, Armendariz R, et al: Current trends in the diagnosis and treatment of carcinoma of the pancreas. Am J Surg. 813–817, 1983.
53. Halpert B, Schmalhorst WR: Carcinoma of the prostate in patients 70 to 79 years old. Cancer 19:695–698, 1966.
54. Hist AE, Bergman RT: Carcinoma of the prostate in men 80 or more years old. Cancer 7:136–141, 1953.
55. Rosenberg SE: Is carcinoma of the prostate less serious in older men. Am Ger Soc 13:791–798, 1965.
56. Hanash KA, Utz DC, Cook EN, et al: Carcinoma of the prostate a 15 year followup. J Urology 107:450–453, 1972.
57. Klein LA: Prostatic carcinoma. N Engl J Med 300:824–833, 1979.
58. Catalona WJ, Scott WW: Carcinoma of the prostate: A review. J Urology 119:1–12, 1978.
59. Kagan AR, Hintz BL: Is there a best management for localized adenocarcinoma of the prostate. Cancer Clin Trials 20:359–363, 1979.
60. Boxer RJ, Kaufman JJ, Goodwin WE: Radical prostatectomy for carcinoma of the prostate: 1951–1976. A review of 329 patients. J Urology 117:208–213, 1977.
61. Bagshaw MA, Ray GR, Pistenma DA, et al: External beam readiation therapy of primary carcinoma of the prostate. Cancer 36:723–728, 1975.

62. Hunt KE, Fry DE, Bland KI: Breast carcinoma in the elderly patient: An assessment of operative risk, morbidity and mortality. Am J Surg 140:399–342, 1980.
63. Kesseler HJ, Seton JZ: The treatment of operable breast cancer in the elderly female. Am J Surg 135:664–666, 1978.
64. Goldenberg IS, Bailar JC, Eishenberg H: Survival patterns of elderly women with breast cancer. Arch Surg 99:649–651, 1969.
65. Henderson IC, Canellos GP: Cancer of the breast. N Engl J Med 302:78–90, 1980.
66. Henderson IC: Chemotherapy in breast cancer: A general overview. Cancer 51:2553–2559, 1983.
67. Kaufman RJ: Advanced breast cancer. Additive hormonal therapy. Cancer 47:2398–2403, 1981.
68. MacMahon B: Epidemiology of Hodgkin's disease. Cancer Res 26:1189–1200, 1966.
69. Lokich JJ, Pinkus GS, Moloney WC: Hodgkin's disease in the elderly. Oncology 29:484–500, 1974.
70. Peterson BA, Pajak TF, Cooper R, et al: Effect of age on therapeutic response and survival in advanced Hodgkin's disease. Cancer Treat Rep 66:889–898, 1982.
71. Foon KA, Zighelboim J, Yale C, et al: Intensive chemotherapy is the treatment of choice for elderly patients with acute myelogenous leukemia. Blood 58:467–470, 1981.
72. Bloomfield CD, Thelogides A: Acute granulocytic leukemia in elderly patients. JAMA 226:1190–1193, 1973.
73. Rosner F, Sawitsky A, Grunwald HW, et al: Acute granulocytic leukemia in the elderly. Arch Intern Med 136:120, 1976.
74. Fernandez G, Schwartz JMN: Immune responsiveness and hematologic malignancy in the elderly. Med Clin N A 960:1253–1271, 1976.
75. Leeper RD, Shimaoka K: Treatment of metastatic thyroid cancer. Clin Endo Meta 9:383–404, 1980.

6. Indwelling Permanent Vascular Access Devices and Their Management

RICHARD BERJIAN, D.O.

INTRODUCTION

Critical to the long-term supportive care of many cancer patients is the need for a constant vascular access modality to sustain the nutritional, hematological, and chemotherapeutic demands of that patient since repeated venipuncture of peripheral veins rapidly exhausts the available sites as localized phlebitis and venous thrombosis can be expected to develop [1, 2].

This chapter will review the choices available to the practicing clinician for methods of 'permanent' vascular access in cancer patients, with particular emphasis on the criteria for selection, the complications associated with use, and recommendations for management.

ANGIOACCESS MODALITIES

Central venous catheterization

With the introduction of percutaneously placed right atrial catheters, the possibility of access to the central venous system made the long-term use of total parenteral hyperalimentation available for clinical application [3]. Because polypropylene plastic catheters tend to age and crack after a period of time, siliconized rubber catheters have been introduced which permit access for longer periods of use [4].

The percutaneous approach results in a short pathway from the skin to the subclavian or internal jugular vein. The risk of ascending infection developing along the catheter from the skin to the venous entry site can limit the long-term usefulness of this technique [5, 6]. The possibility for developing sepsis always exists, even with the strictest maintenance of aseptic conditions [4, 5]. In those patients undergoing bone marrow transplanta-

Higby, DJ (ed), The Cancer Patient and Supportive Care. ISBN 0-89838-690-X.
© *1985, Martinus Nijhoff Publishers, Boston. Printed in The Netherlands.*

tion, one vascular access line is needed for total parenteral hyperalimentation and a second line is required for drug treatment, blood monitoring, and blood product replacement therapy. In the past, this necessitated placement of a second right atrial catheter, doubling the risk of ascending infection leading to sepsis. Cancer patients who are usually immunocompromised and extremely ill while undergoing chemotherapy are especially at great risk for acquiring infections. The administration of broad spectrum antibiotics, cytotoxic immunosuppressives, and steroids to these patients would also predispose to the development of fungal infections [7]. In order to reduce the rate of infection, final in-line filtration of the solution has been utilized, but this has not always been shown to be effective [8]. While a 0.45 micron filter blocks the passage of fungi and large bacteria, a 0.22 micron filter would be needed in order to block the passage of most other bacteria. With the smaller filter, however, an infusion pump would be necessary to provide a constant rate of the infusate. It has been shown that there is a relationship between bacterial colonization on the skin and catheter sepsis when the pathway from the skin puncture site to the vein is short [9, 10]. Thus, most cases of catheter-related sepsis are the result of inadequate catheter care [6, 10, 11].

Broviac/Hickman siliconized rubber catheters for right atrial or inferior vena cava placement

With the introduction of the Broviac and Hickman siliconized catheters, a safer and more reliable means of long-term venous access was made available for a variety of clinical situations [12, 13]. These two single lumen catheters differ only in their inner and outer diameters; the inner lumen of the Broviac catheter measures 10.0 mm, while the luminal diameter of the Hickman catheter measures 16.0 mm. The double lumen Hickman catheter is a combination of both catheters and allows for the administration of total parenteral hyperalimentation through the smaller lumen, while permitting the use of the larger lumen for blood sampling and the administration of blood products, medications, and chemotherapy (Figure 1). These catheters have integrated dacron cuffs permitting ingrowth of tissue around the catheter, which provides fixation as well as a fibrous barrier against ascending infection from the catheter entrance site at the skin.

The procedure for placement is the same for the single lumen Broviac, Hickman, or double lumen Hickman catheter; which catheter is used is determined in part by the diameter of the vein to be used for access. The following description for placement of a double lumen catheter demonstrates our technique for customizing the end of the catheter. The procedure can be performed under local or general anesthesia. Entrance into the large

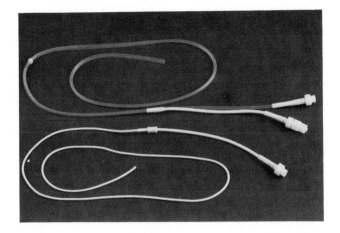

Figure 1. 1) Top Catheter: Double lumen Hickman catheter. 2) Bottom Catheter: Single lumen Broviac catheter.

central veins can be gained using the cephalic veins, external or internal jugular veins, or a tributary of the superficial saphenous vein [14–16]. A percutaneous technique for placement of a siliconized right atrial catheter via the subclavian or internal jugular vein has been reported, but cannot be used for placement of a double lumen catheter [17].

Technique-placement of double lumen Hickman catheter

The patient is placed upon an operating table which is equipped with fluoroscopy for monitoring catheter placement into the right atrium. The sterile skin preparation and draping should allow approach to either the cephalic or jugular veins, since on occasion one may need a vein larger than the cephalic for successful cannulation with a double lumen Hickman catheter. We prefer the external jugular if it can be well demonstrated on physical examination. The choice of incisions for the different veins is identified in Figure 2. In approaching the cephalic vein it is wise not to incise the investing fascia of the pectoralis major muscle until the delto-pectoral groove is clearly identified, since this will avoid a fruitless search for the vein between the muscle fibers of the pectoralis major muscle.

If the cephalic or external jugular veins are of small caliber, graduated vessel dilators are useful for dilating and determining the direction of the vein. When the internal jugular vein is used, the vessel is encircled with silk or rubber 'loops' to control backflow, while a # 40 or # 50 vascular purse string suture is placed at the venotomy site to control the bleeding at the point of catheter entry.

After the selected vein has been isolated, a subcutaneous tunnel is made from the venotomy site towards the sternum at the level of the 4th or 5th

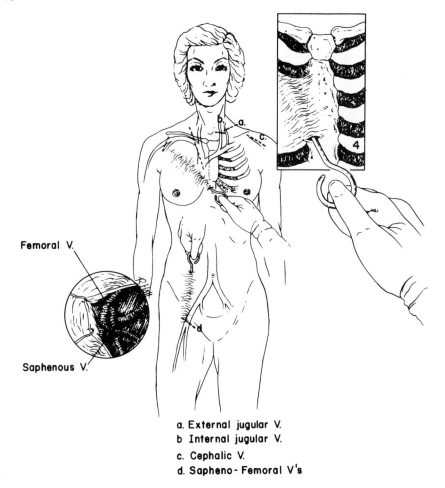

a. External jugular V.
b Internal jugular V.
c. Cephalic V.
d. Sapheno- Femoral V's

Femoral V.

Saphenous V.

Figure 2. Incision sites: a) external jugular vein; b) internal jugulat vein; c) cephalic vein; d) sapheno-femoral veins. [Inset] ribs; site of tunneling insertion at level of 4th interspace.

interspace. Instead of using a long forceps to create the tunnel, we use a long tunneling rod with a small hole drilled at the end through which to thread the tie. This results in a smaller tract and thus less likelihood of trauma and hematoma formation, which may be especially important in thrombocytopenic patients. A more readily available instrument that can be used is a uterine sound. After passing a suture through the end of the catheter or tying it to the sound, the catheter is drawn through the tract.

After choosing an appropriate length of catheter to reach the right atrium (2–3rd interspace), measuring from the smooth rounded portion to the tip, the distal excess catheter is cut and discarded. It is important that the smooth rounded part of the catheter be placed at the ligature site of the venotomy (Figure 3, b. section) to avoid a leakage of blood that would occur

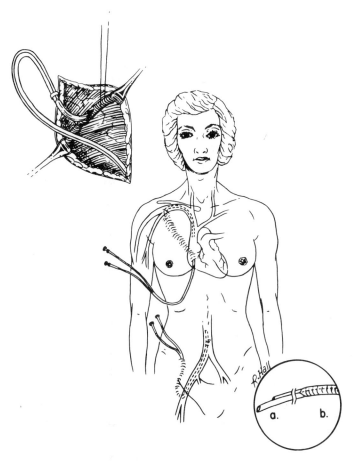

Figure 3. Final position of right atrial double lumen Hickman catheter via the cephalic vein or right inferior vena cava double lumen Hickman catheter via the right sapheno-femoral vein: a) beveled end of catheter with smaller lumen more proximal than larger lumen; b) rounded smooth portion without groove between the catheters for site of venotomy ligature.

along the groove of the fused catheters. Any attempt to encircle a ligature at any other site along the catheter will result in occlusion of the smaller lumen in order to secure hemostasis.

When cutting the excess catheter of a double lumen Hickman, our preference is to cut both ends obliquely (Figure 3, a. section); however, the end of the smaller catheter should be cut approximately 15 mm proximal to the end of the larger catheter. This will reduce the admixture of hyperalimentation solution in blood sample aspirate which is usually drawn through the larger lumen of the catheter. Introduction of this tailored double lumen catheter into a small vein is also easier when only one lumen enters the vein as a leading edge.

In order to confirm the final position of the catheter tip, a radiopaque dye is injected into the larger lumen and the catheter position is viewed by flouroscopy. Following satisfactory placement, the catheter is flushed with heparinized saline (1000 units/500 cc normal saline) and capped with an intermittent infusion cap diaphragm which may be used for injection. A piece of tape is placed around the catheter proximal to the diaphragm, and a small atraumatic clip is placed at this site to occlude the lumen to prevent venous backflow and intraluminal clot formation while the lines are temporarily disconnected. Closure of the skin and subcutaneous tissue over the venotomy site is performed with skin or subcuticular sutures and adhesive skin tapes.

For those patients who have undergone placement of the catheter into the internal jugular vein, a tracheostomy tray should be available at the bedside; catheter migration might occur, and if bleeding should develop along the grooves of the double lumen catheter, this could cause an acute airway obstruction.

Following the procedure, the lines may be used immediately or they can be filled with heparinized saline (100 units heparin/ml) and 'heparin locked'. Patients are instructed in wound care and cleaning and heparin flush should be performed at least every 12 hours when the catheter is not in use.

Catheter removal

When a malfunctioning catheter is to be removed, it is wise to first do an angiogram through the catheter to evaluate the cause of the malfunction prior to removal (See section regarding complications). If a functioning catheter is to be removed because it is no longer needed, a steady pull on the catheter will usually allow it to be withdrawn. If resistance is met, a steady gentle pull should be maintained, avoiding sudden jerking movements, which could cause the catheter to break. Rarely, a surgical 'cut-down' over the dacron cuff sites will be necessary to free the catheter. Those catheters that are infected with drainage exiting from the skin insertion site are more easily removed with constant traction than those which are not.

Complications

Among the complications which might occur, catheter occlusion and development of infection are the most common. There is also the possibility of damage to the catheter, although techniques are available to repair a catheter that has been cut or perforated.

Catheter occlusion

This is perhaps the most common complication associated with placement of the Broviac/Hickman catheter. In one study of 43 patients who received 78 catheter placements for hyperalimentation through a siliconized rubber right atrial catheter for periods ranging from one to fifty-two months (mean duration 12.4 months), occlusive obstruction was the cause for 15 (29%) of the 52 catheters that were removed [13]. However, in another study which reviewed 102 infants who received catheterization of the inferior vena cava through the saphenous or femoral vein, only six patients were reported to have developed vena caval obstruction and thrombosis [16].

When a previously well functioning Broviac or Hickman catheter can no longer be flushed or does not allow the free aspiration of venous blood, the obstructed catheter should be filled with 3 cc of 1:1000 units of heparin followed by 1 cc of normal saline, which is injected using a slightly forceful thrust. If this does not result in easy aspiration of blood or ease of injecting through the catheter, the line should be 'capped' for one hour and the procedure repeated again. If the catheter continues to remain obstructed, an angiogram study should be performed through the catheter to determine the cause of the obstruction, which may be due to an extraluminal caval obstruction, an intraluminal clot, dislodgement of the catheter, or positional obstruction of the catheter due to sharp angulations. Should the catheter be occluded, this will be quickly evident; if the catheter is not functioning due to caval thrombosis, many small collateral veins will appear. If evidence of a superior vena cava occlusion is suspected, bilateral venograms in both arms will document this finding. In these cases, it is usually wise to remove the catheter since it is no longer functional.

Early in our experience, we were confronted with a double lumen Hickman catheter that was partially occluded with a 'ball valve' clot at its tip. A sleeve of clot surrounded the catheter and a long propagated tail of clot extended beyond the catheter. To dissolve this clot and prevent the possibility of a pulmonary embolism developing at the time of removal, a bolus of urokinase was given through the catheter over 10 minutes, followed by a maintenance infusion given every hour for twelve hours. Follow-up catheter angiogram study showed no evidence of the clot, and the catheter was removed uneventfully under local anesthesia. Based on our further experience, we would now recommend using 5000 units of streptokinase (Hoechst-Roussel 'Streptase®') every hour to dissolve an obstructive clot in the catheter. Following this, an angiogram study through the catheter could determine whether any extraluminal clot persists.

More recently, we have uneventfully removed at the bedside a number of single and double lumen catheters that had similar propagated clots causing partial occlusion without the use of streptokinase. The theoretical risk of massive pulmonary embolism still exists, however, and this should be made clear to both the patient and the physician responsible for the patient's care before attempting to remove a catheter under this circumstance.

Infection

Infectious complications from the use of Broviac/Hickman catheters in cancer patients may present as a local inflammation at the catheter exit site or along the subcutaneous tract of the catheter. Blood cultures positive for the same organisms cultured at the skin exist site may also indicate catheter-related infection, and fever may be a late manifestation. Early detection and antimicrobial treatment prior to the onset of constitutional symptoms can avoid a precipitous episode of septic shock. Gram-positive and gram-negative bacterial infections as well as fungal infections can occur in these patients, and despite meticulous sterile care, reports of catheter-related sepsis range from around 12% to 56% [1, 18, 19].

Most *Staphylococcus* infections resulting from catheter placement are believed to be caused by bacteria entering the body at the catheter entrance site in the skin [5–9]. In a recent study, it was reported that six of 27 pediatric oncology patients experienced 14 episodes of catheter-related bacteremia. Blood cultures from the peripheral veins were positive in 12 of the 14 episodes. Antimicrobial therapy via the Broviac catheter cured the infection in 10 of 11 episodes. However, two of these patients required catheter removal because of persistent infection with positive blood cultures [20].

Of the seven patients with proven staphylococcal right atrial catheter infections in Larson's series, four patients had developed infection at the intravenous site and subcutaneous tunnel [6]. In three patients, septic thrombophlebitis involving the cephalic, axillary, and subclavian veins developed. In five of seven patients in whom right atrial catheter infections developed, there was an untreated infection present at the time of catheter insertion and a positive history of sepsis [5]. Abraham et al. recently reported on the safety of the long-term use of 71 silicone elastomer right atrial catheters placed in 57 consecutive patients with acute leukemia [21]. In 38 patients who developed systemic infections, only eight catheter-related infections occurred during 6,779 days of use. These authors concluded that even in this group at high risk for granulocytopenia and sepsis, there was only a small ratio of serious catheter-related complications with no catheter-associated mortality found. Recent reports of catheter-related sepsis now suggest that *Staphylococcus epidermidis* appears to be the most common etiological agent in patients who are granulocytopenic and receiving cytotoxic therapy [22, 23]. In addition to the suggestion of a change in the spectrum of bacterial infections in these patients, the development of fungemia is now also being reported more frequently [24–26].

In those cases where catheter sepsis is suspected, quantitative blood cultures taken from the catheter may show a higher bacterial colony count than blood cultures obtained from peripheral veins [27]. Even if the source of sepsis is not from the catheter tip, colonization of organisms in the catheter tract can occur which can then cause sepsis [20].

Our current recommendations regarding suspected catheter-induced bacteremia at Roswell Park Memorial Institute is to obtain simultaneous blood cultures from a peripheral vein and from the catheter, and then to infuse the appropriate antibiotic therapy through the catheter. This should prove sufficient to eradicate the infection in the majority of cases encountered [20]. Control of the infection and cure of the sepsis is considered successful if the patient becomes afebrile and if blood cultures from the catheter are negative 24 and 48 hours after antimicrobial treatment is discontinued. If persistent positive blood cultures are obtained from the blood drawn through the catheter despite adequate antibiotic coverage, the catheter must be removed and replaced. Replacement of another 'permanent' vascular access should be withheld, if possible, until at least 48 hours after indicated antibiotic therapy has been administered, since this will reduce the likelihood of reseeding and colonization of the new catheter or its tract. During that interval, peripheral veins or temporary percutaneous central vein catheterization may be utilized for maintaining venous access. If nutritional supplementation is necessary during this time, calories can be provided by the administration of fat emulsions in addition to crystalloid solutions by way of peripheral veins.

Catheter damage

To avoid damage to a siliconized rubber catheter, the use of sharp instruments or scissors near the catheter should be avoided. Only smooth edge clamps or clips should be applied to occlude the catheter and the site of occlusion should be covered with a piece of tape to protect the catheter surface. If a perforation or cut occurs more than 4 cm from the chest wall, temporary repair is feasible. Utilizing a sterile field and clamping the catheter close to the chest wall, the catheter is cut at a selected site and a # 14 gauge 2 inch angiocath is inserted into the catheter lumen proximal to the damaged site; the stylet is removed. The angiocath hub can then be connected to the intravenous solution. The portion of catheter distal to the angiocath insertion site should then be saved for later permanent repair.

For permanent repair of the catheter, a kit can be obtained (Evermed, P.O. Box 296, Medina, Washington 98039) which must be sterilized using a steam autoclave. Under sterile conditions, the damaged catheter is prepped with betadine solution followed by alcohol wipes. Sterile gloves are changed; the powder must be removed with alcohol soaked gauze squares to avoid having the powder from the gloves weakening the adhesive used in repairing the catheter. The technique is as follows:

Technique for catheter repair [28] (Figures 4a & 4b)

1. A syringe is preloaded with one ml of adhesive and the plunger is inserted into the syringe. A blunt end needle is attached to the end of the syringe.

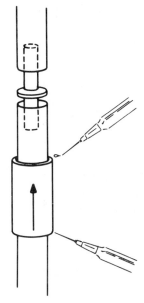

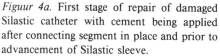

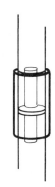

Figuur 4a. First stage of repair of damaged Silastic catheter with cement being applied after connecting segment in place and prior to advancement of Silastic sleeve.

Figuur 4b. Final appearance of Silastic sleeve overlying the connecting segment after application of cement.

2. Using a sharp scalpel or scissor, the catheter is cut just proximal to the area of damage and the distal portion discarded.
   The replacement segment is cut so that the repaired catheter will be between 15–20 centimeters from the chest wall.
3. One end of the connecting segment is inserted into the damaged catheter up to its center ridge. The opposite end is inserted into the replacement piece to again reach the center ridge.
4. The adhesive is applied liberally to the center ridge and a Silastic sleeve is brought to rest over the center ridge. Adhesive is injected under the Silastic sleeve and the catheter and sleeve are rolled between fingers to spread the adhesive. The excess is wiped away.
5. The catheter should not be used for infusion for at least two hours and the joint should be splinted with a gauze covered tongue blade for 48 hours.

Totally implantable right atrial siliconized catheters:
'Infuse-A-Port'® (Infusaid Corporation, 1400 Providence Highway, Norwood, MA 02062) and 'Medi-Port' (Cormed Company, 591 Mahar Street, Medina, NY 14103)

These new single lumen catheter systems can be used for both venous and hepatic artery access (Figure 5). They differ from the Hickman/Broviac

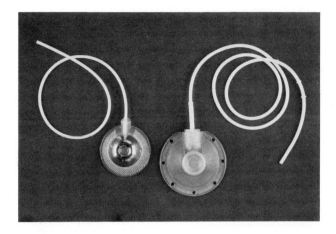

Figure 5. Totally implantable siliconized catheters. As pictured, the Medi-Port catheter (left) and the Infuse-A-Port (right).

catheters because, at their proximal ends, is a contoured disc chamber which is totally implanted subcutaneously. Using a sterile 22 gauge Huber point needle, the disc chamber lying under the skin can be injected [29]. Since the device is covered by the skin and totally implanted, contamination from a skin exit site does not occur as it can with Broviac/Hickman catheters.

There were, however, some factors limiting the use of these catheters. The first was that it was not approved for aspiration and blood sampling. However, both 'Infuse-A-Port'® and 'Medi-Port'®, now outline in their literature a technique for aspiration of blood. Secondly, they are single lumen catheters and therefore not suitable for bone marrow transplant candidates who require double lumen catheters. The third was that if long-term continuous infusion is necessary, problems of infection from a skin entrance site are still possible. Our experience with these catheters is limited; however, it appears likely that it will play a greater role in patients undergoing long-term chemotherapy and in whom blood sampling is relatively infrequent.

Instructions to patient/family for home catheter care

When the patient is discharged from the hospital, it is essential that proper instruction and supervised maintenance care of the catheter by the patient and a responsible family member be approved by the nursing staff. A copy of the teaching plan format is shown (Figure 6) that allows one to follow the steps necessary for successful care of the catheter by the patient.

As part of the 'Patient Education Series', a manual formulated by the Nursing Education Department of Roswell Park Memorial Institute is given

ROSWELL PARK MEMORIAL INSTITUTE
Department of Nursing

PATIENT/FAMILY TEACHING PLAN

Signature – Title-Initials	Signature – Title-Initials

(Addressograph)

PERMANENT RIGHT ATRIAL CATHETER (HICKMAN,BROVIAC)

PURPOSE: To teach safe home management of the permanent right atrial catheter.	Patient	Family Member Name:

CONTENT	INSTRUCTION GIVEN	
	Date & Initials	Date & Initials
1) Basic anatomy and position of catheter		
2) Purpose of the catheter		
3) General safety rules		
4) Signs of infection		
5) Demonstration of: heparin solution instillation		
exit site dressing change		
6) Supervised practice of: heparin solution instillation		
exit site dressing change		
7) Emergency procedures		
8) Anticipatory guidance for patient and family concerns about home management of the catheter		

MATERIALS	MATERIALS GIVEN	
	Date & Initials	Date & Initials
Patient Teaching Booklet – "Home Care of the Permanent Right Atrial Catheter"		

LEARNER OBJECTIVES	OBJECTIVES MET/REVIEW GIVEN				
	Patient			Family	
Upon completion of this teaching unit, the patient/ family will be able to:	Date & Initial	Score*	Review**	Score*	Review**
1) Describe the position and purpose of catheter					
2) State general safety rules					
3) State three signs of infection					
4) Demonstrate competency in: heparin instillation					
exit site dressing change					
5) Describe emergency procedures					
6) Identify a means to resolve concerns about home management of the catheter					

*Score the degree to which the patient/family is able to utilize learning as follows:

SCORE 1 – Safe Technique, Confident Performance, Good Recall
2 – Safe Technique, Lacks Confidence, Moderate Recall
3 – Unsafe Technique, Lacks Confidence, Poor Recall

R.P.M.I.
M-197
Rev. 2/82

**For scores of 2 or 3, review correct information/procedure and place a check (✓) in Review Space

Figure 6. Family/Patient Teaching Plan.

to the patient and the responsible family members as a reference guide. These steps have ensured good patient compliance and have been well received by both the patients and the nursing staff.

ARTERIOVENOUS ANGIOACCESS (SHUNT, FISTULA, GRAFT)

The creation of an arteriovenous shunt or graft is a more technically demanding operation than the placement of a Broviac or Hickman right atrial catheter and is used chiefly in the patient whose angioaccess needs are for renal hemodialysis. The presence of superficial vein thrombosis or occlusive arterial disease can limit the availability of vessels for anastomosis. Complications, including vascular occlusion and the possible loss of digits, limit this modality for vascular access and should be used in the cancer patient only when absolutely necessary. If the cancer patient also requires long-term hyperalimentation, a central venous access site would be needed in addition, which can be another source of potential complications.

While no attempt is made to describe all of the alternative techniques and variations in the performance of arteriovenous shunts or grafts, I will briefly review some of those procedures and their more commonly associated complications. Essential to the success of all of these procedures is the preoperative evaluation of the chosen extremity to determine the patency of the arterial and venous segment. A careful determination of the arterial pulses, including the execution of an Allen Test in order to confirm the presence of blood flow to the superficial palmer arch, should be performed [30].

The superficial veins should be carefully examined because the most preferred veins may have been selectively thrombosed and therefore not usable. Although the choice of extremity should be based upon the quality of the vessels available, the non-dominant arm is usually preferred.

One should choose a site most near the wrist so that if the shunt cannot be constructed or eventually fails, a second can be constructed at a more proximal site. Local infiltration anesthesia has been successful for construction of these procedures at the wrist or antecubital fossa and for the interposition of saphenous vein segments or heterografts. General anesthesia has been reserved for children and uncooperative adults.

External arteriovenous shunt

When the first practical use of hemodialysis was introduced by Kolff in 1944, the first external angioaccess device for an immediate purpose evolved [31, 32]. Glass or metal cannulas were placed in a peripheral artery and vein, and the blood was passed through the artificial kidney. Following dialysis, these cannulas had to be removed because of thrombosis; this limited the number of sessions of dialysis each patient was able to undergo.

The external angioaccess shunt is rarely used today and is limited to: 1) those patients undergoing treatment for acute renal failure, or 2) removal of intoxicants by short-term dialysis. When long-term therapy is contemplated for an immunocompromised patient, external cannulas are not suitable for angioaccess because of the inherent risk of developing sepsis.

Internal arteriovenous fistula (Figure 7)

With the success of the Brescia-Cimino subcutaneous radiocephalic fistu-

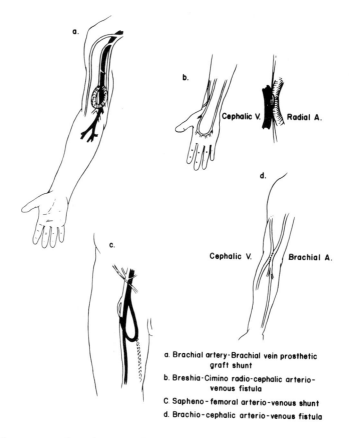

a. Brachial artery-Brachial vein prosthetic graft shunt

b. Breshia-Cimino radio-cephalic arterio-venous fistula

C Sapheno-femoral arterio-venous shunt

d. Brachio-cephalic arterio-venous fistula

Figure 7. Some types of arteriovenous fistulas, shunts, and prosthetic graft shunts.

la [33] in the wrist, patients gained a greater freedom of activity without the presence of any external devices or encumbrances. This now allowed for repeated percutaneous cannulizations of arterialized superficial veins. Using a side-to-side, end-to-side, or end-to-end technique, the radial artery and cephalic vein are anastomosed to form an artificial fistula. The patency of the shunt can be confirmec by auscultation of a bruit or by palpation of a thrill over the fistulas.

Postoperative complications of thrombosis can be reduced by the avoidance of excessive compression with tight bandages. Thrombosis and occlusion of the fistula is usually related to poor venous run-off. The operative correction of thrombosis requires making a venotomy and passing a Fogarty embolectomy catheter (Edwards Labs, Santa Clara, California 92705) for withdrawal of the thrombus [34]. More recently, the use of a streptokinase instillation of 5,000 units/hour has been utilized and has demonstrated some benefit in dissolution of clots and thrombi [35].

Aneurysm formation can occur in both the distal and proximal parts of a side-to-side fistula. This can be most painful and can produce edema distal to the fistula site. Correction is provided by ligating the distal venous limb. Aneurysm formations within the central venous segment are usually not symptomatic and require no treatment if the fistula functions well. False aneurysms can occur at the points of venous connection or at the anastomosis. Symptomatic or enlarging false aneurysms should be repaired early because they can erode through the skin and eventually rupture.

Prosthetic and biologic arteriovenous grafts

Newer graft materials have been developed since Teflon tips were first used in external shunt devices. Biologic materials, eg, autologous vein graft, homologous saphenous vein, cadaveric vein, modified umbilical vein, and xenograft (eg, modified bovine carotid artery), were utilized in the initial stages of arteriovenous grafting [36]. All required a period of time for healing before they could be used. With the development of dacron velour, Teflon, Impra, and Gore-tex (expanded polytetrafluoroethylene), prosthetic material was made available for immediate use [36–39].

Any suitable artery or vein can be utilized for grafting, but the ideal site is in the forearm, since grafts in the thigh may be at a greater risk for causing limb ischemia or development of infection.

Grafts may be straight or looped, but the likelihood of thrombosis in looped graft fistulas is much higher than in straight grafts [40]. This complication is possibly associated with kinking or twisting of the graft during implantation. Other complications associated with arteriovenous fistulas and grafts include extremity ischemia and arterial steal syndrome. The reader is referred to a detailed review of the other choices one may utilize for arteriovenous shunts and fistulas [40]. Wobbes et al. analyzed the results of 100 consecutive cancer patients who received either an AV fistula, saphenous vein autograft, or PTFE (polytetrafluoroethylene) graft for providing vascular access for chemotherapy. The failure rate for the AV fistula reached 44%, while the failure rate for the PTFE forearm graft was 80% [41].

It would appear, however, that in dealing with the long-term treatment of an immunosuppressed cancer patient who is granulocytopenic and thrombocytopenic, the use of arteriovenous techniques for angioaccess is a less appealing modality for unrestricted usage because of its inherent high complication rate.

AMBULATORY INFUSION PUMPS FOR REGIONAL AND SYSTEMIC CHEMOTHERAPY

Hepatic Artery Infusion

The presence of inoperable primary or metastatic carcinoma of the liver is associated with a poor prognosis. Jaffee and associates reported a median survival of 75 days from the time of diagnosis in patients with untreated liver metastases. In primary gastrointestinal malignancies, the duration of survival is dependent upon the extent of hepatic involvement [42].

While systemic chemotherapy administration of 5-fluorouracil (5-FU) for gastrointestinal malignancies has been reported to bring about a 20% response rate (objective tumor regression), early reports by other investigators have suggested that continuous, long-term intra-arterial chemotherapy can achieve higher response rates with less toxicity [43–46]. Subsequent reports have now confirmed objective response rates ranging from 35–80% in the treatment of hepatic metastases using intermittent or continuous hepatic artery infusion of chemotherapy [47–50]. Survival rates in those patients who have an objective response are found to be superior to those who do not and to the survival rates in untreated historical controls [48, 49].

The Central Oncology Group study (reported in 1979) compared the response to intravenous 5-FU with that to hepatic artery infusion of 5-FU in patients with hepatic metastases from colorectal carcinoma, and found no difference in terms of response rate, time to progression, duration of response, or survival rate (51). While the actual response rate was slightly higher in those patients receiving intra-arterial 5-FU, the difference was not statistically significant. More recent studies of long-term hepatic artery infusion of chemotherapy for patients with primary and metastatic hepatic lesions from a variety of tumors have reported response rates of up to 80% with increased survival in those patients responding to treatment [40, 52–55].

Earlier studies utilized percutaneous insertion of catheters into the hepatic artery with a reported success rate of catheter placement up to 85%; however, catheter-associated complications such as sepsis and bleeding at the site of insertion, arterial thrombosis, and catheter displacement limit this technique to a time period of two to three months [50, 52, 56–58]. The more recent development of a totally implantable drug infusion pump (Infusaid Corporation, Sharon, Mass.) in the subcutaneous tissues has made it possible to administer continuous long-term hepatic artery infusion chemotherapy without the many technical problems associated with percutaneous insertion, external catheters, and pumps [59, 60]. Uncontrolled studies by Ensminger et al. [60] and Balch et al. [53] report objective response rates up to 80% (Ensminger) with an increased survival using this implantable pump [53, 61]. Weiss et al. [54] reported that from the time of diagnosis of liver metastases, no significant difference in median survival was found in those patients treated with this technique (21 patients) as compared with those who were declared ineligible for the study and not so treated (10 patients). However, the median survival for the treated group after pump implantation was significantly better (13 months) than the group that was ineligible (4 months) from the time of evaluation for the study. This comparison is not entirely valid because the majority of those patients (9 patients) considered ineligible were excluded from hepatic arterial infusion because of the presence of extrahepatic abdominal metastases.

AMBULATORY INFUSION PUMP DEVICES

Pre-operative Evaluation — Surgical Catheter Placement/Hepatic Artery Infusion

Patients selected for hepatic artery catheter placement and chemotherapy infusion should preferably have tumors confined to the liver. Those patients with tumors involving other organs in addition should not routinely undergo this modality of treatment. Candidates selected should have adequate hepatic reserves based upon laboratory and physical findings. The presence of ascites, jaundice, or portal hypertension is a contraindication to surgery because of the risk of developing hepatic artery thrombosis following catheter placement.

Celiac and superior mesenteric angiograms can provide accurate demonstration of the hepatic vasculature. If any vascular anomalies are present, they can thus be shown preoperatively. Michels reports that only 55% of the cadavers he examined had a conventional celiac trunk with hepatic, left gastric, and splenic arteries [62]. In 12% of cases, the right hepatic artery was found to arise from the superior mesenteric artery, thereby requiring separate catheter placements in the right and left hepatic arteries in order to infuse the whole liver. Documentation of portal hypertension can be obtained during the venous phase of a celiac and superior mesenteric arteriogram. Because the Infusaid system appears to be an improved method for prolonged regional drug delivery, a description has been included as a vascular access modality for specific organ chemotherapy of cancer.

AMBULATORY INFUSION PUMP DEVICES

External ambulatory infusion pumps have been designed with a regulated pressure energy source for the purpose of delivering continuous systemic or regional infusion chemotherapy. The first of these devices to be developed was the 'Chronofusor'® introduced in 1963; however, it is no longer manufactured. This pump had a spring-clock mechanism which was capable of delivering 5 cc of solution every 24 hours, and it had a reservoir capacity of

25 cc. The activating mechanism after priming was a winding key, which when fully wound was operative for 12 hours [63]. The Chronofusor® was carried with a holster draped about the neck, shoulder, or hip.

The Cormed® pump (Cormed, Medina, NY) is a nickel-cadium battery powered infusion pump, which weights 17 oz and delivers from 4–20 cc/24 hours (Model ML6-4) or 10–50 cc/24 hours (Model ML6-6). The collapsible reservoir bag has a 50 cc capacity and the battery can be recharged every seven days. The maximum efficiency of delivery is at 50% of its infusion capacity (10 cc/24 hours; Model ML6-4). The Cormed® is also carried with a holster draped about the neck, shoulder or hip.

The Armed® Infusor (Alza Corporation, California) is another ambulatory infusion pump which uses a syringe reservoir within which the drug is contained in an elastic bag. The energy pressure is created by the stretched elastic which delivers the fluid at a rate of 0.4-2 cc/hour. The efficiency of this unit has been reported to have a variation of drug delivery of up to 0.6 cc/hour [64].

Travenol (Travenol Labs, Chicago) has a similar system which contains a disposable reservoir of 60 cc and releases a fixed volume of 48 cc of fluid over 48 hours. This unit is also clipped to the clothing for carrying.

The Auto-Syringe® (Travenol Labs, Chicago) is a battery driven portable pump that utilizes a standard syringe for a reservoir. Models available differ by only a small degree in size and weight. The delivered volume of solution for the four models ranges from 0.01–100 cc/hour. It can be attached at the belt line around the waist; however, because of its irregular control panel facing, it may tend to get caught in the clothing quite easily.

INFUSAID PUMP

The Infusaid pump is a totally implantable ambulatory infusion device and it is most commonly used for hepatic artery infusion. This pump consists of a titanium shell in which a stainless steel bellows drug reservoir is housed [60] (Figures 8a & 8b). The shell is filled with a volatile fluorocarbon which is compressed when the drug reservoir is filled. The fluorocarbon expands at a controlled rate based upon the body temperature to discharge the reservoir at a flow rate of approximately 3 cc/day [59, 60]. Because it has no buttons and is silent, its automatic operation depends upon refilling the chamber by percutaneous injection through the prepared skin. The 50 cc capacity requires refilling approximately every two weeks. The pump also contains a side port which allows for direct access to the hepatic artery catheter for flushing or for bolus administration of drugs. Because it is buried under the skin, it is unobtrusive and is nonrestricting to the patient.

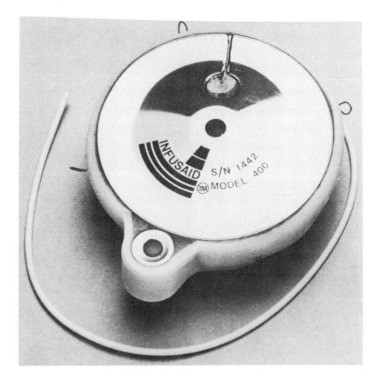

Figure 8a. Infusaid Model 400 implantable drug delivery system.

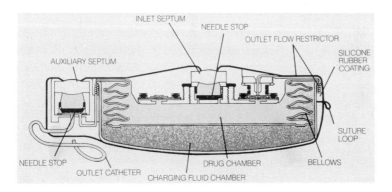

Figure 8b. Cross section – Infusaid Model 400.

Prior to placement of the catheter, 50 cc of sterile saline and 10,000 units of heparin is instilled into the drug reservoir. The unit is brought to physiologic temperature of 38 °C in a sterile water bath and the air is allowed to express itself through the catheter. The pump is implanted in a prepared subcutaneous pocket in the anterior abdominal wall. The Silastic catheter is passed through the fascia and into the abdominal cavity for placement.

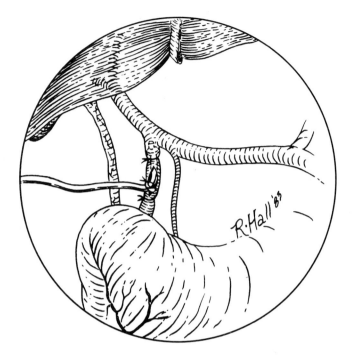

Figure 9. Placement of beaded silastic catheter in gastroduodenal artery for hepatic artery infusion. Note that right gastric artery is not yet ligated.

Operative Technique

The surgical approach to the hepatic artery for catheter placement has been well described by Karakousis et al. [65]. Following exploration of the abdomen to rule out or possibly excise any extra-hepatic metastases, the gastroduodenal artery is isolated after dissection and identification is made of the common and proper hepatic arteries. The right gastric artery is ligated to prevent any drug infusion to reflux into the stomach and duodenum and thereby cause a chemical enteritis. Cholecystectomy is performed to avoid the possibility of developing a chemical cholecystitis.

The gastroduodenal artery is skeletonized and ligated 1.5–2.0 cm distal to its origin from the hepatic artery. The subcutaneous pocket for the implantable pump is made at a convenient site in the upper or lower abdominal quadrant and a suture is placed through to the pump for fixation. The silastic catheter is passed through the abdominal wall into the peritoneal cavity. The hepatic vessels are temporarily occluded and an arteriotomy is made in the gastroduodenal artery; the beaded Silastic® catheter (Infusaid Corporation) is threaded into the artery to reach, but not traverse, the common hepatic artery. With the beaded catheter tip positioned, a silk ligature is placed around the gastroduodenal artery and a second silk ligature is placed around the extra-arterial portion of the beaded catheter (Figure 9). An injection of fluoroscein dye solution into the catheter will confirm the homogenous distribution of dye into both lobes of the liver when viewed under a Woods light or the use of intraoperative nucleotide (1 mCi Tc-99 macroaggregated albumin angiography). Any anatomical variant will require catheter placement in more than one artery if no common channel exists for perfusion to both lobes of the liver. A dual catheter Infusaid pump is now available when two separate arterial sites require infusion. The silastic catheter is then connected to the pump, and meticulous hemostatic and sterile technique is observed during wound closure.

Broad spectrum antibiotics are begun preoperatively and continued for one week following placement. A test for catheter patency can be performed with a radionuclide flow scan of the liver using technetium-99-macroaggregated serum albumin injected into the side part.

Regional chemotherapy infusion can begin 10–14 days following surgical implantation. The pump is filled with a 5-fluorodeoxyuridine (5 FUDR) and heparin solution to result in a delivery of 1000 units of heparin and 0.2 mg/kg/day of 5 FUDR.

To refill the pump, the skin overlying the pump is cleaned with a povidone iodine solution and a 22 gauge Huber-point needle (Vita Needle Company, Needham, Mass.) attached to an empty syringe and inserted in the central septum, and the residual volume drained. (The actual daily flow rate can be calculated from the residual volume). The pump is refilled with drug and heparin solutions accordingly.

Toxicity from infusion chemotherapy may be manifested with elevation of liver enzymes or the presence of jaundice and pain. However, by reducing the drug concentration or withdrawing the drug until the hepatic toxicity has subsided, it is possible to resume intrahepatic drug therapy.

The results and preliminary findings of this form of chemotherapy delivery to the liver await further controlled studies to determine if prolonged regional organ infusion will prove to be more effective than systemic chemotherapy in the treatment of inoperable hepatic malignancies.

SOME COMPARISONS OF EXTERNAL AND INTERNAL AMBULATORY INFUSION PUMPS

A major advantage of the implantable infusion pump (Infusaid) over the external infusion pump systems is that there is no external communication to the skin as a potential source for infection. In addition, there is complete freedom from any external holster or tubing. The necessity for surgical placement of the Infusaid pump, however, and its much higher cost, are an important disadvantage. Also, with this unit, the infusion rate cannot be adjusted and is subject to barometric and thermal influence.

External infusion pumps are currently cheaper and they can be used again in other patients. Catheter placement can be achieved percutaneously without an operative procedure. Patients can interrupt, or in some cases (Auto-Syringe), even adjust the rate of infusion. The obvious disadvantages of these external pumps are the greater risk of infection, the increased risk of arterial thromboses, and the possibility of catheter occlusion and displacement. Perhaps patients who are the most suitable candidates for the Infusaid pump are those with no extra-hepatic neoplasm and who are good surgical risks. Poor risks patients, e.g., patients with documented evidence of extra-hepatic malignant disease, may be suitable for a 2–3 week trial using a percutaneously placed hepatic artery catheter and an external infusion pump to evaluate the therapeutic response of the tumor, without incurring the physiologic stress of major surgery.

With the use of an 'Infuse-A-Port'® or 'Medi-Port'® implantable catheter in the hepatic artery, an external pump can be used for continuous infusion by placing a right angle Huber needle (Cormed, Medina, New York) into the disc chamber and securing the needle to the skin. If the treatment proves beneficial and an implantable pump is desired, the disc chamber can be surgically retrieved, the catheter cut from it and attached to a metal connecting piece, which will attach to the Infusaid pump catheter. The pump is then inserted into the subcutaneous pouch to begin continuous infusion.

Venous Access Surgery In The Immunocompromised Patient — Some Thoughts Regarding Surgical Management

Patients undergoing intensive chemotherapy or bone marrow transplantation become severely compromised in terms of host defense mechanisms and often become anemic, thrombocytopenic, and granulocytopenic. Such patients categorically are at a higher risk for medical and surgical complications during treatment than those patients without neoplasia, who have more normal host defense mechanisms. In the performance of these procedures, the surgeon must be meticulous in his technique and must be constantly vigilant in the maintenance of sterility while draping the patient, especially when the fluoroscopic unit is raised over the sterile field during catheter placement. The effort and expense required to maintain a sterile environment for catheter or shunt placement can be undone by any inadvertent break in technique. In patients who are at the nadir of their immunosuppression following treatment, such as bone marrow transplant patients, the emergence of sepsis can occur rapidly, well before successful bone marrow engraftment has taken place.

In those patients with low platelet counts (<20,000/cu mm), hemostasis can be controlled by ligating all large veins and using the electrocautery sparingly at specific bleeding sites. Only small amounts of tissue should be included in the jaws of hemostatic clamps. Platelet transfusions should be available and should be given prior to surgery to raise platelet counts to at least 50,000/cu mm. In my own experience, however, I have not encountered any unusual bleeding problems when platelets were not available for administration to those patients at the time of surgery.

While the occurrence of catheter-related sepsis is higher in cancer patients who undergo chemotherapy with right atrial siliconized rubber catheters than in patients with peripheral venous catheters, it is even more of a problem in patients undergoing bone marrow transplantation [21]. These severly immunocompromised patients, because of their extended state of granulocytopenia, are even more susceptible to bacterial and fungal infections before engraftment than those patients with neoplastic disease in general [66, 67]. In addition, reports of infection from viral pathogens such as herpes simplex, cytomegalovirus, and varicella-zoster virus have now been well documented in these patients along with infections resulting from other viruses [68, 69]. The therapeutic implications for prevention of these infections in patients undergoing bone marrow transplantation is now a major investigative area of study.

CONCLUSION

With the rapid development of multiple 'permanent' vascular access modalities available to the surgeon, it is now possible to individualize an approach that will successfully support the long-term treatment of the cancer patient. The recent availability of a totally implantable silastic catheter and infusion pump for continuous hepatic artery infusion is an appealing approach to the management of liver tumors, which will soon be undergoing cooperative group studies as to its efficacy. While sepsis is always a constant risk that jeopardizes the usefulness of all of these techniques, a careful adherence to sterile procedures can reduce the reported incidence of this complication to allow for the successful use of any of these approaches.

REFERENCES

1. Band JD, Maki DG: Steel needles used for intravenous therapy – morbidity in patients with hematologic malignancy. Arch Intern Med 140:31-34, 1980.
2. Holland RB, Levitt MWD, Steffen CM, et al: Intravenous cannulas – Surgery of their use in patients undergoing elective surgery. Med J Australia 2:86-89, 1982.

3. Dudrick SJ, Wilmore DW, Vars HM, et al: Can intravenous feeding as the sole means of nutrition support growth in the child and restore weight loss in an adult? An affirmative answer. Ann Surg 169:977–984, 1969.

4. Broviac JW, Cole BS, Scribner BH: A silicone rubber atrial catheter for prolonged parenteral alimentation. Surg Gyn Obst 136:602–606, 1973.

5. Maki DG, Goldman DA, Thame FS: Infection control in intravenous therapy. Ann Intern Med 79:867–887, 1973.

6. Larson EB, Wooding M, Hickman RO: Infectious complications of right atrial catheters used for venous access in patients receiving intensive chemotherapy. Surg Gyn Obst 153:369–373, 1981.

7. Frenkel JK: Role of corticosteroids as predisposing factors in fungal diseases. Lab Invest 11:1192–1208, 1962.

8. Bivins BA, Rapp RP, DeLuca PP, et al: Final in-line filtration: A means of decreasing the incidence of infusion phlebitis. Surgery 85:388–394, 1979.

9. Bjornson HS, Colley R, Bower RH, et al: Association between microorganism growth at the catheter insertion site and colonization of the catheter in patients receiving total parenteral nutrition. Surgery 92:720–727, 1982.

10. Bernard RW, Stahl WM, Chase RM: Subclavian vein catheterizations: A prospective study. Ann Surg 173:191–200, 1971.

11. Brereton RB: Incidence of complications from indwelling venous catheters. Del Med J 41:1–8, 1969.

12. Hickman RO, Buckner CD, Clift RA, et al: A modified right atrial catheter for access to the venous system in marrow transplant recipients. Surg Gyn Obst 148:871–875, 1979.

13. Riella MC, Scribner BH: Five years' experience with a right atrial catheter for prolonged parenteral nutrition at home. Surg Gyn Obst 143:205–208, 1976.

14. Heimbach DM, Ivey TD: Technique for placement of a permanent home hyperalimantation catheter. Surg Gyn Obst 143:635–636, 1976.

15. Weiss SM, Stewart M, Rosato FE: Prolonged central venous catheterization through the saphenous vein. Surg Gyn Obst 154:87–88, 1982.

16. Fonkalsrud EW, Ament ME, Berquist WE, et al: Occlusion of the vena cava in infants receiving central venous hyperalimentation. Surg Gyn Obst 154:189–192, 1982.

17. Kirkemo A, Johnston MR: Percutaneous subclavian vein placement of the Hickman catheter. Surgery 91:349–351, 1982.

18. Rhame FS, Maki DG, Bennett JV: Intravenous cannula-associated infections. Endemic and epidemic hospital infections. In: Hospital Infections, Bennett JV, Brachman PS (eds), Boston: Little, Brown, Little, 1979, pp 433–441.

19. Blacklock HA, Hill RS, Clarke AG, et al: Use of modified subcutaneous right atrial catheter for venous access in leukemia patients. The Lancet, May 1980, pp 993–994.

20. Shapiro ED, Wald ER, Nelson KA, et al: Broviac catheter-related bacteremia in oncology patients. Am J Dis Child 136:679–681, 1982.

21. Abrahm JL, Mullen JL: A prospective study of prolonged central venous access in leukemia. JAMA 248:2668–2873, 1982.

22. Wade JC, Schimpff SC, Newman KA, et al: Staphylococcus epidermidis: An increasing cause of infection in patients with granulocytopenia. Ann Intern Med 97:503–508, 1982.

23. Winston DJ, Dudnick DV, Chapin M, et al: Coagulase-negative staphylococcal bacteremia in patients receiving immunosuppressive therapy. Arch Intern Med 143:32–36, 1983.

24. Singer C, Kaplan MH, Armstrong D: Bacteremia and fungemia complicating neoplastic disease. A study of 364 cases. Am J Med 62:731–742, 1977.

25. Lowder JN, Lazarus HM, Herzig RH: Bacteremias and fungemias in oncologic patients with central venous catheters – Changing spectrum of infection. Arch Intern Med 142:1456–1459, 1982.

26. DeGregorio MW, Lee WMF, Linker CA, et al: Fungal infections in patients with acute leukemia. Am J Med 73:543–548, 1982.
27. Cleri DJ, Corrado ML, Seligman SJ: Quantitative culture of intravenous catheters and other intravascular inserts. J Infect Dis 141:781–786, 1980.
28. Bjeletich J: Repairing the Hickman catheter. Am J Nursing 82:274, 1982.
29. Niederhuber JE, Ensminger W, Gyves JW, et al: Totally implanted venous and arterial access system to replace external catheters in cancer treatment. Surgery 92:706–712, 1982.
30. Allen EV: Thromboangitis obliterans: Methods of diagnosis of chronic occlusive lesions distal to the wrist. Am J Med Sci 178:237, 1929.
31. Kolf WJ, Berk HTJ, ter-Weble M, et al: The artificial kidney: A dialyzer with a great area. Acta Med Scand 117:121, 1944.
32. Alwell N: On the artificial kidney. I. Apparatus for dialysis of the blood in vivo. Acta Med Scand 128:317, 1947.
33. Brescia MJ, Cimino JE, Appel K, et al: Chronic hemodialysis using venipuncture and a surgically created arteriovenous fistula. New Engl J Med 275:1089–1092, 1966.
34. Fogarty TJ, Cranley JJ, Krause RJ, et al: A method for extraction of arterial emboli and thrombi. Surg Gyn Obst, February 1963, pp 241–244.
35. Hargrove WC, Berkowitz HD, Freiman DB, et al: Recanalization of totally occluded femoropopliteal vein grafts with low dose streptokinase infusion. Surgery 92:890–895, 1982.
36. Haimov M, Burrows L, Baez A, et al: Alternatives for vascular access for hemodialysis: Experience with autogenous saphenous vein autografts and bovine heterografts. Surgery 75:447–452, 1974.
37. Menon SMR, Talwar JR, Roy S, et al: Comparison of dacron velour and venous patch grafts for arterial reconstruction. Surgery 73:423–428, 1973.
38. Florian A, Cohn LH, Dammin GJ, et al: Small vessel replacement with gore-tex (expanded polytetrafluoroethylene). Arch Surg 111:267–270, 1976.
39. May J, Tiller D, Johnson J, et al: Saphenous vein arteriovenous fistula in regular dialysis treatment. New Engl J Med 280:770, 1969.
40. Butt KMH, Friedman EA, Kountz SL: Angioaccess. Current Probl Surg 13:1–67, 1976.
41. Wobbes T, Slooff MJH, Sleijfer DT, et al: Five Years' experience in access surgery for polychemotherapy – An analysis of results in 100 consecutive patients. Cancer 52:978–982, 1983.
42. Jaffe BM, Donegan WL, Watson F, et al: Factors influencing survival in patients with untreated heptic metastases. Surg Gyn Obst 127:1–11, 1968.
43. Bierman HR, Byron RL, Miller ER, et al: Effects of intra-arterial administration of nitrogen mustard (Western Society Clin Res). Am J Med 8:535, 1950.
44. Sullivan RD, Miller E, Spikes MP: Antimetabolite-metabolite combination cancer chemotherapy – Effects of intra-arterial methotrexate – intramuscular citrovorum factor therapy in human cancer. Cancer 12:1248–1262, 1959.
45. Brennan MJ, Talley RW, Drake EH, et al: 5-fluorouracil treatment of liver metastases by continuous hepatic artery infusion via Cournand catheter: Results and suitability for intensive postsurgical adjuvant chemotherapy. Ann Surg 158:405–419, 1963.
46. Sullivan RD, Norcross JW, Watkins E: Chemotherapy of metastatic liver cancer by prolonged hepatic artery infusion. New Engl J Med 270:322–327, 1964.
47. Ansfield FJ, Ramirez G: The clinical results of 5-fluorouracil intrahepatic arterial infusion in 528 patients with metastatic cancer to the liver. Progress in Clin Cancer 7:201–206, 1978 (Grune and Stratton, New York).
48. Cady L, Oberfield RA: Arterial infusion chemotherapy of hepatoma. Surg Gyn Obst 138:381–384, 1974.
49. Donegan WL, Harris HS, Spratt JS: Prolonged continuous hepatic infusion – Results with

168

fluorouracil for primary and metastatic cancer in the liver. Arch Surg 99:149–157, 1969.

50. Patt YZ, Mavlight GM, Chuang VP, et al: Percutaneous hepatic arterial infusion (HAI) of mitomycin C and floxuridine (FUDR): An effective treatment for metastatic colorectal carcinoma in the liver. Cancer 46:261–265, 1980.

51. Grage TB, Vassilopoulos PP, Shingleton WW, et al: Results of a prospective randomized study of hepatic artery infusion with 5-fluorouracil versus intravenous 5-fluorouracil in patients with hepatic metastases from colorectal cancer: A Central Oncology Group Study. Surgery 86:550–555, 1979.

52. Reed ML, Vaitkevicius VK, Al-Sarraf M, et al: The practicality of chronic hepatic artery infusion therapy of primary and metastatic hepatic malignancies: Ten-year results of 124 patients in a prospective protocol. Cancer 47:403–409, 1981.

53. Balch CM, Urist MM, McGregor ML: Continuous regional chemotherapy for metastatic colorectal cancer using a totally implantable infusion pump – A feasibility study in 50 patients. Am J Surg 145:285–290, 1983.

54. Weiss GR, Garnick MB, Osteen RT, et al: Long-term hepatic arterial infusion of 5-fluorodeoxyuridine for liver metastases using an implantable infusion pump. J Clin Oncol 1:337–344, 1983.

55. Cohen AM, Greenfield A, Wood WC, et al: Treatment of hepatic metastases by transaxillary hepatic artery chemotherapy using an implanted drug pump. Cancer 51:2013–2019, 1983.

56. Clarkson B, Young C, Dietick W, et al: Effects of continuous hepatic artery infusion of antimetabolites on primary and metastatic cancer of the liver. Cancer 15:472–488, 1962.

57. Sundqvist K, Hafstrom LO, Jonsson PE, et al: Treatment of liver cancer with regional intra-arterial 5-FU infusion. Am J Surg 136:328–331, 1978.

58. Petrek JA, Minton JP: Treatment of hepatic metastases by percutaneous hepatic arterial infusion. Cancer 43:2182–2188, 1979.

59. Blackshear PJ, Dorman FD, Blackshear PL, Jr et al: The design and initial testing of an implantable infusion pump. Surg Gyn Obst 134:51–56, 1972.

60. Ensminger W, Niederhuber J, Dakhil S, et al: Totally implanted drug delivery system for hepatic arterial chemotherapy. Cancer Treat Rep 65:393–400, 1981.

61. Ensminger W, Niederhuber J, Gyves J, et al: Effective control of liver metastases from colon cancer with an implanted system for hepatic arterial chemotherapy. Proc ASCO, 1982, abstract #C-363.

62. Michels NA: Newer anatomy of liver-variant blood supply and collateral circulation. JAMA 172:125–132, 1960.

63. Watkins E, Jr: Chronometric infusor – An apparatus for protracted ambulatory infusion therapy. New Engl J Med 269:850–851, 1963.

64. Dorr RT, Trinca CE, Griffith K, et al: Limitations of a portable infusion pump in ambulatory patients receiving continuous infusions of anti-cancer drugs. Cancer Treat Rep 63:211–213, 1979.

65. Karakousis CP, Douglass HO, Holyoke ED: Technique of infusion chemotherapy, ligation of the hepatic artery and dearterialization in malignant lesions of the liver. Surg Gyn Obst 149:403–407, 1979.

66. Thomas ED, Storb R, Clift RA, et al: Bone marrow transplantation (Part II of 2 part article). New Engl J Med 292:895–902, 1975.

67. Santos GW: Bone marrow transplantation. Adv Intern Med 24:157–177, 1979 (Year Book Medical Publishers, Chicago – London).

68. Meyers JD, Flournoy N, Thomas ED: Infection with herpes simplex virus and cell-mediated immunity after marrow transplant. J Infect Dis 142:338–346, 1980.

69. Yolken RH, Bishop CA, Townsend TR, et al: Infectious gastroenteritis in bone marrow transplant recipients. New Engl J Med 306:1009–1012, 1982.

7. The psychosocial adjustment problems of the cancer patient

JAMES P. RAFFERTY

INTRODUCTION

The adjustment problems of the cancer patient have been discussed in the medical and psychological literature for many years. Attempts have been made to document and verify the diverse opinions and perspectives that have been proposed to explain the coping process of patients with a life-threatening illness like cancer [1–4]. The intention of this chapter is not to offer a comprehensive summary of the available literature nor provide a research-generated description of the adjustment process. This chapter intends to provide a clinical perspective of some of the problems and issues that the author believes are important for primary caregivers who work with cancer patients to consider. This chapter will address these issues as they apply to the seriously ill cancer patient who requires frequent and repeated hospitalizations for treatment and care.

FEAR AND THE CANCER PATIENT

Before discussing how cancer patients cope with their disease, two issues deserve some mention in order to appreciate and comprehend the impact a life-threatening illness like cancer can have on a patient and his family. These issues are: (a) the fear of cancer; (b) the fear of hospitalization.

Fear of What Cancer Means

We are a cancer-phobic society. Perhaps no disease is more feared, nor more continually perceived as synonomous with death than cancer despite all the research and treatment advances. Cancer is a particularly frightening disease because it is viewed as an illness with these three characteristics:
1. A cause that is unknown

Higby, DJ (ed), The Cancer Patient and Supportive Care. ISBN 0-89838-690-X.
© *1985, Martinus Nijhoff Publishers, Boston. Printed in The Netherlands.*

2. A treatment that is seen as generating great discomfort and incapacitation

3. An outcome and long-term survival that is uncertain [5].

Adding to the patient's fear of cancer and uncertainty over its outcome is the firmly held belief of many patients that the course of the disease and its treatment is something over which they have no control. Cancer is often viewed as the 'helpless disease'. Treatment is seen as something that is done to a patient and for a patient, with very little opportunity to actively assist the process. Whether or not a particular patient perceives his disease in this manner, it is important for caregivers to recognize and appreciate the impact that the fear of cancer can have on a patient and his family, for it can greatly effect the manner in which they handle the multiple stresses of treatment and hospitalization.

The specific fears that the diagnosis and treatment of cancer can elicit are numerous: fear of possibly dying; fear of pain; fear of social isolation; immobility; physical restriction, etc. Perhaps the chief fear of the seriously-ill cancer patient is that of emotional abandonment by the patient's doctors and family [6]. Usually this fear is not verbalized directly because it might generate anger, resentment and loss of future support; rather, it is most often expressed indirectly as concern about being medically neglected, not receiving adequate nursing care, or feeling neglected in some other manner by hospital staff. This fear of abandonment will be discussed later in this chapter in the section on depression.

The Fear of Hospitalization

Being seriously ill means to suffer. There must be a modification in certain social roles relative to work and family. The ill person must subscribe to certain rules such as cooperation with physicians and other medical personnel [7]. The very act of being hospitalized is often a stressor which is overlooked by physicians, nurses, medical social workers, etc, who are so acclimated to the hospital environment and its routine and rules that they fail to appreciate how difficult it is for many people to cope with and adjust to this world. Being hospitalized is for many people like entering a foreign country. Hospital employees wear different clothes, speak an incomprehensible language, and follow rules and procedures that are dramatically different from how most patients live.

Not the least of these differences is the hospital's attitude towards privacy. The need for efficiency requires that laboratory tests, surgical procedures, and conferences with physicians be scheduled at the convenience of everyone but the patient. Realistically, it can be no other way. However, efficiency of routine is not incompatible with appreciation for and understanding of the reactions of the patient. Medical rounds, where history and lab data are discussed in detail along with diagnostic and treatment possibilities, may reveal information for which the patient is not prepared or can easily misconstrue. Discussions and disagreements about treatment are often voiced just outside the room of the patient, or in front of other patients and families. The heightened anxiety such encounters can generate are obvious. But the the recognition of the meaning and impact of the hospital environment on patients is often overlooked as caregivers proceed with a routine with which they are comfortable and secure. To consider the impact of hospitalization on patients is not mere compassion, but a medical necessity [8].

A brief note should be made concerning how hospitalized patients define their illness, for it often differs dramatically from how caregivers define it. Patients are often chiefly concerned with and define the seriousness of their illness by their immediate, primary symptoms of pain, social incapacitation, isolation, etc. Medical personnel are frequently more attentive to and concerned with the underlying pathology of the organic illness [7]. What this suggests is a difference in orientation and goals between caregiver and patient concerning what is of principal importance. The caregiver's recognition and appreciation of how the patient perceives his illness lessens the chance that the patient's concerns will go unmet, resulting in increased anxiety and apprehension.

COPING STYLES AND THEIR MEANING

At a time of serious illness, when the patient's emotional resources may be particularly depleted, he or she is expected to function competently regarding decisions about where to seek hospitalization, which physician referral to take, which treatment to accept, and what to tell other family members about the condition. These are decisions of everyday life, but the seriously ill patient or the patient who has just been told of the diagnosis of cancer, may be emotionally incapable of handling them.

Several coping styles will now be discussed with the goal of helping the clinician understand their meaning, and in turn, direct that understanding to the care of patients. Obviously, we cannot speak to the wide variation in successful coping patterns to make unequivocal statements about what is always best or normal for all patients under all conditions. A person's response to the diagnosis and treatment of cancer is highly variable and depends on such factors as age, sex, initial psychological stability, education, socioeconomic level, amount of simultaneous stresses, and availability of social support resources [9].

What is meant by coping? The concept of coping as defined by Lazarus [10] contains two functions, an external (problem-solving) one and an internal (regulatory or palliative) one. The external function of coping is concerned with changing a situation that is stressful or problematic. This can be achieved by changing the reaction to a stressor, e.g. seeking medical advice. The internal function of coping is aimed at reducing subjective emotional components of stress and maintaining a satisfactory internal state for processing information and action [11]. The stress of confronting a life-threatening illness like cancer generally involves both coping functions. The style in which the patient copes with illness actively shapes the course of relationships with family members, physicians, and other supportive resources.

Four affective components of coping with cancer will now be discussed in further detail: denial, intellectualization, guilt, and depression. The goal of the discussion will be to elucidate how these components serve both a problem-solving and a regulatory function for the patient.

Denial

Denial is a defensive response to a life-threatening illness that has received quite a bit of attention in the literature. Denial is how one simplifies and adjusts initially to a traumatic stress. Its aims are to maintain the status quo, to withdraw from psychological pain, and to pretend that things are as before. Weisman [12] provides the following clinical insights. Rarely does a patient deny the fact of his disease for very long after the diagnosis. Rather, denial is directed towards the implications of what being seriously ill means. For clinicians who interact with cancer patients, denial is most usefully understood when viewed not as a static, solitary act, but as a process that exists in a social context. That is, a patient denies something, to someone, for some reason, at some particular time.

When faced with the crisis of a serious and debilitating illness, the patient needs to maintain some semblance of normalcy within his relationships. The patient may try to keep the important relationships in his/her life stable by protecting them from emotional change. The patient attempts to maintain a simplified, yet constant relationship with important others. These efforts are often directed toward avoiding discussion or expression of feelings that might alter these important relationships. Frequently, the most valued relationships for the patient are his physician and selected family members.

How often has a physician, in discussing treatment or prognosis with a cancer patient, sought to elicit the patients's fears and concerns, but observed the patient as seemingly unconcerned or apparently responding appropriately, only to find out later from someone else that the patient is indeed greatly distressed and upset? What is happening here? In many cases the patient perceives the physician as such a valued and important part of his care that he denys the uncomfortable expressions of emotion so as not to jeopardize that relationship. The patient may fear that the physician will not stay involved with the patient if treatment fails and the disease progresses; to express his true concern and frustration might have the effect of causing the physician to emotionally distance himself. Such a risk is too great. However, the cost to the patient is often further emotional isolation, increased anxiety and uncertainty or depression.

Understanding that denial in its social context is an attempt to maintain the status quo with the patient's most valued relationships has important implications for how the clinician works with the patient and family. The clinician's goal becomes one of not trying to make the patient face the seriousness of the illness and the possibility of death, but rather, helping the patient realize that no matter what the outcome, the physician will maintain active involvement in the care of the patient, which means attending to the physcial and psychological discomfort of the patient and family. It means believing that no matter how debilitated and deteriorated the patient's status, there is never 'nothing more to be done'. In the acutely terminal phase of cancer, perhaps too much talk and attention is given to the psychological problems of the patient and not enough to the patient's physical comfort [13]. There is always something more than can be done in terms of patient or family comfort, especially the self-evident problems and management of physical distress.

The patient's resistance to expressing distressful reactions, understood as a means of maintaining support from valued others such as the physician, suggests that the reassurance of continued involvement with the patient, regardless of the patient's progress, is a most necessary component of medical care. This reassurance emanates not from what the physician says, but from the physician's competence in coping with the physcial and emotional problems of the patient [14]. It requires an ability on the part of the physician to deal constructively with his own anxiety, frustration, and helplessness in working with seriously ill, often terminally ill, cancer patients [15]. Further understanding of how the physician can achieve a productive ability to cope with the personal stress of working with the seriously ill cancer patient is discussed by the author elsewhere [16].

Intellectualization

A disease like cancer threatens the patient's sense of having meaningful control over his own destiny. Patients who focus more on what they 'know' is happening to them rather than on how they 'feel' about what is occurring are searching for control. It is important for many patients to attempt to master their disease by actively participating in their care and searching for some meaning in what has happened to them. Knowledge is often sought to gain control, as if knowledge was power. Knowledge reduces uncertainty and makes events more predictable even if less hopeful. Knowledge also is often used by the patient or his family to find 'loopholes' from a diagnosis that engenders overwhelming fear and anxiety.

Patients who value knowing versus feeling as a coping style may appear to the physician as overly-concerned with the minute aspects of their treatment. These patients can be misperceived as not having sufficient trust in the expertise of their physicians, or as interfering with their treatment by requesting knowledge about alternative therapies or procedures. Intellectualization can be useful and realistic as a means of mastering the patient's multiple fears and concerns. The desire for information and understanding of the disease and treatment process is most apparent in the parents of a child with a malignancy. Parents become resident experts on medication dosages, side effects, lab values, etc., as a means of controlling the intense helplessness they experience in caring for their child. Information and participation in the child's care regulates the intensity of the fears the parents have. In adult cancer patients the need for control and mastery is no less reasonable. It is a indication of their own need to understand what is happening to them rather than a reflection of mistrust in their physician. When clinicians realize that intellectual understanding is an important and useful coping strategy, there is less tendency to avoid requests for information, less resentment when these requests are continually repeated, and less concern that the requests reflect lack of trust in the physician's competence and lack of regard for the physician's skill.

Guilt

Most people look for a cause or reason for the events that happen to them. Yet so often the cause of a disease like cancer is unclear. It becomes difficult for the patient to understand why he/she has been stricken with such a disease. The tendency to find cause for what happens to us is so great, that cancer patients often lay blame on themselves. (When this is realistic, as in the case of a smoker who develops lung cancer, guilt can be even more devastating). Self-blame is often evoked in attempting to answer the question: 'Why me?' The patient can reach the conclusion that the disease is punishment for some transgression. Such guilt is often so intolerable that is may be expressed as blame for how the hospital, physicians, or nurses have treated the patient. This is especially the case when the patient's complaints seem non-specific and appear to be generalized to 'the' doctors or 'the' hospital, or when the patient's complaints appear to be expressed at little inconveniences in the hospital routine (when meals are served, when physicians make rounds). The goal for the caregiver who suspects that a

patient's hostility is a function of self-blame for being ill is to show acceptance and understanding of the overwhelming frustration and anger associated with the disease. It is of little help to a guilt-ridden patient for the
caregiver to explain or rationalize away the patient's projection of blame,
for such explanations communicate to the patient the unreasonableness of
his concerns, fostering further self-blame. When the caregiver is able to
avoid personalizing the patient's complaints, he can recognize that allowing
patients to ventilate reduces their sense of weakness and powerlessness and
helps them achieve a sense of control (the caregiver, of course, must determine first whether the patient's complaints are justified).

Guilt defies accurate definition. It can represent a constellation of feelings
where the predominant affect is not self-condemnation and blame, but
anxiety based on anticipated failure in interpersonal relationships. All relationships are imperfect. Because a significant and valued relationship never
provides all one hopes for, it can contain elements of sorrow and guilt [14].
Terminally-ill patients frequently review their past and present relationships
and often recognize and evaluate their failures and incompleteness. Clinicians do patients a disservice if they perceive guilt as always fantasized,
unreal, intrapsychic, and something that should be avoided and forgotten
about; sometimes the patient may need to recognize, admit and be forgiven
for the source of his/her guilt. We need to appreciate the moral and spiritual
perspectives of our patients and realize their importance for psychological
adjustment and functioning. Helping the patient reappraise his self-blame as
signifying a reasonable response to some sort of uncomfortable feelings
involving spouse, children, etc. can provide tremendous emotional relief.
The goal for the physician is to recognize this possible source of self-blame
and make the appropriate psychological or spiritual referral.

Depression

That many patients would respond to the diagnosis and protracted treatment of cancer with depression is intuitively obvious. The important clinical question is not if the patient experiences depression, but how he handles
it when it occurs. Many factors can contribute to a patient's depression:
feelings of personal weakness, lack of control, feeling different or abnormal,
etc. Depression in many cancer patients is not simply a lowered mood in
reaction to the fact of having a disease, but a response to feelings of alien-
ation, dependency, and helplessness at the way their lives have changed.
How the patient handles these feelings is related to the habits developed to
handle stress in the past.

People need others at a time of crisis in their lives and a serious illness
like cancer is such a crisis. Temporary regression to the point of depression
in a cancer patient might be considered a normal, healthy response. The

important clinical question is: when is depression destructive? Dependency on family and/or hospital staff is the most direct solution to feelings of helplessness and depression and can be characterized by an inability to make decisions: a need to lean on others for functioning; increased demand for attention; overwhelming self-criticism, etc. Remembering that the hospital is one of the few places where an individual forfeits control over virtually every task to which he/she is accustomed, the first assessment must be: wherein does the problem lie: 1) the immediate environment (hospital)? 2) the patient's previous coping history? 3) the patient's interpersonal relationships? 4) some combination of these?

The second area to assess is whether the patient's depression is a constructive plea for help ('Help me solve a problem') or a destructive regression ('Do something/everything for me'). A constructive plea for help, when met, usually decreases a sense of helplessness and thus decreases depression. A destructive regression to the degree of 'Do everything for me' requires an immediate plan of action because it so directly reinforces inadequacy and lack of confidence. A realistic plan of action should include all disciplines that interact with the patient and follow these general guidelines: 1) identify specific behavior to be changed, rather than psychological aspects of personality; 2) set small, attainable goals that serve to increase self-esteem and lower a sense of helplessness; 3) set clear expectations among all disciplines involved; 4) refrain from trying to logically reason the patient into changing (it doesn't work and just frustrates everyone involved); 5) focus on positive accomplishments (catch the patient doing well).

ISSUES IN HELPING: HINTS FOR CAREGIVERS

Telling The 'Truth' To The Dying Patient

The pendulum has swung in the past twenty years or so from withholding information from patients to providing them with detailed information on all possible complications of their disease and treatment. Much of this swing in the attitude toward providing information to patients comes from the patient's own desire to be more actively involved with treatment and from the social and legal issues involved with informed consent. Information can be conveyed either directly or indirectly through anxiety, uneasiness, or avoidance. We often modulate the information we communicate to seriously ill patients by either withholding negative information or by communicating with the patient in such a manner that tells the patient very little [17]. The dichotomy between 'telling' and 'not telling' seems to be a false one. The critical issue is 'how' to tell.

The stress of uncertainty at not knowing is as damaging as negative information. Yet to overwhelm the patient with negative details of the illness and prognosis does little to help the patient adjust to the dilemma. The critical issue for the clinician is to understand the function of information. Cassell [18] stipulates that information concerning a patient's illness and prognosis should not only reduce uncertainty, but also be the basis for some type of action, and that these two functions are inextricably related. Cassell further describes three criteria the clinician can use as guidelines in determining when and how to discuss negative medical information with a patient. These guidelines can be posed in the form of three questions: 1) does the information reduce uncertainty, now or in the immediate future? 2) does the information improve the patient's ability to act now or in the near future? 3) does the information improve the amount of trust and confidence between physician and patient? No information should be imparted unless the physician is prepared to answer the questions raised by the information and to assist and teach the patient how to act and function against the consequences of the information. The conveying of negative information to a seriously ill patient must always rest within the context of the physician/patient relationship. In determining when and how to tell negative information to the patient, the sensitive clinician can, in addition to addressing the three questions described above, look to the patient for clues about what information is needed. It is just as important to let the patient tell us what they need and realize that what is needed now may change as the disease progresses, hospitalization is prolonged, or pain increases.

The Psychological Meaning of Hope in Terminal Illness

The concept of maintaining hope in the seriously ill flows directly from an understanding of what it means to convey negative information to a patient. Frequently negative information is perceived as destroying hope and withholding such information is seen as a prerequisite for maintaining hope, confidence and compliance in both the treatment and the physician. Hope can be defined from many different perspectives.

From a psychological perspective, hope is a learned response. It is not maintained by unrealistic reassurance, sermonizing about the 'will to live', nor by withholding unpleasant, sad medical information. As a learned response, hope stems from having achieved a series of successful experiences. We are hopeful about the future because we have been successful in achieving something of value in the past. For example, a student is hopeful about passing coursework and accomplishing something of value professionally because he had a series of successful experiences in achieving academic success in the past. Hope in the future is maintained because the student has, and is, successfully accomplishing something.

Hope in seriously ill cancer patients is maintained when they have reasonable and realistic goals to achieve. These goals can be as simple as attempting to gain enough physical strength to walk unassisted to the bathroom, or as complex as achieving sufficient nutritional status and pain management to return home. Three important guidelines should be kept in mind: 1) the goals must be ones the patient wishes to achieve, not ones the hospital staff thinks the patient ought to achieve. This requires some comprehensive understanding of the patient's lifestyle and support systems. 2) the goals must be addressed before the patient is so debilitated and weakened that he/she cannot possibly achieve any reasonable goals. This requires identifying and addressing the issue of when the medical goal should no longer be physical cure, but physical and psychological care. 3) terminally ill patients often do not have the same 'will to live' as acutely ill patients do. If the goal of the hospital staff and family is to motivate the terminally ill patient to 'get well", it places an unnecessary and unrealistic burden and expectation on the patient's already limited resources.

Assessing The Vulnerable Family

A discussion of how the family responds to a member with cancer should most reasonably be intertwined throughout an examination of how the patient reacts because the family is frequently not the refuge of the sick, but the unit needing care [19]. For sake of clarity only, the family's reponse is treated as a separate discussion.

What puts a family at risk for a maladaptive response to a serious illness in a member? Generally the family of a cancer patient can be considered at risk if: 1) they experience stress events with great frequency and/or great severity; 2) family members define minor threats as crises and have limited crisis-meeting resources [20]. Limited crisis-meeting resources were evaluated in a study of vulnerability in cancer patients [21]. The study suggested six features that distinguish a patient and family at risk for psychological disruptions: 1) a pessimistic view of life with frequent regrets about past family events; 2) a history of depression; 3) a tendency toward feelings of worthlessness and destructiveness; 4) a family history replete with psychological problems and reported current marital conflicts; 5) the anticipation that support and assistance with their problems will not be available; 6) lower socioeconomic status. The signs of vulnerability are not always conspicuous and often require an adequate social history to verify.

What about the family who is not a candidate for intense psychological and social disruption, but for whom the presence of a seriously ill member remains intensely problematic? For these families the crisis of a life-threatening illness like cancer is a turning point in the family's life cycle. Issues such as: 1) how to tolerate the emotional and physical separation from loved ones and 2) how to negotiate the temporary or permanent loss of the key supportive role of the sick member (breadwinner, parent, etc.) are just two examples [22]. What makes this turning point a difficult transition is that often family members react to a sick member in extremes. Either they are overly sympathetic and supportive of the passive-dependent nature of the sick member's illness or they demonstrate great intolerance of any dependent behavior as if illness was viewed as a sign of weakness [20]. Illness can also cause considerable strain on a family because the size of the modern nuclear family is such that fewer people are available as resources to take on the tasks of the sick person. If an extended family is available, they often serve the role of primary emotional supporter. If an extended family is not available, the family often engages the hospital staff as another support system to assist in the emotional care of the sick member.

Barriers to Effective Communication Between Patient and Family

Two primary barriers to effective communication between a seriously ill patient and his family are: 1) the family's attitudes toward how they should interact with seriously ill patients and 2) their lack of appreciation for what talking accomplishes.

Cancer frequently leads to crucial interpersonal difficulties for all involved because of the misunderstanding of what it means to effectively communicate with a seriously ill person [23]. People often cease to communicate openly when they are frightened or concerned. Because family and friends try to take their cues from the patient and have been socialized to believe that the discussion of negative emotions is detrimental to patients, a conspiracy of silence can develop whereby neither patient nor family can express and receive support for the many emotions and feelings they have. Seriously ill patients quickly learn that certain emotional reactions (sadness, tears, anguish, etc.) create empathy in family members and hospital personnel, whereas emotional reactions such as bitterness and anger alienate both personal and professional relationships. The patient quickly learns to avoid expressing the latter. This inhibition of negative affect and the accompanying lack of understanding and support can be a major cause of the depression that is seen in seriously ill patients.

The reactions of family members is determined by: 1) the feelings each family member has about the patient: Is it a conflictual relationship? Is it a relationship based on mutual trust and openness? 2) the family member's attitude toward the illness: Does the illness create additional disharmony and lack of support? Does it generate a pooling of supportive resources? 3) The beliefs each member has concerning what is appropriate behavior to display in front of the patient: Does the family member believe that a constantly cheerful, optimistic attitude devoid of any recognition of negative emotions is the best way to support the patient? Does the family member understand the importance of addressing the variety of uncomfortable emotions that are present with someone who is seriously ill?

The patterns of communication among family members tends to continue in the same style as prior to the illness. Assessing previous ability to communicate openly and honestly is an important clue as to how the family will interact with the sick patient. With a prolonged and debilitating illness, certain feelings are intensified while others are suppressed. For example, negative feelings or feelings with negative overtones like anger, frustration, helplessness, etc. are generally softened or diverted from the ill person. A shifting negative feelings family member that doesn't visit or in some way of expression of onto another (the member enough breaks the family norms) or the suppression of negative feelings because it might depress the sick person, leads to an inability to respond in a flexible manner to the concerns and worries of being seriously ill.

During the ordeal of a life-threatening illness, what benefit can there be in family members 'just talking' about the emotional impact of the disease with the patient? How can talking be helpful? Talking and interacting emotionally with the patient about concerns and feelings of being ill can serve two important functions: 1) it is a means of maintaining relationships at a time of great uncertainty and 2) because the crisis of serious illness is so threatening, the patient often has an intense need to clarify what is happening to him emotionally. Talking, therefore, is a means of validating the patient's feelings and reassuring him/her of their normalcy, thus enhancing the patient's self-esteem.

The goal of the physician in this regard is an educative one. By addressing with family members some of the issues they may need to discuss, and by reassuring them that suppressing feelings is not a healthy way to help the patient maintain a positive, hopeful attitude, the physician can redirect the emotional focus of the family's interactions away from avoidance and detachment and toward a cooperative relationship that emphasizes both problem-solving and expressive functions of coping. Too often communication and questions among family members are directed at the wrong caregiver (e.g. clergy, medical social worker, etc.) due to either an incorrect assumption about the caregiver's area of competence or because of lack of accessibility and availability of the treating physician. It makes for good medicine as well as good patient care to provide adequate access to and time with the physician.

CONCLUSION

This paper provides an overview from a clinical perspective of some of the psychological problems in seriously ill cancer patients. Guidelines for how the clinician can effectively address these problems are given.

By way of a concluding comment it should be mentioned that a number of barriers often impede the physician from effectively incorporating a psychosocial component to his care of seriously ill patients [24]: 1) a lack of teamwork or compartmentalization among disciplines due to the rigid vertical structure of the hospital system; 2) scarcity of time due to a system that rewards physicians for 'getting things done' and keeping the organization running smoothly; 3) the increasing stereotype of the physician as solely a disease-oriented technician; 4) lack of training to adequately prepare physicians to care for the multiplicity of needs of the seriously ill. No matter what the impediments, good medical care of seriously ill patients mandates availability and accessability to psychosocial aspects of the disease in making treatment decisions.

REFERENCES

1. Cullen JW, Fox BH, Isom RN (Eds): Cancer: The Behavioral Dimensions, Raven Press, New York, 1976.
2. Wortman CB, Dunkel-Schetter C: Interpersonal Relationships and Cancer: A Theoretical Analysis, Journal of Social Issues, 35(1):120–155, 1979.
3. Sobel HJ (Ed): Behavior Therapy in Terminal Care, Ballinger, Publishing Company, Cambridge, Massachusetts, 1981.
4. Cohen J, Cullen JW, Martin LR (Eds): Psychosocial Aspects of Cancer, Raven Press, New York, 1982.
5. Sontag S: Illness as Metaphor, Farrar, Straus, and Giroux, New York, 1978.
6. Weisman AD: Coping With Cancer. McGraw-Hill, New York, 1979.
7. Robinson D: The Process of Becoming Ill, The Trinity Press, London, 1971.
8. Kornfeld DS: The Hospital Environment: Its Impact on the Patient, Advances in Psychosomatic Medicine, 8:252–270, 1972.
9. Falek A, Britton S: Phases in Coping: The Hypothesis and Its Implications, Social Biology, 21(1):1–7, 1974.
10. Lazarus RS: Psychological Stress and Coping in Adaptation and Illness, International Journal of Psychiatry In Medicine, 5:321–333,1974.
11. Coyne JC, Lazarus RS: Cognitive Style, Stress Perception, and Coping, Handbook on Stress and Anxiety: Contemporary Knowledge, Theory, and Treatment, Kutash II, Schlesinger IB (Eds), Jossey-Bass Publishers, San Francisco, 1980.
12. WeismanAD: On Dying and Denying, Behavioral Publications, New York, 1972.
13. Lack SA: I Want to Die While I'm Still Alive, Death Education, 1:165–176, 1977.
14. Roberts FJ: The Doctor's Attitude To The Dying Patient, New Zealand Medical Journal, 87(607):181–184, 1978.
15. Barton D: The Caregiver, Death and Dying: A Clinical Guide for Caregivers, Williams and Wilkins Company, Balitmore, 1977.
16. Rafferty JP: The Personal Stress of Working with the Seriously Ill: Impact on the Caregiver, Progress In Cancer Control III: A Regional Approach, Mettlin, C., Murphy GP (Eds), Alan R. Liss, Inc., New York, 1983.
17. Barton D: Dying, Death and Bereavement as Health Care Problems, Death and Dying: A Clinical Guide for Caregivers, Williams and Wilkins Company, Baltimore, 1977.

182

18. Cassell EJ: Telling the Truth to the Dying Patient, Cancer, Stress, and Death, Tache J, Selye H, Day SB (Eds), Plenum Medical Book Company, New York, 979, pp 121–128.
19. Giacquinta, B: Helping Families Face The Crisis of Cancer, Cancer Pathophysiology, Etiology and Management, Kruse LC, Reese JL, Hart LK (Eds), C.V. Mosby Publishing Company, St. Louis, 1979, pp 452–456.
20. Francis GM, Munjas BA (eds) Manual of Sociopsychologic Assessment, Appleton-Century-Crofts, New York, 1976.
21. Weisman AD: Early Diagnosis of Vulnerability in Cancer Patients, American Journal of Medical Sciences, 271(2):187–196, 1976.
22. Moos RH: Coping With Physical Illness, Plenum Medical Book Company, New York, 1977.
23. Dunkel-Schetter C, Wortman CB: The Interpersonal Dynamics of Cancer: Problems in Social Relationships and Their Impact on the Patient, Interpersonal Issues in Health Care, Friedman HS, Dimatteo MR (Eds), Academic Press, New York, 1982, pp 69–100.
24. Benfeld DG: Inhumanity is The Enemy, Akron Beacon Journal (Sunday edition), August 26, 1979.

8. Legal and Paralegal Issues and Cancer Patient

PETER A. REESE and WILLIAM A. PRICE

INTRODUCTION

The legal and paralegal problems which confront the cancer patient stem from the potential disability, incapacity, expense, inconvenience, and even death which neoplastic disease entails. All issues are complicated by the uncertainty which necessarily accompanies treatment and convalescence from any serious illness. The subject is broad, and this chapter is an attempt to outline major areas which should be considered by the cancer patient and his or her family. The physician should be conversant with these areas so that he/she can at least indicate to the patient those areas which should be explored.

Every situation is unique, and hard and fast rules cannot be given. In any legal affair, the law pertaining to an area may be different amongst the fifty states. In addition, the law is not static, and new statutes and court decisions are likely to eventually alter any treatise on this subject. Therefore, it is wise to seek legal counsel when a life threatening disease is diagnosed.

RECORD KEEPING

Though this topic seems mundane, it is of great importance. Information which may be necessary to properly manage the patient's affairs during the course of his/her illness should be readily available. It may be very difficult, time consuming and expensive to obtain items later on when the patient is incapacitated or deceased. All patients should be advised to spend some time 'getting their affairs in order' whenever it is possible to do so prior to therapy.

Record items of particular concern are listed in Table 1 (which may be duplicated for the patient's use).

Higby, DJ (ed), The Cancer Patient and Supportive Care. ISBN 0-89838-690-X.
© 1985, Martinus Nijhoff Publishers, Boston. Printed in The Netherlands.

Table 1.

---

a) Birth certificates, marriage licenses, social security account number.

b) Bank books and checking accounts, time deposit accounts, safety deposit box locations and contents.

c) Investment information such as stocks, bonds, brokerage account reports and receipts documenting transactions.

d) Real estate information such as deeds, tax bills, tax searches and surveys, leases, evidence of purchase costs and expenses for improvements.

e) Ownership information of personal property. Automobile registrations, appliance owners manuals and warrantees, receipts for purchase prices of various household items.

f) Homeowner or tenant insurance policies. Auto policies. Life insurance, health insurance with as much account information as is feasible to accumulate.

g) Wills, powers of attorney, trust instruments. Records and documents of any organization which the patient serves as an officer.

Consideration should be given to the proper location, custody, and availability of all documents. Where are they? Who has access? Who knows what and where they are? A responsible person or persons should always be chosen as custodian. It may be wise to entrust an attorney with legal documents. Other items may best be kept in a safety depository. The proper decision will depend on individual circumstances. However, care must be taken to assure that materials are available when and where they are needed. For instance, it is of little value to include burial instructions in a will if the persons responsible for funeral arrangements are unaware of the contents. It is often the case that wills are not seriously studied until several months after an individual's demise.

A vast additional area of record keeping requirements is opened up if the patient is an owner of a business. While it is likely that larger operations will possess orderly records, the same is not always true of the small business. Therefore, it is wise for the patient who is a substantial owner of a modest enterprise to spend time straightening out its records. Professional assistance from an accountant should be considered.

PLANNING

The ability to plan properly for future events depends heavily on the individual's knowledge of his or her condition, and whether the disease has affected mental competency to make decisions. If a patient is unable to manage his or her own affairs, then friends, family, or professional counsel must take charge. The difficulty with which such intervention is undertaken will depend on individual situations; however, considerable stress to both patient and the intervenors is to be expected. Any actions should be taken in consultation with the treating physician.

Even when the patient is able to function in a logical fashion under the stress and trauma of a life threatening disease, good plans are difficult to formulate in the atmosphere of uncertainty associated with prognosis of many forms of neoplasia. The physician must base estimates of the future degree of disability, quality of life, and duration of survival of a particular patient on personal experience and statistical data accumulated in the treatment of patients with similar afflictions. While such prognostication has great value, it is better suited to making statements about groups of patients than to prediction of an individual's outcome. (The situation is reminiscent of the statistician who drowned in the stream which only averaged a foot deep). In any group of cancer patients, 'miracles' will happen. Some individuals will be cured of a disease which carries a lethal prognosis, while others will fail in treatment of relatively good prognosis situations, or will perish or suffer terrible side effects from straightforward and commonplace diagnostic and therapeutic procedures. Therefore, an individual plan must take note of these uncertainties.

SURROGATES

The Power of Attorney

A power of attorney is usually embodied in a written document which allows another person to act on behalf of the patient. A power can be extremely useful in situations which require prompt action which is impossible or inconvenient for the patient to undertake on his own. If such incapacity is anticipated, a power of attorney should be considered.

Almost every facet of legal activity is a potential subject for a power of attorney. Standard form documents usually contain a check lists of powers which are extremely broad. Probably the most often used power allows banking transactions to be conducted by the surrogate. It is always wise to inquire of the particular institution as to the form and content of the document required. Due to the common law 'at will' revocability of powers of attorney, many banks require notice of revocation to the bank before the power may be terminated. This places the grantor of the power at risk, rather than the bank, when the person possessing the power attempts to use it beyond the time desired by the grantor.

Committees and Conservators

When a person is mentally incompetent, a committee or a conservator may be appointed to conduct his/her affairs. In such cases, the individual cannot grant a valid power of attorney by reason of the incompetency. The appointment usually involves a judicial proceding to determine the necessity of an appointment and the suitability of the person or persons to be appointed. This process is governed by the laws of individual states and should not be attempted without legal counsel.

The estate tax is a levy on a person's right to transfer assets at the time of death. The gift tax is designed to work with the estate tax to prevent the avoidence of estate taxation by giving away assets during a person's life. While estate and gift tax matters primarily involve federal statutes and their interpretation, many states also have similar taxes. Therefore, a given estate or gift may be doubly taxed, depending on the state of residence of the individuals involved in the transaction. This diversity amongst various states makes it difficult to lay out general guidelines for tax planning as to whether getting before death is preferable to leaving as an inheritence. It is wise to consult professional counsel on the legal situation in a particular state.

While it is hazardous to state general rules, estates in excess of $300,000 probably will benefit from competent professional planning. The current state of federal taxation involves scheduled increases in the threshhold levels for filing returns from $275,000 in 1983 to $600,000 in 1987. The size of estate which will pass without tax is also scheduled to increase gradually to $600,000 in 1987. At the present time, substantial tax benefits can result from survival to the first day of the next year; while this fact is not usually of much use, it can become important in rare circumstances where decisions regarding life support are made. These increases have effectively eliminated the Federal estate tax as a consideration in planning many estates, although individual state tax provisions must still be confronted.

If one is fortunate enough to have sufficient assets to require estate planning to avoid taxes, there are many mechanisms available to aid in tax savings. The most commonly used mechanism is annual giving in amounts less than the level which is taxed. Presently, an individual is allowed to give any other individual $10,000 per year without any Federal tax consequences. This amount is doubled if the donor's spouse joins in the gift. For example, a man can give $10,000 to each of his three children and six grandchildren each year. Thus he can divest himself of $90,000 per year and pay no taxes. This amount is $180,000 if his wife joins him in making the gifts. Thus it is possible for a cancer patient to gift substantial sums to his heirs without tax. Many other more sopisticated mechanisms exist to ease the tax burden in the United States. These include matrimonial deduction family trusts which avoid double taxation in passing assets from one spouse to the other and then to children. The purchase of private annuities, creation of charitable trusts, and low-interest or interest-free loans can remove large sums from an estate, thereby avoiding taxation at death. The use of gifts to the cancer patient, equalization of spousal estates, and tax exclusions for sale of residence can also produce substantial savings. All of these approaches require professional assistance to ensure legal compliance and to prevent penalty assessments.

INSURANCE

Once the diagnosis of cancer has been made, it may be quite difficult to obtain life insurance at reasonable rates. Physical examinations and disclosure of existing conditions are generally required prior to issuance of a policy of any size. This is to be expected as cancer patients are a high risk group: however, it does not affect previously acquired benefits. The patient should be very careful to preserve any insurance coverages already in force. Particular care should be taken to pay premiums and comply with terms and conditions of policies.

Some insurances are obtained via group plans at the individual's place of employment. Care should be taken with respect to employment termination or leave taking so as not to jeopardize any benefits.

Many retail credit purchases require life insurance, and some other debt situations, such as margin stock market accounts, provide insurance coverage as part of mandated service charges. It is usually unwise to pay off such charges any faster than necessary.

SELF-PAUPERING (Giving Everything Away)

Individuals of modest or moderate means may wish to protect their assets from dissipation by major medical costs which accompany illness. Sometimes an attempt is made to qualify for various forms of public assistance, including Medicaid, by giving all assets to relatives or friends, with the understanding that assets will be returned as needed by the donor.

There are many problems involved in this tactic, not the least of which is that authorities may consider it a fraudulent transaction, and deny *all* benefits. There must also be a considerable length of time between the gift and eligibility for benefits. Situations will vary: however an eighteen month to three year waiting period is the norm.

Another problem involves good faith and trust between the donor and the recipient of essentially all of the former's worldly assets. This is a traumatic step, giving away everything which a person has struggled for years to accumulate. It is likely to be accompanied by considerable anxiety. Later on, friction may develop between the parties as a result of the changed relationship. Resulting disputes will be very unpleasant and stretch the fabric of the most cordial of interpersonal bonds. In addition, all assets will now be subjected to the risk of attachment by the creditors of the recipient. For instance, the recipient might be involved in a serious automobile accident which results in a staggering judgment being levied against him/her. The ultimate outcome could be the loss of all the donor's assets through the unintentional acts of the recipient. The self-paupering strategy is almost never indicated.

RIGHTS OF PATIENTS

Many legal rights and benefits are available to cancer patients, as the following examples demonstrate.

— Your cancer may leave you with a temporary or permanent impairment (i.e. throat cancer and speech). What are your rights to continued employment? How is a promotional opportunity affected?
— A child under treatment for leukemia may have special educational and transportation needs. How must the school district respond?
— A senior citizen living in a nursing home develops cancer. May the nursing home refuse to accommodate unique treatment conditions?

People of all ages survive cancer treatment and lead highly productive lives. Some may undergo periods of disability, especially during treatment stages. And even though a cancer patient may possess all of his or her capabilities, the perception of an employer, for example, may be otherwise.

Employment Rights

For example, the New York State Human Rights Law, like similar laws in most states, prohibits discrimination against an individual because of a disability, in hiring, in discharge, and in the terms and conditions of employment – including promotions. This same Human Rights Law also prohibits discrimination, based on disability, in credit, in publicly-assisted housing, in union membership, and in all places that any member of the general public might go in order to live, travel, or do business of any kind.

As long as an individual is capable of performing 'the essential duties' of a job, an employer cannot refuse employment or provide less favorable pay and working conditions, or deny equal promotional opportunities. Similarly, an employment agency or labor union must treat all individuals equally. Indeed, no inquiry may be made which directly or indirectly expresses a limitation based upon a disability, unless the disability involves a 'bona fide occupational qualification'. This also applies to apprenticeship and other training programs.

If an individual affected by a disability is also a woman, or is a member of a racial or ethnic minority group, or is over 40 years old, the chance that they will experience job discrimination may be greater. However, various federal and state laws also prohibit employment discrimination based upon sex, race, nationality and age.

Finally, the Federal Rehabilitation Act of 1973 prohibits discrimination against any otherwise qualified handicapped individual in connection with almost *any* program or activity receiving federal contracts or financial assistance. This statute alone reaches many major employers in any community.

Wherever an employer has limited a qualified employee in any way that adversely affects status or opportunity because of disability – including job assignment, tenure, compensation, sick leave, training, fringe benefits and employer-sponsored social programs – almost all statutory remedies provide at least 'make-whole' relief, such as back pay, reinstatement, promotion and constructive seniority. Additionally, under some laws, damages may be available for the emotional distress which resulted from the discriminatory action.

Under certain conditions, individuals may bring private lawsuits, in either federal or state court, to enforce these rights. In most cases, the filing of a written complaint with the proper federal or state agency is a *precondition* to the right to bring a lawsuit. Further, since this 'administrative complaint system" is designed to create an opportunity for early conciliation and settlement, there will be a filing *time limit* – usually 180 to 300 days from the date of the discriminatory incident. Failure to comply with the intricacies of such preconditions and time limits can foreclose a most valuable remedy. On the other hand, sometimes an unnecessary administrative complaint can create lengthy delays or precludes access to the greater damage remedies available in court actions.

Accordingly, the patient who suspects discrimination should *always follow two cardinal rules:*

One: Consult an attorney before taking an action, formal or informal.

Two: See an attorney *immediately,* even if there is merely the suspicion of discrimination by your employer.

Besides safeguarding legal rights, the attorney will provide sound advice on how to document and react to any given job circumstance where future legal action is a possibility.

Basically, each child undergoing cancer treatment is entitled to a free public education tailored to *individual* educational needs 'regardless of the nature or severity of the person's handicap' and 'as adequately as the needs of non-handicapped persons are met'.

Both state and federal statutes and agencies provide for special education programs – including instruction at home, in hospitals, and in supplementary, remedial resource rooms at school – in order to meet the unique needs of a child with a 'handicapping condition'. This extends to pre-school, elementary, and secondary education. Special education rights and resources also embrace 'related services', such as transportation, psychological services, counseling, and physical therapy. Either the school or the parent may refer the child for initial evaluation, the first step in obtaining special services.

A private or parochial school child is also entitled to services from public agencies. The kinds of services will depend upon the development of an 'Individual Education program' (IEP), which occurs within 30 days of a determination by the public school system that the child needs special education or related services. A representative of the private school is to be involved in the IEP process. Thereafter, where the private school is unable to provide necessary home or hospital instruction, for example, the public schools must provide the service. Of course, the private school is not obligated to meet special in-school educational needs, and withdrawal to a public school may be necessary. On the other hand, the private institution may not exclude a qualified child who can undertake the existing curriculum 'with minor adjustments'.

Rights to Special Programs. All children with handicapping conditions must have access to special educational and related services 'appropriate to insure a free public education'. Services deemed necessary under the IEP must be provided by the local public school system either directly, or by referral to a neighboring public program at the expense of the local agency. The local school system may even be required to develop new special education programs.

Rights to Regular Programs. Conversely, a child may well be able to participate in the regular school program despite disability; the law protects these children against wrongful segregation into special programs. Under applicable laws and regulations, handicapped children must be placed in the 'least restrictive environment' offering a maximum opportunity for an education with non-handicapped children. If this is not achieved without extra remedial support, then the local agency is required to provide supplementary services, such as resource rooms. This also applies to non-academic and extra-curricular activities.

Enforcement. Parents who feel that their children have been deprived of required programs have many procedural rights during an initial administrative process involving at least three possible stages: (1) eligibility evaluation, (2) IEP development and initial placement, and (3) a due process hearing to resolve disputes between the agency and parents. For example, the school system cannot place the child in a special program without parental consent. The parent must be involved in the IEP process. Although the agency can itself use the due process hearing to override a refusal of consent, the parent can appeal to the state or even the federal agency – and ultimately to the courts. Moreover, the parent has the right to an independent evaluation of the child, usually at public expense, and/or a hearing before an impartial hearing officer.

This same due process hearing may also be utilized to challenge a failure to provide needed programs and related services. Again, the parent may finally resort to a law suit. Throughout, the parent may be represented by an attorney and expert witnesses. If a court action is necessary, and is successful, all attorney fees and expert expenses may be awarded to the parent by the court.

Especially in the case of evaluations and placement decisions, the special education decision-making process can move very fast. There are a series of time deadlines, as well as many procedural rights which can and should be used to great advantage at all stages. If a dispute is anticipated, or if the parent lacks confidence in the school officials who will control the process, act *at the outset* to retain an attorney with expertise in educational law. Your own lawyer will readily refer you to such a specialist.

Senior Citizen's Rights

Two key principles should by now be very clear: It is illegal to discriminate against disabled people, and any business or institution which receives any government funding will be subject to many laws and regulations designed to enforce the rights of the disabled. A third principle is also obvious: You will probably need an attorney, perhaps even a specialist, in order to gain the full benefit of your rights.

Nowhere do the above principles apply with greater force than in the area of senior citizens rights. Nowhere is the field more complex – and more neglected. Nowhere are so many areas of the law so interrelated: pension planning; wills and estate taxation, mental competency and conservatorships; medical and Social Security benefits; nursing home negligence and medical malpractice; and, of course, the protections of human and civil rights legislation.

A good example is the obligation of a nursing home to accommodate the unique treatment needs of a cancer patient. Can the facility (a) refuse admission; (b) refuse to meet treatment needs; and (c) seek to discharge the patient?

It is likely that state and federal law will be applicable because the nursing home receives Medicare reimbursement and was probably constructed with grants or tax write-offs under various federal programs. The facility will also be supervised by a state agency.

There are three basic types of nursing home facilities, defined in terms of available medical and nursing care. The highest level of care is offered by a 'skilled nursing facility', including a registered nurse on duty at all hours. A secondary level is the 'intermediate' care facility, where the availability of skilled care is largely limited to an oversight role, such as administration of oral medications. The lowest level is the basic residential facility, offering little more than custodial and personal hygiene care.

Where cancer treatment is limited to hospital visits and easily administered medication, an intermediate care facility should prove adequate. However, when treatment needs become more complex, the patient may be forced to transfer to a skilled nursing facility. Under federal patients' rights rules, a nursing home may seek to transfer or discharge a patient because of 'medical reasons'. Indeed, the more qualified and intensive care offered in a skilled facility may well benefit the patient.

If the patient does not need skilled nursing 'on a daily basis', Medicare may not pay for the skilled nursing home care. In addition, under Medicare, continued hospitalization must be the only alternative to skilled inpatient nursing care.

If there is no medical rationale which warrants in-hospital treatment as opposed to skilled nursing care, then a skilled nursing home can be required to accept or retain the patient. The home cannot refuse to meet treatment needs which would ordinarily fall within the scope of services for which skilled nursing homes are licensed. There may be an inherent conflict between the hospital and the nursing home, each with an interest in shifting the patient back to the other facility for long term care. Where the skilled facility, the hospital, and/or the attending physicians disagree over the medical treatment which is necessary, legal action may be taken to hold the patient in the highest level of care until the dispute is resolved. In practice, this is a rare situation in which the opinion of the doctor will usually be controlling.

The patient's family should monitor the nursing home and its staff to insure the quality of care. If it is felt that proper care is not being administered, the family and patient may, among other things, complain to the state supervisory agency, withhold regular payments to the nursing home, and sue for negligence.

Almost any nursing home will be subject to basic federal rules governing non-discrimination on the basis of a handicapping condition. The patient may not be denied an opportunity to receive benefits and services equal to those offered non-handicapped persons. The benefits and services must be as effective as those provided to others and must not be provided in a manner which limits the participation of the handicapped patient.

CHOOSING AND WORKING WITH AN ATTORNEY

This chapter reviews only a few of the legal issues that may affect a cancer patient. There are many specific questions which are not answered in this chapter. What should be done if there is suspicion of medical malpractice? If a patient drives a car while affected by prescription drugs, can he/she be convicted for a Driving While Impaired (DWI) offense? (The answer is probably yes, if the patient was warned of the potential effect on driving ability.) What impact will illness have upon a partnership agreement? Will business credit be restricted? What about obligations to creditors? The impact on pension rights? Divorce agreements? College financial aid?

In our complex highly specialized culture, ready access to preliminary legal advice can bring great benefits. Everyone, whatever their health status, should have a continuing and trusting relationship with an attorney. Million dollar verdicts and public interest lawsuits may attract all the media attention, but more remarkable is the time, money and aggravation that can be saved when normal problems are anticipated and discussed at the earliest possible stages with an attorney.

Some general rules for choosing and working with an attorney follow.

a) *Free First Interview*

Most attorneys do not charge for an introductory discussion of a legal question. However, do not 'shop around' by phone. The opportunity for face-to-face judgment will be lost to both of you, and the attorney will be very uncomfortable about advising a stranger during a first phone interview. Only a personal interview can give the attorney a proper 'feel' for your situation.

b) *Benefits of a Continuing Relationship*

Once your attorney knows the circumstances, he or she can become a continuing source of good advice. Then a simple phone call will often produce the sense of direction needed for the patient to deal with a problem. In very serious matters, the need for calculated action geared to future legal consequences will be recognized early, when it will count the most. In law, as in medicine, the most effective conduct is preventive in nature. And as with doctors, one can achieve much more with an attorney who is trusted.

c) *Honesty*

It is best to be straightforward with one's attorney. The revelation of all circumstances, especially anything that may work against the case, is important. Any painful facts will certainly emerge sooner or later, and a lawyer's best advice will be wasted if he is not appraised of these issues initially. Difficult problems can usually be handled by careful strategy and good preparation. If an attorney represents a client in an uninformed fashion, the case will be jeopardized and money wasted.

d) *Referral to a Specialist*

Although many attorneys can offer sound general advice in most matters, there are specialized areas such as tax planning, employment law, and education rights where only a specialist will be truly competent. Moreover, the preparation and trial of large damage cases, in areas such as product liability and medical malpractice, often require expensive expert testimony. the average attorney cannot afford to finance such a case on a contingency basis, so there will be occasions when the best service an attorney can offer will be a referral to another law firm with appropriate expertise and resources.

e) *Fees and Retainer Agreements*

One should never hesitate to discuss fees and expenses – at least by the end of the first interview. The attorney may ask for a 'retainer fee' before proceeding. This is a partial up-front payment of some portion of the total fee. The client is always entitled to an estimate of the total fee, as well as other expenses. The attorney will usually charge on the basis of a precise hourly rate, unless a flat fee is set for all legal work to be performed on the case. Negligence cases usually involve written contingency fee agreements, where the fee will be an exact percentage of any final damage award, and will be remitted to the attorney upon settlement or verdict.

Remember: Unless the attorney is working for a flat fee or under a contingency agreement, the client is entitled to periodic billings which record specific services performed on an hourly basis. Also remember that while lawsuits to enforce statutory rights may at first appear prohibitively expensive, many statutes, coupled with the Civil Rights Attorney's Fees Awards Act and the Equal Access to Justice Act will provide for all attorney fees and expenses in a winning case – paid by the losing party.

CONCLUSION

The patient with cancer faces several issues having to do with the law and society. As in any other area of life, planning at a time when the whole situation can be judged objectively is vastly superior to dealing with each crisis as it comes up. Many patients with malignant disease can look forward to a few months or even a few years of relatively unimpaired life, even when the ultimate prgnosis is grave. It is a terrible tragedy when most of that time must be devoted to dealing with financial and legal issues because coherent planning and sound advice was not obtained at the outset.

The authors, both lawyers, recognize that the following suggestion may be seen as self-serving and be met with skepticism; however they believe that one of the best services the physician can render to his/her patients with cancer is to urge them to form a reltionship with a lawyer as soon after the diagnosis as possible for the purposes of planning and anticipating problems. Furthermore, the conscientious physician should stand ready to communicate with the lawyer in areas where the two professionals can, working together, best serve the patient/client and his/her family.

REFERENCES

1. Schlesinger, Sanford J, Wolf, Ferome L: Planning for terminally-ill client's estate requires review of assets, recent transactions. Estate Planning, pp 290–297. September 1980.
2. Mundt, William F: Client with limited life expectancy still has opportunity to do estate planning. Taxation for Lawyers. pp 162–167. November-December 1980.
3. American Civil Liberties Union Handbooks, The Rights of the Elderly, The Rights of the Handicapped, The Rights of Hospital Patients.

9. The Role of Clergy in the Supportive Care of Cancer Patients

LEWIS R. BIGLER

INTRODUCTION

It would be possible to address the role of the clergy in the care of the cancer patient in a specific, practical manner, or one which would be more philosophical. The material presented here is hopefully both direct and philosophical at the same time.

To be a clergyperson working with cancer patients takes a life of extraordinary dedication to the truth. Although we are all dedicated to the truth in cancer care, the clergyperson for cancer patients must have a special dedication, which involves a life of continuous, never-ending, and stringent self-examination.

We all know the world only through our living in it, through our being an experiential part of it. This is true of caretakers, as well as for the person who receives care. Our focus must not be limited to only the patient and family, but also upon those who are providing the treatment and care.

The clergy working with cancer patients/families must understand themselves before they can understand their patients. At the least, they need to understand their own life plan and philosophy before they can begin to understand that of the patient. It is easy to get into a situation where one is working out his own philosophy of life with the patient as the guinea pig. While the clergyperson may be served by this approach, the patient will be victimized.

Clergy who are going to work with cancer patients (and what parish pastor is not going to come into contact with cancer patients in his ministry?) must have, therefore, as part of their training, an understanding of their own perception of cancer and what cancer does to people.

Many clergy examine the world and the people in that world, or focus on biblical material and theological reflections, but have not looked at the dynamics of their own relationship to cancer. These types of clergy are

Higby, DJ (ed), The Cancer Patient and Supportive Care. ISBN 0-89838-690-X.
© *1985, Martinus Nijhoff Publishers, Boston. Printed in The Netherlands.*

always competent, but seldom wise; we need both wise and competent people working with the cancer patients and their families.

The life of wisdom must combine contemplation and action. We must contemplate and act *with* the cancer patient. On the other hand, we cannot permit ourselves to act without contemplation of ourselves in relationship to this illness.

In hospitals, contemplation is not held in high regard. In my first experience in a children's hospital, the resident on my assigned floor would wryly suggest that he had done all that medical science could do for a particular child and perhaps I could go in and 'use a little prayer' – maybe the 'almighty' would be willing to provide some 'answers'. Prayer is seen over and over again as a 'spiritual tool', a means to an end, rather than as an instrument of contemplation which is then to be followed by action. Medically trained psysicians/scientists seem to suggest that the clergy 'pray too much' and 'act too little'. But is it not unnecessarily restrictive to use only a part of the resources available in the care of other human beings?

Fortunately, such attitudes seem to be changing, at least in some circles. We are beginning to realize that what needs to be addressed is as much inside the patient and family as on the outside.

A life of unrestricted dedication to the truth means a willingness to be personally changed by the encounters we have with our patients, with physicians, and others. Otherwise, we live in a closed system, the very system which we are often accused of being a part of: our own religious world that does not include the physicians' world of action. We are seen as being in the world of the 'spiritual', while the physician sees himself in a world of scientific 'realities'. Clergy need to be involved in the whole aspect of patient care with a sense of being in both worlds, the world of contemplation and the world of action.

OPENNESS AND CHALLENGE

The 'healing of the spirit' as an aspect of supportive care, does not take place until it includes the desire and drive towards truth, which in turn must include openness and acceptance of challenge.

Openness in the pastoral care of the cancer patient and family is not only to be encouraged, but insisted upon. The patient must be urged to verbalize his thoughts and feelings.

Of all of those (whatever their spiritual, psychological, emotional, intellectual or physical orientation) who develop the disease of cancer, few are consciously looking for a challenge to their faith, their belief system, or their ideas and feelings about the situation they are in with their disease. They certainly do not expect the clergyperson to provide an education or a discipline to their lives and conditions. Rather, they simply seek relief and release from the stress of the situation they now face.

Clergy must be constantly aware that when patients realize that a challenge is being offered as part of support, many will react with avoidance. The clergy must lead them toward a realization that the only real relief lies in the challenge and discipline offered. This delicate process may often be prolonged and, in fact, may be unsuccessful; some patients may never permit themselves to become involved in such a care/support system. Clergy continue to see many who desire only a modified kind of support and do not wish challenge and discipline. If there is not a previous condition of openness or at least the possibility of such a condition, only limited support can be offered or accepted. The patient may dictate what is acceptable, which is often only encouragement of the clergy to be 'with them' (for whatever reason). More than 50% of our patients will never verbalize in specific terms what it is that we have done together.

One technique is to encourage patients to become open by asking them to put into their own words (free association) whatever they are thinking about, or to tell of their dreams and/or fears.

Communication through physical clues must be noted. The clergyperson must not presuppose that he knows anything that the patient does not communicate. Intuitiveness and experience must guide the questions. If the patient is open, it is easier to move in the direction of providing substantial support. If the patient does not respond to this approach in a positive manner, the clergyperson is not any further behind; it simply becomes necessary to proceed more slowly.

Sometimes a patient will respond to the above by relating that he has things on his mind. This is a signal to encourage him in that case to speak of that which he feels most reluctant to share.

Sometimes the patient will do so, but many times will choose to share something else less threatening. In this case, the patient should be encouraged for his openness and the suggestion made that perhaps he will feel desirous of sharing the more threatening thought at a time in the future. On return visits, of course, further opportunities are offered for such openness.

Patients, rather than address their real fears or needs, may talk about 'everything under the sun'. They may speak of children, family needs, and concerns of employment, even though they may have been told that very day that there is little prospect for control of the disease. An attempt may be made to transform the time with the clergyperson into a social hour of light talk and pleasant recollections. Sometimes this may be an unconscious attempt to test the clergyperson before trusting him with more serious material. Other times, it simply reflects a deeply rooted pattern of life, one which dictates that the deepest fears and needs be kept inside, behind a socially acceptable front.

For patients to be open to the challenges offered by the clergyperson as part of supportive care, it is necessary for them to be able to see their lives realistically so that inspection of that life can be accomplished with the help of the clergyperson and perhaps others, e.g., family members. It does little good to have the clergyperson merely report to the patient in general terms his analysis of the situation and what he thinks should be done.

HONESTY AND REALITY

Dedication to honesty and reality means the attitude of always seeking to hear what others say and what others understand is being said; to hear not only what is said in words, but what those words mean through inflection and context. The clergyperson must always be searching for ways to reflect the truth, and reality (as it is experienced) to hold it up for the review of others in a loving and caring way.

This kind of honesty is part of the support offered by the clergy. It is not painless, BUT IT IS MORE POSSIBLE IN THE HOSPITAL SETTING, INVOLVING LIFE AND DEATH, THAN IN EVERYDAY LIFE. People often lie to avoid the pain and discontent of challenge and discipline. Therefore, it is not unnatural for a patient to lie when confronted by life-threatening disease. Lying, at least partially, is an attempt to get around the valley of the shadow of death because we *do* fear evil. To walk through that valley of the shadow of death and to fear *no* evil for God is with us, is a very appropriate message to these patients. Lying is an attempt to circumvent legitimate suffering, challenge and discipline. Such behavior denies the reality of the situation and is therefore, mentally unhealthy and spiritually empty.

Circumvention of the truth is an attempt to find a shortcut to avoid working through the disruption caused by truth. As clergy, we are dedicated to growth and meaning in people's lives (and in their deaths, as well). We must always seek ways to foster this progress. As such, we are in favor of legitimate shortcuts to get there. (Note: we are speaking of "legitimate" shortcuts; many shortcuts are not).

What the clergyperson offers is a legitimate shortcut to personal strengthening and growth, but it is often ignored by other caregivers. There is fear that the discussion of serious matters will foster dependency or result in resignation or weakness on the part of the patient. However, this attitude often covers up the real fears on the part of the caregivers. A prime example is the tendency to not tell the patient or the family of the fatal nature of the disease, or some other threatening information about it. The clergyperson, by fostering personal strength and growth, creates a situation in which it is easier for the patient to receive the truth. For example, sometimes when our assistance is requested by caregivers or family members, the desire is for the patient to accept his illness, or at least accept the offered treatment, and we are asked to change the patient's depressed attitude, anger, denial of reality, or effect some other change. Usually the family or staff have exhausted their own resources in trying to help the patient, and now they turn to the clergyperson to find the solution. But, often the request is to effect this change without confronting the basic roots of the problem. We may be told that the patient has shown this pattern before, but there isn't time now to address this habit of behavior. The clergyperson is requested to make the patient see reason and accept what is 'best for him'. The requesting person (physician, other caregiver, family member) does not want to be involved in the supportive treatment; they merely want the clergyperson to take care of the problem of the patient's compliance. Others, with even less openness, come to the chaplain professing a willingness to 'do anything', but when it is explained that the patient needs the care of the whole family and all must examine their relationships together (challenge and discipline), they cannot find the time or expend the energy to become involved in this sort of exercise, which involves self-examination and 'turning their own lives inside out' by altering habits and relationships. Wanting 'painless' assistance, wanting 'answers' rather than challenge and disipline, they turn for help elsewhere. Later, they will console themselves by stating that 'everything possible' had been done for the loved one; they 'even' asked the chaplain, social workers, psychologists, and many, many others and 'nobody was able to help him!'

This is basically false, of course. Our very difficult task in supportive care is to keep the truth before them. The challenge to us is to guide our patients and their families toward adjustments, from their personal background and their own perception of legitimate and painful challenges. The two most common lies that we will hear and must always anticipate are: (1) we really love the patient, and (2) we were always loved by the patient. It may be that this love actually was present, but when love was not present, there is the strong need of family to convince themselves and others of the opposite. The work of our supportive care, in this case, involves the confronting of lies with truth and honesty, but doing that at the speed which the patient and family are able to take. Yet, we must never shrink from our responsibility. It is as inappropriate for us to 'force' a patient too fast toward truth as it is to not confront or challenge him with discipline at all.

We must keep an environment of honesty and reality about ourselves if we are going to help the patient to honesty and reality. If we become enmeshed in the business of interlocking lies, i.e., lies that we have told and lies that have been told to us by others, then we are in for trouble. The lies of the patient can only be uncovered and healed in an atmosphere of utter honesty. To accomplish this, the first step is to bring to the patient an atmosphere of openness and truthfulness so the patient can enter into this situation with our love and care. How can we expect a patient to endure the pain of confronting their own lies and reality unless we are willing to do so ourselves?

WITHHOLDING THE TRUTH

Physicians, as well as clergy, are not unaware of the criticism that they 'withhold truth'. Lying can take a lot of different forms. One kind of lie is when we make a statement that simply is not true. This is the bold-faced lie that simply says that one does not have any problems and everything will be fine in the future. The second is a statement we make that is not in and of itself a lie, but one that leaves out a significant part of the truth. We can tell a patient that 'we got all of the tumor'. At the same time, we may not tell that there is a virtual certainty that residual disease will eventually recur. Neither lie is excusable, but the second type is more widely used. We are faced with this kind of withholding of truth in our ministry in supportive care, but we cannot provide support if it is condoned.

The second kind of lie, sometimes called the 'white lie', is just as destructive to supportive care as the 'bold-faced lie'. If a group of caregivers withhold information essential to the understanding and making of decisions about one's care and health, they have lied and not provided supportive care.

It is often a temptation to lie by withholding essential information because it is more difficult to detect and confront, and therefore, even more dangerous than telling an out-and-out lie.

'White' lying is considered medically acceptable in some circles because 'we don't want to hurt people' or 'we don't want them to give up hope'. For health care personnel to feed their patients the 'junk' of white lies is seen by some as not only acceptable, but also loving and caring. On the surface these justifications seem very altruistic, but result in superficial relationships and an atmosphere of distrust. For a husband and wife who have lived together through all kinds of good and bad news for fifty years to suddenly take a position of protection by lies, is destructive to the supportive process.

DEPRIVATION

Although such withholding and lack of openness is often rationalized on the basis of 'loving relationships' and the 'protection of those we love from unnecessary worries', such 'protection' is not necessary. The patient usually knows anyway that he is very sick, that the family members are very nervous, and that the doctors are avoiding him. The patient is deprived of the knowledge he might gain about his illness and what he can then contribute to its treatment, about what needs to be done about money, decisions about the children. etc. The patient is deprived of the reassurances which might be received if these topics had been openly discussed. The patient is deprived of the role model of openness and honesty that is necessary for continuing supportive care. The patient is provided instead with a role model of partial honesty, incomplete openness, and lack of courage. At the same time, he is encouraged to be open, to be honest about what he wants and feels, and to be brave in the face of illness. The result is anger.

For some people, the desire to protect the patient is motivated by misguided love (as mentioned above). For others, the desire to protect the patient serves more as a cover-up, a rationalization, and/or a desire to avoid being challenged or disciplined. They wish to maintain authority over the patient by saying to him in effect, 'you leave these decisions to us and you just get well'. We say to the patient that he must see us as strong and loving caretakers – 'Trust us, we know what to do.' 'It is good that you trust us since we are the experts.' 'Don't challenge our wisdom and experience.' It allows the family members and the staff to feel strong and enables them to encourage the patient to feel safe. This attitude supports the self-delusion that by maintaining a superficial approach, things will automatically resolve themselves and produce less stress on the caregivers as well as the patients (as long as no embarrassing questions are asked).

Does a real conflict arise if one uses total honesty? Are not these patients very vulnerable and in need of protection? For example, every surgical procedure involves dangers and threats to the patient's life and integrity. One cannot even undergo anesthesia without some risk. The idea of death as a consequence of a medical intervention is extremely threatening. And certainly many patients, especially children, do not have the capacity to perceive this with much perspective. They are seriously threatened by the prospect of serious illness or death. However, if the threat is really that great, the patient is going to be dealing with it whether we talk about it or not. On the other hand, if the procedure is basically sound, then the family and staff would indeed be doing the patient a disservice if they said that death was the greatest fear to be faced. (Note: The concluding appraisal of Informed Consent).

When we are ministering to persons with all of these pressures on them, it is necessary that we do not prematurely share our own thoughts, opinions and insights with patients in the earlier stages of care because they may not yet be ready to receive or deal with what we see as the needs and concerns; they are still attempting to learn how to work with more preliminary feelings.

We must be careful that our own interpretations or knowledge of something (surgery, hospital procedure, the truth about God) are not imposed upon the patient until he is prepared to receive them. This is not lying, but simply a recognition that the unconscious may not hear things for which it is unprepared. When it is ready, it will hear what is said.

THE SELECTIVE WITHHOLDING OF TRUTH

The selective withholding of one's opinion must be practiced from time to time as part of the supportive care process. If people were to always speak their minds on all issues that affect the patient, they would be considered abrasive and would be deemed untrustworthy. This is especially true when we are part of a larger organization such as a hospital. There is simply no way around the fact that if we are going to be effective in an organization, we must at least partially become an 'organization' person. This means that at times we will need to merge our personal opinion and identity with that of the organization.

On the other hand, we do not want to become the kind of person who 'does not make waves', but is always on the side of the organization. We will then have lost our personal integrity and become a total organizational cog. Rather, there must be a role for the preservation of the integrity of one's identity balanced with the needs of the organizational good. Exercising the continuing balance we need in providing supportive care is a great challenge.

RULES

We will express opinions, feelings, ideas, and even knowledge of the disease from time to time, and these will affect the human affairs of our patients. What are the rules to live by?
(1) Never speak a falsehood.
(2) Bear in mind the fact that withholding the truth is ALWAYS POTENTIALLY LYING. In each instance where truth is withheld, a significant moral decision has been made.

(3) The decision to withhold the truth should never be based upon our own personal needs or the needs of a third party. Among those temptations is the need to hold power and to be liked.

(4) The decision to withhold truth must always be entirely based upon the needs of the person(s) from whom the truth is being withheld.

(5) The assessment of another's total needs is an act of responsibility which is so complex that it can only be done when one operates with genuine love for the other.

(6) The primary factor in the assessment includes an understanding of that person's capacity to utilize the truth for his own spiritual growth.

(7) It should be borne in mind that the process of making such a decision includes our tendency to underestimate rather than overestimate what other people can handle.

The ministry to cancer patients in need of spiritual supportive care from us is a never-ending burden of self-discipline, which is why most people opt for a life of rather limited honesty and controlled openness with patients. The result is relative closedness and hiding. Yet, the rewards of this difficult life of honesty with patients and families are rich.

Open people will continually grow, becoming better able to establish, maintain and care for intimate relationships than closed people. Because they are never speaking falsely, they can be secure that they have done nothing to add to the confusion of the people ministered to. In fact, as we provide a source of illumination and clarification, we are then free to be ourselves. We will not have to construct new lies to hide the old ones. The discipline necessary for honesty is far less than the energy required for secretiveness.

DISCIPLINE OF THE DISCIPLINE

There must be FLEXIBILITY AND JUDGMENT in the care of patients. We alone hold total responsibility for what we do. We must, however, also be free to reject responsibilities which are not ours. We must be able to help our patients to live joyously in the present moment and not expect that all gratification is in the near future ('when you get well'). Discipline itself must be disciplined. This discipline of self is a form of balancing our caregiving actions.

'Discipline of the discipline' seems to imply rigidity and inflexibility. To illustrate the process of flexibility implied in discipline, I will describe an approach to one of the universal and yet most misunderstood of all of the problems facing the patient: anger.

Anger is an emotion which is bred into us by countless generations of human sinfulness (or, by another interpretation, a survival advantage). We experience anger whenever we find another person or thing encroaching upon our territory, taking power from us or otherwise threatening us. Anger is the instrument we have learned to use to fight back, to survive when attacked.

Usually, cancer is seen as a thing, a disease. However, for some patients, the disease becomes focused in the person of the nurse, the physician, and/or others. The big question, 'Why me?' and the second biggest, 'What do we do now?', are based in the attempt to understand the truth of the situation we are in. We have spent so much of our lives staying out of trouble, but now, it seems we are caught. Is it something or someone who has caught us? Is it God? Is it a careless person who did not care for us correctly? A missed diagnosis? Or is it our own fault for being unobservant or careless for missing what is now so obviously important?

The quiet acceptance which is often beheld in cancer patients results from a conditioning which suggests there are times when it is not wise or appropriate to respond to the threat of the disease with anger. Therefore, the patient directs his energy into other activities such as in the initiation of new and experimental treatments. Judgment has taught us to regulate our emotions. If one is going to learn to live with cancer, to survive, one is nurtured to express anger only when it is beneficial, when one chooses to express it, or when it is justified or needed. This comes out in a passive manner – late night buzzer ringing, poor coping with pain, unrealistic demands on staff, shortness with family, etc.

Some variety in expression of anger is also significant in how it is channeled. Patients learn to be 'good' to get good, responsive care. Sometimes it is best to express anger only after much deliberation and self-examination, while there are other times when it is best to express it right away. Sometimes the patient will express anger coldly and calmly. Other times, it comes forth loud and hot.

A 70-year-old professional man expressed irritation and withdrew from his wife after a final attempt was made to surgically open his esophagus and to bypass the tumor in his stomach. He used his anger to say goodbye. He removed all except his nurses from his list of friends. His wife was abused so as to make sure that even she would be relieved to let him go. But, she responded by preaching platitudes at him about continuing care and new hopes. His reply was that he just wanted to 'go home'. She tells him how good the care is in the hospital. He responds with silence or with sardonic and vitriolic comments about promises not fulfilled. With the chaplain, he was pleasant, but broke all visits short by asking for prayer after a brief greeting and before any meaningful dialogue could take place. The only breakthrough that was possible came when the chaplain directly appraised the appropriateness of his anger. He responded with a flood of pain-filled words, tears, and then again, silence. He then relaxed and slept.

The patient is not often able to appraise the appropriateness of his anger. In fact, he is almost totally inexperienced in this sort of self-assessment. The patient may state that he has never been sick in his life, that he has always been well. This often reflects the confusion resulting from the anger he feels and the frustration of not knowing how to respond to it.

We all learn that we ought to regulate our anger and other emotions. We know that we must make some choices about when and how to express anger. Will it be helpful, appropriate, worthy of our self-image? Caregivers and family members also do not want to face these angers. Therefore, instead of guiding the patient to channel anger into creative expressions, they tend to encourage suppression of the anger.

In my experience, in order to function in the face of the seriousness of cancer, the patient must be able to accommodate that disease into his life-style. There needs to be deliberation and self-evaluation by the patient before he is able to appropriately express the anger in a way which advances him on the pathway of living. The chaplain must talk with the patient about what is felt, the sense of loss of control, the sense of isolation, the experience of loss of body image and self-assuredness, and many other issues. Rather than a figurative 'pat on the head' and offering the platitude that the patient is brave, or encouraging the patient to suppress his anger and frustration as something the staff cannot tolerate, there must be a mechanism for its truthful expression and a way of working it through in dialogue, acting it out, and having that acting out taken as a serious, non-verbal expression of where the patient is in his own life.

Some patients need to be guided into expressing that anger right away, right at the moment that they feel it. Others seem to need some time to release it slowly and deliberately.

Part of the guidance provided by the clergyperson is in enabling the patient to learn when and how to match his anger to the right expression for that particular moment. This includes permitting the patient to express anger at us, through personal attacks, corporate attacks, or glancing innuendos.

Every patient has some defect in the complex system of expression of anger, of channeling anger into productive paths. Therefore, one of the chaplain's responsibilities is to allow patients to make their response systems more flexible. The more crippled by anxiety, guilt, and insecurity our patients are, the more difficult this process is in their lives.

GIVING IN

Supportive care demands the flexibility of striking a balance between all the conflicting needs, goals, duties, and responsibilities of the patient and the consequences of treatment for his physical illness. He must learn to 'give in'. There must be a willingness to compromise some of his duties in order to accommodate others. This balance is a discipline because it is the act of giving up something that is precious in order to gain something else which is also precious (health or life). The act of giving in on anything in life is very painful. Yet, we can help our patients learn that the pain of giving in to something wanted in exchange for something required in order to maintain life's balance, is worth it. In cancer treatment, one must continually give up parts of himself. The only alternative is to die (which may simply be another means of balancing or giving in).

Most people choose the alternative of suffering some pain in order that balance may be restored to their lives. Those who are not willing to give in to this pain may eventually or subconsciously contemplate suicide. If we think this is strange, that is because we do not understand the depth of their pain. In any form, giving in to reality is the most painful of all human experiences.

One day, I was called to assist with a patient who had attempted to commit suicide the night before by jumping out a window that was too small for him to fit through, and he was too incapacitated to move through even if it had been large enough. As we talked with each other, I began to see with clarity his anger and his frustration at loss of control that lay behind it all. He was now unable to do much since his disease had advanced so far. He had already lost one leg and had gone through a cordotomy to bring his severe pain under control. There was still pain. In our dialogue, he related to me that he had been a top executive with a powerful corporation until about a year before. He told me many instances of his ability to request or demand things from his employees and to have them accomplished with dispatch. In fact, he had become accustomed to much power and authority over people. Now he was not even able to get to the bathroom without long waits and insistent ringing of his call-button. He could see his life slowly being eaten away by his disease. He had also become enraged at the way his wife was treating him with 'cheer-up' messages that he was looking well that day and that things were going to be better with the next treatment or procedure. He wanted his wife to stop being so unrealistically optimistic and his nurses to be more responsive to his immediate human needs.

Everyone seemed to be oriented towards his long-range cure, but he knew that was not a reality. What he needed was some here-and-now reality acceptance by those around him. He needed some real concern for his present situation, concern for his immediate needs. Giving in was something he wanted to do, but even he did not know how to accomplish it; he needed the assistance of his wife, his nurses, and probably his physicians. We were eventually able to bring the various caregivers and family members to the realization that giving in was not bad, but in fact was a reflection of his own emotional and spiritual needs. Once the family and others joined him in learning how to give in and live, life became more meaningful for him again. He was able to return home and be with his children and grandchildren. He died there in relative peace, free of all but low-level pain, some 16 weeks later. He gained control over his own life and its living. He was able to talk directly with those who were nearest him when he was angry and to appropriately express that anger.

It was necessary for him to tell his wife, with anger, how frustrated he was with her cheer-up messages. However, this also freed her to tell him that she was not ready to give up on him yet, that she would be alone when he died and she had not yet worked that through in her life. She heard his isolation and she shared her own fears with him. They were both able, with guidance from staff, to work out these realities between them so that they could express their anger in appropriate ways and to direct it at appropriate objects, to share the anger and to work through the burdens of life with joy.

REPENTANCE AND REBIRTH

The big question is always, 'Why me?' To have to give up parts of one's self and one's life seems to be a kind of cruel joke on the part of God and, therefore, we are not sure we can ever accept it. In our western world, the human person is considered 'holy'. Death is an insult to the gift of life, even though that is the opposite of our experience of reality. It is the giving in to the self which is most lasting and may be carried on into eternity. It is death and the threat of death that gives life and living their meaning. This 'secret' is a central tenet of religion.

This need to balance our desire for stability and assertion of the self, with the desire for new understanding and knowledge, can only come by giving in to the self, putting the self aside so we can make room for incorporating new material into the self. It reflects the Christian tenet that in order to gain one's life, one must be willing to lose it. For all that is given in to, there is much more gained.

The giving in to self is not a self-enlarging process. The pain of giving in is the pain of death; however, it is only through a death of the old that there is room for the birth of the new. The pain of death is therefore the pain of birth. In order to have a new and better understanding of life and our place in it, we must be willing to give in to the old ideas and understandings.

Christians believe that with the event of death there is the event of birth into a spiritual existence. Our life time certainly is a series of simultaneous deaths and rebirths. As one experiences more births, there will be more deaths. More pain potentially brings more joy – more joy, pain.

Once suffering in our patients is completely accepted, it ceases to be meaningless. This changing from suffering into meaning requires the continuing practice of discipline. This mastery comes with spiritual maturity. For example, things that are of great pain to the child are of no consequence to the adult who has learned to master this world.

Among patients, there is a general lack of the competency needed to change meaningless suffering into meaningful suffering without the nurture of someone else. Spiritually evolved people, through their discipline, mastery and love, have this competence, and their love leads them to answer the call of the patient.

Spiritually developed people have power, and to exercise this power is to make decisions; decisions are painful. To make decisions, there must be awareness of all the truth available. The more truth, the more pain there is in making decisions. The less knowledge we have, the easier it is to make those decisions (or so it seems). The best decision makers are those who are willing to suffer the most over their decisions, but who are still able to make the decisions which must be made regardless.

DISCIPLINE AS A SYSTEM

Discipline, then, is a system of techniques for dealing constructively with pain, and living in the face of pain rather than denying it. We must bring to the cancer patient the skills to solve life's issues. This involves guiding them through the delaying of gratification, assuming (and giving up) responsibility, dedication to the truth in the context of reality, and finally, of balancing all of these issues.

Discipline refers to the system techniques that have been found most helpful in helping families and patients to cope. These techniques are very much inter-related. When working with patients, many techniques may be used at the same time, and therefore, each is not easily isolated and identified. In the care of patients, the strength, willingness, and energy to use these resources are provided by love.

This brief analysis of supportive care by clergy and others who are willing to invest in the life of the patient with their concern is not exhaustive. Much more could be said. As for prayer and meditation, and other 'religious' activities (perhaps sharing some elements with biofeedback, yoga, and psychotherapy), they are not in themselves techniques of supportive care, but are rather aids to the basic elements. Any of these tools are certainly useful, but are not essential. What I have attempted to address are those elements of discipline which are essential. They enable the user to find a higher level of spirituality in the supportive care of his patients.

TO AVOID CHALLENGE

For caregivers involved in treatment of patients, it is a temptation to avoid challenge. That avoidance has been deemed 'natural', as if it is unchangeable. (It is also natural to forget to brush one's teeth until our teeth hurt). Just because something is 'natural', does not mean we should not attempt to change it.

Discipline is a way of overcoming the unacceptable parts of what is 'natural'. It is a way to make the 'unnatural' become 'second nature'. All self-discipline might be defined as teaching ourselves to do what is not 'natural', but is appropriate.

Discipline includes putting ourselves under the scrutiny and discernment of other human beings, our colleagues as well as our patients. We live and work in a community. To enter the fellowship of the hospital and submit oneself to the critique of the medical community is an act of great human courage. The patient is never free of the community of faith, the community of his family and of his world, etc., even as he enters the community of medical care. So too, the caregiver must recognize that he is under the discipline of the whole community.

SYNOPSIS

Healing must include all aspects of the human being, physical, emotional, intellectual and spiritual. Healing is not complete until openness to challenge becomes a part of the way of life. Spiritual wholeness might be defined in terms of this openness to all that is available. We cannot be spiritually whole until we can be forthright with ourselves, with each other, and with God. The patient must see this forthrightness in all who care for him, as well as in his God. The supportive role of the clergy is to see that this openness is brought to bear on his parishioner/patient.

As the patient comes to the medical community, the spiritual community, the whole community, he may request relief, but is in need of challenge and discipline. Many patients stay in treatment, but withdraw from participation in that treatment. Others attempt to manage their treatment to such a level that the caregiver is reduced to the level of a technician. The patient who can be brought to see the challenge in his situation approaches treatment with the potential of being healed in a more than physical way.

We share together the responsibility of teaching one another that the real relief will come only through challenge and discipline. This balance is fragile and achieving it is often lengthy and frequently not as successful as we would like.

For the patient to be made open to challenge, our own views of reality must truly be open for revision and change. But such change must be shared with others or we fall short in our ability to give supportive care. The hospital staff, the family and other key persons must be involved. To hold 'press conferences' where we announce our decisions (whether they be the physicians with medical decisions or the patient with family decisions) is empty. We must all be involved in this challenging process.

For chaplains and other caregivers to provide supportive care means to live a life of total dedication to what truth means in the face of the need for honesty in communicating. It is a continuous and never-ending process of self-monitoring to assure that we are communicating and not just speaking words. We must reflect as accurately as possible truth and reality as we know it and as the patient can comprehend it.

Such truth and honesty does not come painlessly. People lie to avoid pain and the consequences of pain. In a way, our supportive care process is a shortcut, a path to the goal for meaning in life and death. It is easier to get there with the support of others than without it. The short cut of course must always be legitimate. Cheating is not legitimate, and indeed, empty and terrifying to many.

CONCLUSION

We have a tendency to ignore legitimate shortcuts such as supportive care as described above, and resort to illegitimate ones because we know that it takes energy, commitment, and honesty to go through the supportive care experience. We all want patients to get through the disease in the best possible manner. However, it takes dedication to truth and honesty if we are going to get them through this time with growth, purpose, and meaning. It will require readjustment of our own protective mechanisms and the behavior patterns we are used to. How can we expect to bear the pain of confronting reality unless we are willing to share that pain with one another?

NOTE ADDED BY EDITOR: I apologize both to the author and the reader for my editorial decision to alter the author's non-sexist language to the more traditional usage of the masculine instead of the more cumbersome masculine/feminine complex pronouns. I take this step solely in the interests of improving the ease of reading the text.

A GUIDED READING LIST

Paul Ahmed (ed. of Coping with Medical Issues): Living and dying with cancer, 1981, Elsevier-North Holland Inc., New York.

Aaron T. Beck, Harvey L.P. Resnik, Dan J. Lettieri: The prediction of suicide, 1974, The Charles Press, Bowie, Maryland.

Ernest Becker: The Denial of death, 1973, The Free Press, Macmillan Publishing, New York.

Richard G. Benton: Death and dying, principles and practices in patient care, 1978, Van Nostrand Reinhold Company, New York.

Margaretta K. Bowers, Edgar N. Jackson, James A. Knight, Lawrence LeShan: Counseling the dying, 1975, Jason Aronson, New York.

Leo F. Buscaglia: Personhood: The art of being fully human, 1978, Charles B. Slack, Thorofare, New Jersey.

James P. Carse: Death and Existence: A conceptual history of human mortality, 1980, John Wiley & Sons, New York.

Barrie R. Cassileth: The Cancer patient: Social and medical aspects of care, 1979, Lea and Febiger, Philadelphia.

Park O. Davidson, Sheena M. Davidson (editors): Behavioral medicine: Changing health lifestyles, 1980, Brunner/Mazel Publishers, New York.

Herman Feifel: New meanings of death, 1977, McGraw-Hill Book Company, New York.

Jeome D. Frank: Persuasion and healing: A comparative study of psychotherapy, 1973, The Johns Hopkins University Press, Baltimore/London.

Alfred P. French: Disturbed Children and their families: Innovations on evaluation and treatment, 1977, Human Sciences Press, New York.

Erna Furman: A child's parent dies: Studies in childhood bereavement, 1974, Yale University Press, New Haven/London.

Charles A. Garfield: Psychosocial care of the dying patient, 1978, McGraw-Hill Book Company, New York.

Ira O. Glick, Robert S. Weiss, C. Murray Parkes: The first year of bereavement, 1974, John Wiley and Sons, New York.

Jane Goldberg (editor): Psychotherapeutic treatment of cancer patients, 1981, The Free Press, A Division of Macmillan Publishing Co., New York.

Charles E. Hollingsworth, Robert O. Pasnau: The family in Mourning: A guide for professionals (Seminars in Psychiatry, edited by Milton Greenblatt), 1977, Grune & Stratton, New York.

Patricia H. Kennedy: Dying at home with cancer, 1982, Charles C. Thomas, Springfield, Illinois.

Robert Jay Lifton: The broken connection, 1979, Simon and schuster, New York.

James J. Lynch: The Broken heart: the medical consequences of loneliness, 1977, Basic Books, Inc., New York.

John A. MacDonald: When cancer strikes, 1979, McClelland and Stewart, Toronto, Canada.

WL Northridge: Disorders of the emotional and spiritual life, 1961, Channel Press, Great Neck, New York.

Colin Murray Parkes: Bereavement: Studies of grief in adult life, 1972, International Universities Press, New York.

John K. Pearce, Leonard J. Friedman: Family therapy: Combining psychodynamic and family systems approaches, 1980, Grune & Stratton, New York.

Ernest H. Rosenbaum: Living with cancer (Mosby Medical Library), 1982, New American Library, New York.

Theodore Isaac Rubin: Reconciliations: Inner peace in an age of anxiety, 1980, The Viking Press, New York.

Margaret Raymond, Andrew Slaby, Julian Lieb: The healing alliance: A new view of the family's role in the treatment of emotional problems, 1975, w.w. Norton and Company, New York.

William T, Sayers: Body, Soul, and Blood: Recovering the human in medicine, 1980, Asclepiad Publications, Inc., Troy, Michigan.

Bernard Schoenberg, Arthur C. Carr, Ausin H. Kutscher, David Peretz, Ivan Goldberg (editors): Anticipatory grief, 1974, Columbia University Press, New York/London.

Bernard Schoenber, Irwin Gerber, Alfred Wiener, Ausin H. Kutscher, David Peretz, Arthur C. Carr (editors): Bereavement: its psychosocial aspects, 1975, Columbia University Press, New York/London.

Edwin S. Shneidman: Death and the college student, 1972, Behavioral Publications, New York.

Edwin S. Shneidman: Death: Current perspectives, 1976, Jason Aronson, Inc., New York.

Jean Tache, Hans Selye, Stacey B. Day: Cancer, Stress, and death (Sloan-Kettering Institute Cancer Series, Series editors: Robert A. Good, Stacey B. Day), 1979, Plenum Medical Book Company, New York/London.

Cameron K. Tebbi: Major topics in pediatric and adolescent oncology, 1982, G.K. Hall Medical Publishers, Boston, Massachusetts.

Donald A. Tubesing, Sally G. Strosahl: Survey research report, 1976, Wholistic Health Centers, Chicago, Illinois.

Donald A. Tubesing: Wholistic health: A whole-person approach to primary health care, 1979, Human Sciences press, New York.

Jan Van Eys: Humanity and personhood: Personal reaction to a world in which children can die, 1981, Charles C. Thomas Publishers, Springfield, Illinois.

Robert M. Veatch: Death, dying, and the biological revolution: Our last quest for responsibility, 1976, Yale University Press, New Haven/London.

John G. Watkins: The therapeutic self: Developing resonance – Key to effective relationships, 1978, Human Sciences Press, New York.

Avery D. Weisman: Coping with cancer, 1979, McGraw-Hill Book Company, New York.

Avery D. Weisman: On dying and denying: A psychiatric study of terminality, 1972, Behavioral Publications, New York.

Granger E. Westberg (editor): Theological roots of wholistic health care, 1979, Wholistic Health Centers, Chicago, Illinois.

Cynthia B. Wong, Judith P. Swazey: Dilemmas of dying policies and procedures for decisions not to treat, 1981, G.K. Hall Medical Publishers, Boston, Massachusetts.

Gerald H. Zuk, Ivan Boszormenyi-Nagy (editors): Family therapy and disturbed families, 1975, Science and Behavior Books. Inc., Palo Alto , California.

In Addition:
' Deciding to Forego Life-Sustaining Treatment: Ethical, Medical and Legal Issues in Treatment Decisions'. President's Commission for the Study of Ethical Problems in Medicine and Biomedical and Behavioral Research, Superintendent of Documents, U.S. Government, Washington, D.C., 1983.

and

'Making Ethical Decisions: The Ethical and Legal Implications of Informed Consent in the Patient-Practitioner Relationship'. President's Commission for the Study of Ethical Problems in Medicine and Biomedical and Behavioral Research, Superintendent of Documents, U.S. Government, Washington, D.C., 1982.

10. The Oncology Nurse: An Emerging Role in Research and Holistic Cancer Treatment

KATHLEEN KILLION and EILEEN POWELL

INTRODUCTION

From the date of diagnosis, the nurse oncologist plays an important role in the care and management of the oncology patient. This role is broad and involves all aspects of treatment – from the various diagnostic procedures needed for a definitive diagnosis, to being a constant person throughout therapy for not only the patient, but also the family.

Some of the duties of the nurse oncologist discussed here include: 1) clinical assessment of physical and psychological status of the patient; 2) educator and informational source to the patient and his/her family; 3) liaison for medical and other related personnel as a member of the health care team; 4) collection of data and implementation of protocol requirements; and 5) administration of chemotherapy and skillful performance of minor technical procedures.

Before a detailed discussion of the above, it is important to note that the object of treatment of oncology patients is not only disease-directed, but should be holistic as well. The nurse oncologist can make the difference. The 'Joint Practice' method of delivering care to cancer patients provides quality and well-organized care and management [1]. A report from the Veteran's Administration concludes, 'We have observed that persons with cancer, including the entire family unit, are faced with multiple complex problems which we believe are better met through combined education, experience and skills of the nurse and physician collaborating in joint practice' [1]. This collaboration requires mutual commitment, respect, and trust between the nurse and physician. These components are also seen in the relationship developed between the nurse oncologist and the patient and his/her family.

Higby, DJ (ed), The Cancer Patient and Supportive Care. ISBN 0-89838-690-X.
© 1985, Martinus Nijhoff Publishers, Boston. Printed in The Netherlands.

ASSESSMENT

One of the most vital tasks required of the nurse oncologist can be termed 'assessment'. The cancer patient under active treatment is extremely labile in terms of both psychological and physical status. After the initial history and physical examination, physician contact tends to be relatively brief and directed towards determining objective changes and dealing with these. Physician visits are often quite formalized, in which specific questions are asked by the doctor and answers to these questions given by the patient. Although the physician may provide the patient with an opportunity to vocalize other concerns, his/her demeanor, his/her status and often his/her 'busyness', tend to make the patient uneasy about discussing more nebulous concerns; often the patient will preselect what he/she thinks the physician should know about.

The nurse oncologist, who usually spends more time with the patient, whose status and demeanor invite discussion, and who has become a 'friend', is in a position to elicit other concerns from the patient. In this role, the nurse can often deal with patient concerns more effectively and can call to the physician's attention those issues which may need his/her intervention.

The nurse also may be the major contact for family members who often wait outside while the patient is being evaluated by the physician, but who prequently are with the patient during the administration of chemotherapy or during the performance of a procedure.

The family members may have information which the patient does not, and may in fact reveal that the patient's behavior has changed, that he/she is not compliant with the regimen prescribed, or that his/her activity level has altered substantially.

Especially with respect to hospitalized patients, the nurse also may detect more subtle changes because of his/her more prolonged and more frequent contact with the patient, which may have a great deal of importance with respect to the medical management plan.

It is because the nurse is in a position to know the patient in a more complete way that he/she can decide what is really happening. It is important for the nurse to cultivate the ability to determine whether he/she is hearing reality-based complaints rather than those based on the frustration of having a devastating illness. It is important to have a person who can consistently be there to assess changes, whether they be in the patient's physical condition or in the way he/she is handling his/her illness. Emotional changes can shed light on physical changes. The patient that is usually argumentative and uncooperative in his/her daily routine who becomes complacent and quiet, may also be the patient that used to rest quietly through the night, but now is awake with every bed check. This patient may be physically too exhausted to fight back, or emotionally preparing to die. It is the nurse oncologist that must look into the many reasons for the changes in behavior. He/she must decide, with the help of family, staff personnel, and the physician, whether these changes are appropriate or whether the patient needs some help with handling his/her feelings.

Emotional adjustment to the diagnosis of cancer can and often does mimic the stages described by Kubler-Ross in her work, 'On Death and Dying'. It is helpful to staff and family to have a member of the health care team familiar with the stages described [2, 3]. Not every person goes through all the stages exactly as they are described, but most persons do at some time during their treatment, display feelings and emotions that can be related to this natural reaction to potential and actual loss. It is important for patients to know that there is no right or wrong way to deal with the serious situation they are faced with and that with the help of trained personnel they can learn to cope satisfactorily with the disease.

The tone of a patient's feelings can often times be directed by the persons involved with his/her care. If the care is given haphazardly and is not goal-directed, a patient may sense that he/she is 'unimportant' to the health care team. Conversely, if his/her care is organized, goal-directed, and positive, his/her confidence in the system can help him/her overcome some of the feelings of hopelessness that are certain to occur.

SPECIALTY SKILLS

Nurses have expanded their roles and have become an essential component of the medical oncology team. With the increased use of clinical trials in large teaching institutions, it has become a major responsibility of the nurse oncologist to prepare and administer chemotherapeutic agents. This task, as well as many others, has developed from sheer necessity. In a typical medical oncology treatment unit, a small number of attending physicians (perhaps with interns, residents, and fellows rotating on a monthly basis) deal with a large number of patients. The nurse oncologist is often the one person who is familiar with each patient with respect to the details of his/her regimen. As a result of his/her stable role in the health care team, he/she has become highly skilled and developed a strong theory base for the preparation and administration of the many antineoplastic agents in use.

Chemotherapy administration begins with patient and family teaching. The physician is responsible for the initial explanation of the patient's condition and his/her plan for therapy. When cancer treatments are planned and explained, patients have either just been confronted with the diagnosis of cancer or have been told that they have a recurrent disease which requires treatment. Anxiety and fear are often very high in these people, thus interfering with their comprehension of the explanation delivered by the physician. Therefore, it becomes the duty of the nurse oncologist to continue to convey information and assist the patients and family to understand therapy. Patients undergoing treatment will depend upon and appreciate the extra time spent by the nurse to explain different aspects of their therapy. The schedule of the proposed protocol, how the treatment is given, the equipment used to administer therapy, and what may be done to lessen or control the possible side effects from therapy, are all parts of protocol information that the patient should understand prior to instituting therapy [4].

Experience has shown us that patients who understand their treatments and know what to expect will adjust and cope better with their disease and its treatment.

The scope of chemotherapy administration in the treatment of cancer is broad, ranging from the chemical composition of the compounds to the expected time it takes for a given tumor to demonstrate response.

The actual preparation of the compounds, involve knowledge regarding correct diluent for each agent, being aware of the alcohol content of some preparations, the time necessary to administer an agent, and the direct effect each drug will have on the patient's veins. The experienced nurse oncologist understands and respects the importance of vein selection, especially in patients who will receive extended therapy. Cancer patients quickly realize that their veins are a precious commodity. If permanent right atrial catheters are used, proper procedure regarding their use and care is also the province of the nurse oncologist.

When the antineoplastic agents are administered, the nurse oncologist must be familiar with the drugs. He/she must be able to identify which are vesicant or potentially harmful if infiltrated. He/she must be thoroughly confident in the quality of venous access so as to prevent possible extravasation. If a drug extravasation is suspected, approved and effective treatment must be administered swiftly and competently to avoid further infiltration and possible tissue damage.

When administering any medication, there are four observations which must be made. These have been termed the four 'rights' [5]: the right drug, the right dose, the right route, and the right patient. Antineoplastic drugs are toxic, and if given incorrectly or in the face of myelosuppression, acute consequences may arise. As a safeguard to him/herself and to others that may indirectly come in contact with these agents (eg, as other staff members, housekeeping or maintenance personnel), the nurse oncologist must be aware of and practice the recommendations for safe handling of chemotherapeutic agents. Much investigation is being conducted to determine the possible risks of chemotherapy exposure to persons preparing and disposing of these agents.

In several large cancer centers, it has also become the responsibility of the nurse oncologist to perform minor procedures such as bone marrow biopsies and aspirations and intrathecal administration of chemotherapy. Nurse oncologists, with the guidance of physicians, have accrued much experience and expertise in the accomplishment of these procedures. The nurse who performs several such procedures in the course of his/her weekly routine develops technical skills which often surpass those of the physician, and it becomes a great comfort to the leukemic patient who undergoes several bone marrow examinations and lumbar punctures to know that a familiar person with a 'skillful hand' and supportive attitude will be performing the procedure.

RESEARCH

The type of institution where the nurse oncologist functions will determine the extent of research-oriented responsibilities he/she has. In large research centers, there are nurses whose main duties focus on research and its components.

Large collaborative groups (eg, CALBG, ECOG, SWOG, etc) are an integral part of oncology research. By using a large number of patients, adequate information is obtained in a short time. In order for this method to work, consistent, concise and reliable feedback from the individual data collectors is necessary. The careful management of medical data for oncology research can only be done by someone with medical background and a broad knowledge base in oncology. The nurse oncologist who specializes in data mangement increases the efficiency, accuracy, and completeness of data used in these and other studies.

One of the first stages of protocol-related work is to determine whether the patient is eligible for registration on a particular study. This can be tedious and time consuming, but eligibility assures that the patient meets the criteria needed to qualify him/her for entrance into the specific study, in addition to assuring that the eventual treatment selected is appropriate.

As the field of oncology becomes more complex, the accepted modalities for treatment change and become more specific to individual diseases and their status. The difference between accepted methods for treating Hodgkin's disease in stages I and II are dramatically different from those used in stages III and IV, or for the relapsed patient. These determinations can only be made if proper staging and evaluation are done prior to the initiation of treatment. In many centers, the nurse oncologist, because of his/her familiarity with protocol requirements, is often the person relied upon to see that all required studies are completed.

He/she is also the person available to explain the testing procedures that are necessary to the patients and to their families. This is often where the relationship between the two has its beginnings.

The management of chemotherapy is also a part of the research component of the nurse oncologist's duties. Preliminary information must be given to the patient prior to obtaining the informed consent needed to initiate treatment with investigational drugs. This information, although supplied by the physician, is often reinforced and expanded by the nurse. The actual handling and administration of the chemotherapeutic agents is overseen by the physician, but carried out by the nurse, who has responsibility to deliver the ordered treatment with a minimum of acute complications.

It is important to note that accurate recordkeeping, in reference to dosages of chemotherapeutic agents, the presence of toxicities and severity, with a precise grading scale that is accepted throughout the medical community, and the response rates and durations, are the means used to evaluate protocol studies. When studies are done on a collaborative basis, it is imperative that the information be reliable in order to effectively utilize this information.

Historically, it has been shown that nurse oncologists greatly increase the completeness and reliability of such information [6]. Even in small centers and private practices nurse oncologists are often responsible for adherence to protocol requirements and recordkeeping.

EDUCATIONAL CONSIDERATIONS AND FUTURE TRENDS

The educational requirements of the nurse oncologist are not as yet dictated by any standards. Many of the nurse oncologists of the past fifteen years have acquired their knowledge and expertise at their place of employment through supervised learning experiences, attending physician work rounds and x-ray rounds, etc, and in the process, gaining understanding of the disease process, the appropriate diagnostic work-up, treatments and their complications, and follow-through management and observation.

Effective nurse oncologists have a strong medical/surgical knowledge base from which to build, which is necessary to assimilate effectively the principles of cancer care.

In approximately the past ten years, in-service education programs have become more formalized, offering the professional nurse an avenue to broaden his/her scope of oncology nursing. The extent of published literature on cancer nursing, authored by nurses as opposed to physicians, has increased greatly both in quantity and diversity of subject matter, thus helping to increasingly define this new nursing specialty and provide a growing educational reference base.

The field of medical oncology has expanded greatly and the future role of the nurse oncologist will likely become more encompassing and important as time goes on. Trends in oncology care and management are shifting from large centers to individual practitioners who use centers for consultation and information regarding modalities of treatment, probably because in addition to the increasing number of medical oncologists, patients prefer not to travel long distances for their management. It will become increasingly important for the nurse oncologist to be qualified and available to function competently in association with private oncologists.

The need to create formal educational programs adhering to established standards, cumulating in certification for performance and overall professional excellence is apparent for this specialty of nursing.

RESPONSIBILITIES

Being responsible is defined as: 1) being liable to be called upon to answer for one's acts or decisions (answerable); 2) able to fulfill one's obligations (reliable, trustworthy); 3) being able to be a free moral agent; 4) involving accountability for important duties [7]. The responsibilities of the nurse oncologist involves all these aspects. However, first before one is able to be responsible, some degree of self-knowledge is essential. Oncology is a very demanding field. The issues of life and death, quantity versus quality, and personal ethics are encountered on a daily basis. Because the nurse oncologist has arisen from the ranks of the 'nurse', there are a multitude of issues to be explored.

Oncology is an ever-changing field due to ongoing research. Basic research is constantly being integrated into patient care, resulting in conventional treatments, research protocols and the cures which are seen today. A nurse oncologist must necessarily be involved with research-related tasks. Some are benign, such as data collection. But others involve 'invasive' procedures such as serial blood sampling or protocol required diagnostic procedures and sometimes seem of questionable worth. Occasionally these leave the nurse oncologist with ambivalent feelings, as does the administration of toxic treatments prescribed for patients in whom response is unlikely. Not every one can work their way successfully through this. It is imperative that the nurse oncologist be able to see beyond immediate patient comfort and also be sufficiently knowledgeable so that he/she can effectively participate in ethically ambiguous decisions. Longevity and experience seem to be the most effective teachers.

A nurse who has no oncology experience can hardly be expected to know how he/she might deal with these issues. It is the 'responsibility' of the nurse oncologist to offer these issues as 'food for thought' to the nursing personnel so that when a situation does present itself, there has been some cognizant effort made to deal with the questions. Also, it is important for the nurse oncologist to try to guide fellow nurses through the difficult path of ethical decisions he/she has gone through. Not every person can accept the rationale that has proved itself to others and that is evidenced by the fact that every nurse cannot deal with oncology patients on an effective level.

The nurse oncologist's first responsibility is to his/her patients. Even though the research-oriented approach is necessary in dealing with cancer and its treatment, it is imperative to remember that every patient is an individual with their own needs and limits. The nurse oncologist shares the responsibility to see that every patient be dealt with on this level. In order to treat a patient successfully, a holistic approach must be employed. In a team effort, this aspect may tend to become submerged, and the nurse oncologist must see that disease-directed efforts be organized, thoughtful, and appropriate to the individual patient.

The therapeutic unit consists not only of the patient and staff members, but also the patient's family. In the last ten years, many treatment regimens have shifted to being administered on an out-patient basis. For this to be effective, there must not only be patient cooperation, but family support. The nurse oncologist can be a 'significant other' to families as well. He/she is the person who can and should assess situations at home to decide if ancillary personnel such as social workers, visiting nurses, or psychologists are necessary. The nurse oncologist often must educate the patient's family with respect to disease-related physical limitations, treatment regimens, and also some expected emotional changes. It is important for families to be informed of side effects from treatments such as nausea and vomiting, alo-pecia, and sterility so that they can be realistically dealt with. The patient's emotional lability is more easily tolerated if the family understands that it may be treatment related and is usually transient. The stressors that affect oncology patients and their families are great in number, but can often be controlled with proper education and counseling, both before and during treatment. The nurse oncologist has the opportunity and is usually available to meet these needs.

CONCLUSION

As stated previously, nurse oncologists arise from the ranks of nurses.

Often, moving up the ladder or specializing in nursing means losing some of the satisfaction gained from 'taking care' of patients on a day-to-day basis. There is, however, compensatory satisfaction gained from working in this area. Being able to fulfill responsibilities to the optimum, means seeing patients functioning on a high level through all phases of treatment. It means helping families deal with the horrendous word 'cancer' as a strong family unit, allowing others to help where they can. It can also mean seeing that the dying patient and his/her family have improved quality of life in the final days, and seeing the family more effectively deal with the death of a member. Witnessing all this carries a great deal of satisfaction, and this enhances one's feeling of self worth, which completes the cycle and enables the nurse oncologist to go on learning, teaching, and practicing.

REFERENCES

1. Ryan LS, Edwards RL, Rickles FR: A joint practice approach to the care of persons with cancer. Oncology Nursing Forum 7(1):8–11, 1980.
2. Fergusson JH, Andronkites A: Communicating with families of children with cancer. Aspects of Oncology Nursing, Adria Labs, December 1981.
3. Hippard V: Psychological aspects of oncologic nursing. Aspects of Oncology Nursing, Adria Labs, September 1981.
4. Donely PJ: The oncology research nurse. Aspects of Oncology Nursing, Adria Labs, June 1982.
5. Walton M: Professional: Cost and quality. Nursing Clinics of North America 8(4):685–689, 1973.
6. Hubbard SM, Donehower MG: The nurse in a cancer research setting. Seminars in Oncology 7(1):9–17, 1980.
7. Webster's New World Dictionary – College Edition. World Publishing Company, 1968.

READING LIST

Grant MM, Padilla GV: An overview of cancer nursing research. Oncology Nursing Forum 10(1):58–67, 1983.
Henke C: Emerging roles of the nurse in oncology. Seminars in Oncology 7(1):4–8, 1080.
Heuther MA, Powell AH, Vaughan BA, Evans DF, Cole SW: Team services of a clinical specialist group. Nursing Vlinics of North America 8(4):691–701, 1973.
Reiter F: The nurse clinician. American Journal of Nursing, February 1966, pp 274–280.
Starch P: Factors influencing the role of the oncology nurse specialist. Oncology Nursing Forum 10(4):54–58, 1983.

11. The Doctor and the Cancer Patient: Sources of Physician Stress

DONALD J. HIGBY

INTRODUCTION

The relationship between doctor and patient is an extremely complex one. The physician who specializes in the care of cancer patients is subject to frequent personal stress arising from this relationship, tensions from different directions which do not usually affect his colleagues in other medical disciplines to nearly the same extent. These stresses arise from the doctor's personality, his training and life experience in medicine, the conflict between the role of physician and that of clinical investigator, and the inadequacies of the traditional contract (the doctor-patient relationship) in satisfying the needs of both doctor and patient in the circumstance where the patient has cancer.

This essay is an examination of these ongoing sources of professional stress.

THE PERSONALITY OF THE PHYSICIAN

Krakowski has proposed a psychoanalytically-based formulation accounting for why an individual chooses to become a physician [1]. Attraction to medicine is in part the result of a greater than normal fear of death and personal dissolution acquired during childhood. The development of this fear is in part predisposed when the individual fails in some way to meet expectations regarding physical abilities. This results in a curiosity about the workings of the body.

Generally, fathers of physicians are characterized as strong, aloof, and remote, whereas mothers are strong, close, and warm. Often, the physician-to-be has experienced severe illness in himself or a close 'other', or has witnessed the dying of another during childhood.

Higby, DJ (ed), The Cancer Patient and Supportive Care. ISBN 0-89838-690-X.
© *1985, Martinus Nijhoff Publishers, Boston. Printed in The Netherlands.*

The decision to become a physician is often present at an early age, and on a primitive level, it represents a reaction formation to fear of death resulting in a need to fight illness in others.

Krakowski points out that the individual who will become a physician faces symbols of death during the course of his training and makes attempts to desensitize himself. Desensitization can take the form of compulsivity; the attitude of 'scientific' objectivity; ways of developing distance from patients (eg, the morbid verbal shorthand used by physisians in training when discussing patients). Since the physician in training has to face his own fears of death, especially when his patient is dying, he must be able to rationalize that what he is doing is all that can be done. This posture leads to further compulsivity, further sacrifice of the non-medical part of life, and eventually influences the choice of a subdiscipline. Physicians may enter non-clinical specialities in order to escape from the confrontation with illness entirely. Physicians who enter surgical specialities may be literally defending themselves against their fears with a knife. Non-surgical clinical specialities may be populated by individuals who have reacted to the conflict by emphasizing the more cerebral aspects of medicine. They see themselves as scientists, thinkers, planners, and mediators. (It is interesting that the rise in randomized prospective clinical trials parallels the growth of the subspecialty of medical oncology, whereas surgical cancer literature is still fairly heavily invested with the more classic approach to medical investigation involving analysis of cases and conclusions which are not only derived from inductive, but deductive reasoning).

Krakowski surveyed 100 physicians and found that 21 had manifestations of depressive illness. He noted that physicians reacted to stress in ambivalent ways. Stress arising from personal problems resulted in anxiety and depression; stress arising from professional causes resulted in increased work (compulsive behavior). Of the classic findings of a compulsive personality, 80% of the physicians surveyed had at least three of five criteria and 20% had four of the five traits (ie, sufficient for diagnosis).

The personality factors of caregivers that are usually associated with the most effective and committed helpers are often the very factors that make the caregiver most prone to emotional exhaustion and the least likely to seek and/or accept help [2–3]. Unresolved guilt is often the result of this stance when the desired result (eg, cure of the patient) is not accomplished. Characteristics of idealism and perfectionism so common in young physicians are indicators that mature and adaptive mechanisms for coping with failure are underdeveloped [4]. That such is likely is further suggested by the fact that most young physicians have successfully surmounted progressively difficult challenges, and personal failure is not only a rare experience, but is extremely threatening since by the time the individual has traversed medical training, it means the inability to pursue one's life goals.

Thus, the forces which lead a person to choose medicine, the actual process of undergoing medical training, and the failure of the new physician to have developed methods for adequately coping with frustration, all combine to create in a physician a situation in which his needs are modestly reinforced by success and markedly threatened by failure. A satisfactory balance is usually the case in most specialties where most of the patients respond to treatment. Cancer medicine, however, reverses the ratio between success and failure and severe stresses result in the physician practicing an oncological specialty.

Physicians in most other specialities have, besides more frequent successful outcomes among their patients, other reinforcers of their self image: making intellectually challenging diagnoses; being able to totally heal many patients; enjoying the resultant gratitude of patients, family and community; and the respect of colleagues in the helping professions. The oncology specialist seldom makes diagnoses; his treatments are toxic and often fail to save the life of the patient. Patients who undergo marked toxicity which comes repeatedly with visits to the physician are not as expressive of gratitude as most patients, and since a large fraction of the oncologist's patients do eventually die, there are frequent situations where there is great ambivalence about how far to carry medical measures. Because of this ambivalence, the resulting disagreements between the oncologist, the other caring personnel (housestaff, nurses, other physicians), and the patient's family are much more frequent than in other patient encounters and thus the overwhelming professional balance in such that the rewards which satisfy most physicians are markedly diminished where oncologists are concerned and the failures, real or perceived, are more common.

SOURCES OF STRESS IN THE INTERACTION BETWEEN THE PHYSICIAN AND
THE PATIENT WITH CANCER

There have been several investigations which shed light on some of the stresses which are encountered by physicians caring for cancer patients. Small, et al [5] studied the stresses in physicians as they cared for patients with ovarian cancer in different stages. The physician, who is socially and personally required to play the role of an omnipotent figure, finds himself helpless when his patient is terminal. This in turn leads to anxiety, loss of self-esteem, and depression. The physician also may be subject to survivor guilt after the patient has expired.

In Zahler's study [6], pediatric interns were interviewed within 36 hours of the death of their patients. When there was time for some interaction between physician and patient/family prior to death, the degree to which the interns related to the patient was proportional to age and state of consciousness (the older and more communicative, the better the relationship). The relationship with the child also influenced the relationship with the parents. When children became terminally ill, however, there was frequently active avoidance of the parents together with some degree of withdrawal from the patient. Furthermore, seven of the thirteen interns studied were noted to be obviously distressed during the time they cared for a terminally ill child.

Artiss and Levine on the basis of their interaction with physicians in training through a seminar designed to help them cope with cancer patients [7] described several forms of reaction to stress: anger towards staff physicians because they were seen as 'heartless', 'callous', etc.; denial that there were any problems; verbal disapproval or disparagement of psychiatry; joking about the situation with each other; being 'too busy' or 'always forgetting' to attend the seminar. All of these reactions were seen as ways of displacing or avoiding the feelings described above.

Not only is the communication between doctor and patient impaired by such reaction to stress, but in addition, there are different expectations on the part of doctor and patient with respect to cancer.

Turnbull stated that it was unusual for the expectations of physician and patient to match [8]. The patient perceives the fact of having cancer as something which will be painful, will result in loss of body function, which will impair social relationships, etc. The physician, on the other hand, helped by the depersonalizing qualities of modern hospitals, sees the fears and concerns of the patient which are directed towards him as being inappropriate, since he cannot help and should be using his time for people he can help.

As Almy states, the patient seeks relief of symptoms, anxiety, and uncertainty whereas the physician seeks diagnosis, intervention and disposition [9].

Along these same lines, Pfefferbaum using a questionnaire method graded the relative importance of several issues which might be of concern to the cancer patient [10]. The questionnaires were administered to adolescents with cancer as well as physicians caring for these patients. Although both patient and physician agreed on the importance of many concerns, it was interesting that physicians felt the patients were much more concerned than they really were about how to talk to friends about their disease; about knowing someone else who had had cancer; about how cancer would affect their future role as a husband or wife; and about their appearance. On the other hand, patients were much more concerned than physicians thought they were about what to expect if the cancer spread, how cancer could be prevented, what causes cancer, and the chances that the cancer would reappear after treatment.

It is noteworthy that patients with cancer (in this case, adolescent patients) are almost entirely focused on the behavior and origins of their own cancer. The physician, on the other hand, feels that the patient is most concerned about more long range issues. These different perceptions are obviously explainable, but it is evidence that there is a failure to communicate about deep-seated emotional issues.

Thus, it is apparent that the actual interaction between patient and physician when the patient has cancer, is a source of stress and frequently associated with avoidance behavior in the physician.

THE CONFLICT BETWEEN THE ROLE OF CLINICIAN AND THE ROLE OF INVESTIGATOR

Probably in no other area of clinical specialty medicine is the conflict between the role of clinician and the role of investigator so marked as in the oncology specialties. The proper role of oncology (as opposed to those elements held in common with other medical specialities) is the delivery of treatment for malignant disease. Yet, there is no treatment for any malignant disease which could not be improved upon substantially in terms of side effects, toxicity, or efficacy. The common cases seen by most clinical specialists can be treated with very high response rates and very low serious toxicity. The opposite is true for the common diseases seen by the cancer specialist, eg, bronchogenic carcinoma. The frustrations of the oncologist in delivering therapy of high toxicity and relatively low efficacy obviously provokes in him a desire for improved treatments.

The cancer specialist practices in an atmosphere of ubiquitous group studies, protocols, federal programs designed to unify and coordinate the investigative aspects of oncology, and literature abounding in new drugs, approaches, and diagnostic studies which are unavailable to the cancer specialist for his patients. The fascination of the lay public and press with cancer and its treatment aggravates this situation. The oncologist in practice spends a fair amount of time telling patients why the latest reported 'cure' is not appropriate for them. In addition, the literature on cancer treatment is voluminous and much of it is of marginal utility. The cancer specialist because of the state of flux of his specialty, must educate himself much more intensely and learn to evaluate the literature much more scrupulously. It is possible to treat satisfactorily the bulk of patients presenting with, for example, endocrinologic disorders in the manner taught ten years ago. This is in no way true about oncology.

Physicians are advised 'be not the first by whom the new is tried nor be the last to set the old aside'. They learn that the first rule of medicine is 'do no harm'. Neither can be followed by the cancer specialist. If he first does no harm, he cannot treat; if he is very conservative in adopting new therapy, applying new methods, etc, he will soon be out of date and no longer effective as an oncology specialist. On the other hand since many of the new 'breakthroughs' reported turn out to be blind alleys, the opposite problem, namely the investment of time, learning and funds in a new technology which will soon be sidelined, must also be avoided.

The cancer specialist then, because of the pressures mentioned above, must resolve in himself the conflict between being a dispenser of medical lore and developing new and better ways to treat his patients. The physician's response to this may be to reject any participation in clinical studies rationalizing that the extra paperwork, the extra expenses to the patient, and the low yield all make this not worthwhile. The opposite extreme, where every patient is fitted into some sort of protocol, also is a response to the same kind of stress.

The numerous attempts by cooperative groups, centers, and even the National Cancer Institute to enlist private oncologists in clinical studies and the notable lack of success of these attempts (eg, the very small fraction of cancer patients in the United States who are registered on protocol studies) suggest that cancer specialists in private practice for any number of reasons cannot reconcile the role of doctor with that of investigator. In our own experience, this does not seem to be an expressed antipathy towards clinical investigation. Most physicians we have approached about collaborative studies indicate that they are most willing to participate. However, only when there is literally *no added burden* to the physician can we accrue patients to our studies in a satisfactory way. This usually means that nurse clinicians and/or medical oncology fellows must establish liasons with the personnel in the doctor's office so that they can be on hand when the protocol patient visits his physician and see to it at that time that flow sheets are filled out, etc.

This behavior seems so consistent that it may be necessary for the physician in private practice to distance himself in some way from the role of investigator in order to maintain his self image as 'physician'. Since his livelihood and his emotional support are related to the posture of dispensing knowledge, perhaps there is a subconscious rejection of admitting that either of two treatments may be equivalent or that the treatment that will be given is selected not because of knowledge and experience, but by randomization.

The 'academic' physician in the clinical research center, on the other hand, is in a position where his livelihood depends on the rate and quality of research produced. A bed devoted to simple cancer patient care is a threat to a grant, a slowing down of the rate of data accumulation, etc. Furthermore, the academic physician surrounds himself with housestaff, nurse clinicians, and data managers which allow some psychological distance from the patient or at least greater freedom in the role the physician wishes to select. He can, for example, leave the collection of informed consent to the house officer; the administration of chemotherapy to the nurse clinician; the flow sheet compliance to the data manager, etc. while he pursues his basic investigations in the laboratory. Also, of course, he may cultivate and nurture his image as physician by appearing at the bedside of the patient, offering reassurance, dropping a few words of wisdom to the assembled house officers, and in short, leaving the 'dirty work' to others.

Another type of stress arises from this role conflict. Cancer specialists frequently have to decide, when planning the course for their patient, whether to send the individual to a center where important investigational work is being done or to keep the patient under their own care where they may be able to administer a therapeutically equivalent program. The treatment of acute myelocytic leukemia, Hodgkin's disease, etc. are cases in point. A competent cancer specialist in a fully equipped hospital can probably deliver therapeutically equivalent treatment to the majority of such patients as can a major cancer center. Yet, further advances in the understanding of those relatively rare diseases will require more access to such patients by clinical investigators.

There seems to be no ready solution to this dilemma without a fundamental change in how medicine is practiced in this country. The cancer specialist obviously does not want to see himself in the role of a triage officer. The patient does not desire to travel a long distance and (often) be subjected to the apparent or real depersonalization that is associated with many centers. Nor does the third party insurer desire to pay for expensive diagnostic tests which probably would not be ordered with the same degree of avidity by the private cancer specialist. At the same time, the investigational center often *must* have previously untreated patients under the care of center physicians in order to pursue promising lines of therapeutic research.

Krant [11] argues that the moral tensions involved in the above are not amenable to resolution insofar as a single physician is concerned. If the physician's loyalty is to the individual patient's good and only to that good, then the physician cannot enter a patient into a study; he can only suggest that the patient may wish to volunteer for an experiment. To completely avoid any coercion, there must not be a real or imagined reward or punishment associated with the patient's volunteering or failing to volunteer for a study. In some centers, associated in the public mind with 'experimentation', the patient who accepts his physician's recommendation to go to the center may already be in a situation of coercion. He knows that he cannot have the advantage of the center's expertise unless he agrees to participate in a study for which he is being referred.

Krant feels that the physician in charge of the patient should not be the same individual as the experimenter and in fact the two individuals should not even be in an interdependent relationship. Only then can the caring physician assist the patient in decision-making, including helping him say 'no' if that is what he wants to do. Contrast this with the situation existing in many research centers where the caring physician is often a house officer whose future depends upon the good graces of his superiors, many of whom are conducting clinical investigations.

Burkhardt [12] maintains that '... in controlled trials, statistically significant results cannot be obtained if individual ethics are consistently applied'. The controlled trial is justified only as long as the two arms are seen as therapeutically equivalent. Once the trial is underway, the physician must offer the best treatment he can according to his best judgment. As a result, he may object to 'blinded' studies, which in any event cannot easily be performed with respect to therapeutic research. If the study is not blinded, he will almost certainly develop a preference for one arm or another based on numerous factors other than the measured factor on which the study is based. Thus, logically the only studies that can proceed to statistically significant conclusions are those in which in fact the two arms are therapeutically equivalent.

Some would argue of course that a well trained physician will not make a judgment about a treatment until a clinical trial demonstrates statistical significance. This of course requires that the physician ignore his past experience, his intuitions, and the non-measurable evidence that he amasses in the conduct of a clinical trial.

Numerous problems with therapeutic trials as currently performed have been noted [11–13] and some remedies proposed [14–17]. But the fact remains that the classical role of the physician, many of the elements of which are desired and expected by the patient and in fact are therapeutic, demands that the physician apply knowledge to a particular case (art) whereas the role of clinical investigator assumes that the needed knowledge does not exist and must be gained by induction (science). The subterfuges and rationalizations, the proliferation of human subject protection rules, informe consent documents, internal review boards, etc. relating to the issue of clinical investigation indicate very clearly that this is a major and ongoing source of stress for all oncology specialists, whether in private practice or in academia.

SYNOPSIS

The personality of the physician vis-a-vis the patient with cancer, the dynamics of the atypical relationship between the cancer patient and the cancer specialist, and the imperfect and often investigational nature of cancer treatment, all militate to undermine and threaten the traditional doctor-patient relationship, which is normally a source of reward for the physician and a major source of solace and support for the patient. There is evidence that this state of affairs brings about stress in the physician to which he not infrequently responds in ways which may be ego protective, but which may also distance him from his patient. This may in turn result in reactions in the patient, eg, non-compliance, hostility, and even turning to unorthodox sources of 'treatment'. What is desired by the patient is the knowledge, skill, and advice of the physician *expressed* and the compassion and support during the times of greatest stress. What the patient often receives is knowledge and skill with minimal *expression* and a withdrawal during times of greatest stress.

THE DOCTOR-PATIENT RELATIONSHIP

Paternalism (an action taken by one person in the best interests of another without the other's consent [18]) lies at the heart of the classic doctor-patient relationship [19]. Up until only recently, this was to some extent justifiable because the physician did in fact possess the knowledge to prescribe what was best, medically speaking, for the patient; and treatment while less effective, was often less risky. As medicine has become much more complicated and interfering with respect to the life of the patient and as the general education level of the population has risen, this strong paternalism has come into question. The physician cannot be the best judge of the entire field of the patient's interests taken as a whole and in fact with respect to some modern medical procedures, both diagnostic and therapeutic, may not be able to judge the appropriateness of the procedure for the patient with respect to non-medical but extremely important concerns.

A modification of this relationship, a weaker paternalism, implies that the physician acts in the best interests of the patient *with his consent,* but not necessarily with his *informed* consent. However, even this approach has come into question [20].

Several attempt at reformulating the relationship which should exist have been made. Among these are the *contractual* [21], in which the patient contracts with the physician for a service; the *economic,* in which the physician is placed in the role of a merchant with a saleable product to deliver [19]; and the *religious,* where the relationship is defined as a covenant [22]. However, these models are generally recognized as very imperfectly reflecting the complex and rich relationship between the doctor and the patient [19].

A model which has gained wide support is that of *patient autonomy* [21–23]. In the extreme form, the patient is the sole decision maker regarding medical intervention. All that is required is that the patient be competent to make a judgment, not that the judgment be related to his best interests, however defined. While this model has been applied in dealing with burned patients in whom survival was unprecedented [14] and may in fact have relevance in the 'treatment' of certain types of malignant disease, eg, metastatic bronchogenic adenocarcinoma, it must be recalled that when the patient is called upon to make an 'autonomous' decision, he is in fact not 'normal', but rather, ill, often angry, and under pressures which do not usually exist when he exercises normal decision-making [25–26]. The question may also be raised as to whether the information necessary for a patient to autonomously make a decision can indeed be transmitted adequately in many cases [27]. Would it be 'right' to simply stand by and allow a young woman with a small breast mass to avoid biopsy and possible further treatment because she does not wish to face the future if she must lose a breast? Or should the physician exercise persuasion, enlist the help of the husband, other women who have been through the procedure, etc? Obviously, the latter is paternalistic and pressures are brought to bear to change the patient's mind about her initial decision.

Thomasma, recognizing many of the difficulties with the paternalistic model and the autonomy model, proposed a *conscience* model [19]. This encompasses the following:
a) the doctor and the patient must be free to make informed decisions
b) doctors are morally required to pay increased attention to patient vulnerability
c) physicians must use their power responsibly to care for the patient
d) physicians must have integrity
e) the physician must have a healthy respect for moral ambiguity.

While this model has several attractive features, it does combine features of the classic paternalistic model and the autonomy model. Furthermore, it presumes a great deal of the character of the physician. With respect to item 'e', for example, it has been shown that physicians in general act by an implicit rather than an explicit ethical code [28] and do not as a rule seek help from expected sources regarding ethics.

Pellegrino has advanced an *existential* model of the doctor-patient relationship [29]. A person in the state of health is in equilibrium between his capacities and his goals. In other words, he is 'becoming himself'. Illness disrupts this process of becoming since it greatly curtails the freedoms necessary to *act* as a fully human person. The patient, unless he chooses to ignore the illness, must seek the help of another person who professes to possess the knowledge and power to heal. This imperative of seeking to restore the equilibrium is an existential one and related to the imperative of becoming oneself.

The healing relationship, then, is inherently an unequal one. The healer professes that he has authentic knowledge and skill and that he will put them at the service of the patient and will act in the patient's best interests to restore as completely as possible, the patient's wholeness.

What is implicitly professed by the physician is, unfortunately, seen differently by patient and physician. The former wants both technical competence as well as compassion whereas the latter often sees the act of profession as one of technical competence only. As a result, patients will probably always seek alternatives to allopathic treatment since they can evaluate compassion, but cannot always evaluate technical competence.

PROBLEMS WITH THE PROPOSED MODELS OF THE DOCTOR-PATIENT
RELATIONSHIP WHEN THE PATIENT HAS CANCER

We have seen, and physicians are generally innately aware, that the physician-patient relationship is an immense source of personal and professional satisfaction, stimulation, and sense of self-worth. That many physicians are 'married' to their profession, have little in the way of deep outside interests, are most content when actively practicing, continue to 'see patients' even when their administrative or research responsibilities may be overwhelming, voluntarily shorten periods of convalescence from illness to get 'back in harness', and sometimes practice far into their dotage, cannot be explained by mere monetary gain and certainly cannot be explained by the prestige they enjoy in possessing the title of 'doctor'. (I am referring primarily to physicians engaged in patient care specialties as opposed to those who do not have therapeutic relationships with patients – the latter usually have 'opted out' at an early stage of career development from the doctor-patient relationship). Yet the doctor-patient relationship regardless of formulation, is almost always stressed when the patient has cancer. With respect to the paternalistic formulation, the physician is frequently confronted with situations where he does not know what is best for his patient, but must pretent that he knows. With respect to the patient autonomy model, the diagnosis of 'cancer' causes a far more serious stress on the patient's decision making ability than do most other diagnoses. With respect to the conscience model, the physician's actions of conscience may often in retrospect be perceived as 'wrong' in that the patient is not responding to treatment. Finally, with respect to the existential model, the patient with cancer often cannot be returned to a state of 'wholeness' and the physician's profession of knowledge and ability to heal is seen as false by both parties.

238

CONCLUSION AND COMMENTS

The relationship between doctor and patient when the patient has cancer, is qualitatively different from that existing when the patient has another disorder. The cancer specialist also is faced with the fact that the usual ratios pertaining to successful and unsuccessful outcomes with respect to his patients in the long run tend to be heavily weighted toward the unsuccessful. Although many oncologists find personal solutions to the stresses they face, these may often be unsatisfactory with respect to the patient and society. There are no easy solutions which result in satisfaction to all concerned regarding the problems described. The factors which lead an individual to become a physician cannot be altered. The total field of expectations that the patient has of the physician cannot in practice be met in many circumstances. The state of the art with respect to cancer treatment requires a considerable passage of time (or an exceptional breakthrough) before cancer treatment is analogous to therapies for other diseases.

This review of stresses which exist in the physician who cares primarily for cancer patients is not meant to imply that a simple solution is possible. However, it is hoped that the delineation of these issues may help cancer specialists gain insight into their own reactions and perhaps, from this self-examination, allow them to at least identify and respond to habitual behavior patterns which are not in their own best interests or those of the patient.

REFERENCES

1. Krakowski AJ: Stress and the practice of medicine. II. Stressors, stresses, and strains. Psychother Psychosom 38:11–23, 1982.
2. Rafferty JP: The personal stress of working with the seriously ill: Impact on the caregiver. In: Progress in Cancer Control III: A Regional Approach, Murphy GP, Mettlin C (eds), New York, Alan R. Liss, Inc, 1983, pp 279–286.
3. Freudenberger HJ: Staff burnout. J of Social Issues 30:159–164, 1974.
4. Rafferty JP: Problems in developing support groups for health care professionals who work with the seriously ill. Buffalo, New York Roswell Park Memorial Institute, 1981, unpublished.
5. Small EC, Anderson B, Watring WG, Edinger DD, Mitchell GW: Ovarian carcinoma: Management of stress in patients and physicians. Gynecol Oncol 15:160–165, 1983.
6. Zahler OJ, McAnarney ER, Friedman SB: Factors influencing pediatric interns' relationships with dying children and their parents. Pediatrics 67(2):207–216, 1981.
7. Artiss KL, Levine AS: Doctor-patient relations in severe illness: A seminar for oncology fellows. New Engl J Med 288(23):1210–1214, 1973.
8. Turnbull PRG: The relationship of the surgeon to the patient with advanced malignant disease. New Zealand Medical Journal 92:354–356, 1980.

9. Almy TP: The healing bond: Doctor and patient in an era of scientific medicine. Am J Gastroent 73:403–407, 1981.
10. Pfefferbaum B, Levenson PM: Adolescent cancer patient and physician responses to a questionnaire on patient concerns. Am J Psych 139:348–351, 1982.
11. Krant MJ, Cohen JL, Rosenbaum C: Moral dilemmas in clinical cancer experimentation. Med Pediatr Oncol 3:141–147, 1977.
12. Burkhardt R, Kienle G: Controlled clinical trials and medical ethics. The Lancet (December 23 and 30), 1978, pp 1356–1359.
13. Little JM: Human experimentation and the physician-patient relationship. Surgery 93(4):600–602, 1983.
14. Gehan EA, Freireich EJ: Non-randomized controls in cancer clinical trials. New Engl J Med 290:198–203, 1974.
15. Byar DP, Simon RM, Freidewald WT, et al: Randomized clinical trials: Perspectives on some recent ideas. New Engl J Med 295:74–80, 1976.
16. Simon R, Weiss GH, Hoel DG: Sequential analysis of binomial clinical trials. Biometrika 62:195–200, 1975.
17. Gehan EA: Design of controlled clinical trials: Use of historical controls. Cancer Treat Rep 66(5):1089–1093, 1982.
18. Childress JF: Paternalism and health care. IN: Medical Responsibility, Robinson WL, Pritchard MS (eds), New Jersey, Human Press, 1979, pp 15–27.
19. Thomasma DC: Beyond medical paternalism and patient autonomy: A model of physician conscience for the physician-patient relationship. Ann Intern Med 98:243–248, 1983.
20. Ackerman TF: Fooling ourselves with child autonomy and assent in non-therapeutic clinical research. Clin Res 27:345–348, 1979.
21. Veatch RM: Professional medical ethics: The grounding of its principles. J Med Philosophy 4(1):1–19, 1979.
22. Ramsey P: The Patient As A Person. New Haven, Yale University Press, 1970, pp 5–32.
23. Childress JF: Priorities in Biomedical Ethics, Philadelphia, Westminister Press, 1981, p 14.
24. Imbus SH, Zawacki BE: Autonomy for burned patients when survival is unprecedented. New Engl J Med 297:308–311, 1977.
25. Lain-Entraglo P: Doctor and Patient, New York, McGraw-Hill, 1969, pp 101–147.
26. Bradley P: A response to the march 1979 issue of the Journal of Medicine and Philosophy. J Med Philosophy 5:213–214, 1981.
27. Barber B: The ethics of experimentation with human subjects. Scientific American 234(2):25–31, 1976.
28. Balkos GK: The ethically trained physician: Myth or reality? Canad Med Assoc J 128:682–684, 1983.
29. Pellegrino ED: Towards a reconstruction of medical morality: The primacy of the act of profession and the fact of illness. J Med Philosophy 4(1):32–56, 1979.

Index of Subjects